Neonatal Hematology and Transfusion Medicine

Editors

ROBERT D. CHRISTENSEN
SANDRA E. JUUL
ANTONIO DEL VECCHIO

CLINICS IN PERINATOLOGY

www.perinatology.theclinics.com

Consulting Editor
LUCKY JAIN

September 2015 • Volume 42 • Number 3

ELSEVIER

1600 John F. Kennedy Boulevard • Suite 1800 • Philadelphia, Pennsylvania, 19103-2899

http://www.theclinics.com

CLINICS IN PERINATOLOGY Volume 42, Number 3
September 2015 ISSN 0095-5108, ISBN-13: 978-0-323-40264-4

Editor: Kerry Holland
Developmental Editor: Casey Jackson

Clinics in Perinatology (ISSN 0095-5108) is published quarterly by Elsevier Inc., 360 Park Avenue South, New York, NY 10010-1710. Months of issue are March, June, September, and December. Business and Editorial Offices: 1600 John F. Kennedy Blvd., Ste. 1800, Philadelphia, PA 19103-2899. Customer Service Office: 3251 Riverport Lane, Maryland Heights, MO 63043. Periodicals postage paid at New York, NY and additional mailing offices. Subscription prices are $285.00 per year (US individuals), $445.00 per year (US institutions), $340.00 per year (Canadian individuals), $545.00 per year (Canadian institutions), $420.00 per year (international individuals), $545.00 per year (international institutions), $135.00 per year (US students), and $195.00 per year (Canadian and international students). International air speed delivery is included in all Clinics subscription prices. All prices are subject to change without notice. **POSTMASTER:** Send address changes to *Clinics in Perinatology*, Elsevier Health Sciences Division, Subscription Customer Service, 3251 Riverport Lane, Maryland Heights, MO 63043. **Customer Service: Telephone: 1-800-654-2452** (U.S. and Canada); **1-314-447-8871** (outside U.S. and Canada). **Fax: 1-314-447-8029. E-mail: journalscustomerservice-usa@elsevier.com** (for print support); **journalsonlinesupport-usa@elsevier.com** (for online support).

Reprints. For copies of 100 or more, of articles in this publication, please contact the Commercial Reprints Department, Elsevier Inc., 360 Park Avenue South, New York, NY 10010-1710. Tel. 212-633-3874; Fax: 212-633-3820; E-mail: reprints@elsevier.com.

Clinics in Perinatology is also pubilshed in Spanish by McGraw-Hill Interamericana Editores S.A., P.O. Box 5-237, 06500 Mexico D.F., Mexico.

Clinics in Perinatology is covered in *MEDLINE/PubMed (Index Medicus) Current Contents, Excepta Medica, BIOSIS and ISI/BIOMED.*

Contributors

CONSULTING EDITOR

LUCKY JAIN, MD, MBA
Richard W. Blumberg Professor and Executive Vice Chairman, Department of Pediatrics, Emory University School of Medicine; Executive Medical Director, Children's Healthcare of Atlanta Faculty Practices, Atlanta, Georgia

EDITORS

ROBERT D. CHRISTENSEN, MD
Divisions of Neonatology and Hematology/Oncology, Department of Pediatrics, University of Utah School of Medicine; Director of Neonatology Research, Women and Newborn's Program, Intermountain Healthcare Salt Lake City, Utah

SANDRA E. JUUL, MD, PhD
Chief, Division of Neonatology; Professor, Department of Pediatrics, University of Washington School of Medicine, Seattle, Washington

ANTONIO DEL VECCHIO, MD
Director, Department of Women and Childrens Health, Di Venere Hospital, Bari, Italy

AUTHORS

GIUSEPPE BUONOCORE, MD
Full Professor of Pediatrics, Department of Molecular and Developmental Medicine, University of Siena, Siena, Italy

PATRICK D. CARROLL, MD, MPH
Women and Newborn's Program, Intermountain Healthcare, Salt Lake City, Utah; Regional Medical Director-Pediatrics and Neonatologist, Neonatal Services, Dixie Regional Medical Center, St George, Utah

GAETANO CHIRICO, MD
Neonatology and Neonatal Intensive Care Unit, Children's Hospital of Brescia, Spedali Civili of Brescia, Brescia, Italy

ROBERT D. CHRISTENSEN, MD
Divisions of Neonatology and Hematology/Oncology, Department of Pediatrics, University of Utah School of Medicine; Director of Neonatology Research, Women and Newborn's Program, Intermountain Healthcare Salt Lake City, Utah

ANTONIO DEL VECCHIO, MD
Director, Department of Women and Childrens Health, Di Venere Hospital, Bari, Italy

EMOKE DESCHMANN, MD
Department of Neonatology, Astrid Lindgren Children's Hospital, Karolinska University Hospital, Stockholm, Sweden

ERICK HENRY, MPH
Women and Newborn's Program, Intermountain Healthcare; The Institute for Healthcare Delivery Research, Salt Lake City, Utah

CASSANDRA D. JOSEPHSON, MD
Professor, Department of Pathology and Laboratory Medicine, Center for Transfusion and Cellular Therapies, Children's Healthcare of Atlanta, Emory University, Atlanta, Georgia

SANDRA E. JUUL, MD, PhD
Chief, Division of Neonatology; Professor, Department of Pediatrics, University of Washington School of Medicine, Seattle, Washington

JOYCE M. KOENIG, MD
Professor, Pediatrics, Molecular Microbiology, and Immunology, E Doisy Research Center, Saint Louis University School of Medicine, St Louis, Missouri

AKHIL MAHESHWARI, MD
Professor of Pediatrics, Molecular Medicine, and Public Health; Pamela and Leslie Muma Endowed Chair in Neonatology, USF Health Morsani College of Medicine, Tampa, Florida

PAOLO MANZONI, MD, PhD
Division of Neonatology and NICU, Sant'Anna Hospital, Azienda Ospedaliera Universitaria Città della Salute e della Scienza, Torino, Italy

MARIO MOTTA, MD
Neonatology and Neonatal Intensive Care Unit, Children's Hospital of Brescia, Spedali Civili of Brescia, Brescia, Italy

ROBERT SHEPPARD NICKEL, MD, MSc
Assistant Professor, Department of Pediatrics, Children's National Health System, The George Washington University School of Medicine and Health Sciences, Washington, DC

ROBIN K. OHLS, MD
Professor of Pediatrics; Director of Neonatal Research, Division of Neonatology, Department of Pediatrics, University of New Mexico, Albuquerque, New Mexico

SHRENA PATEL, MD
Division of Neonatology, Department of Pediatrics, University of Utah, Salt Lake City, Utah

SERAFINA PERRONE, MD, PhD
Department of Molecular and Developmental Medicine, University of Siena, Siena, Italy

GILLIAN C. PET, MD, MS
Neonatology Fellow, Division of Neonatology, Department of Pediatrics, University of Washington, Seattle, Washington

COSTANTINO ROMAGNOLI, MD
Neonatal Intensive Care Unit, Division of Neonatology, Department of Pediatrics, Catholic University of the Sacred Heart, Rome, Italy

MATTHEW A. SAXONHOUSE, MD
Associate Professor; Co-Director of Neonatal Thrombosis Center, Division of Neonatology, Levine Children's Hospital at Carolinas Medical Center, University of North Carolina School of Medicine, Charlotte, North Carolina

MARTHA SOLA-VISNER, MD
Associate Professor of Pediatrics, Division of Newborn Medicine, Boston Children's Hospital, Boston, Massachusetts

KATHERINE SPARGER, MD
Department of Pediatrics, Massachusetts General Hospital, Boston, Massachusetts

MARIA LUISA TATARANNO, MD
Department of Molecular and Developmental Medicine, University of Siena, Siena, Italy

HASSAN M. YAISH, MD
Division of Hematology/Oncology, Department of Pediatrics, University of Utah School of Medicine, Salt Lake City, Utah

MOMOKO YOSHIMOTO, MD, PhD
Assistant Research Professor, Pediatrics, Wells Center for Pediatric Research, Indiana University School of Medicine, Indianapolis, Indiana

Contents

> Certain groups of neonates are at high risk of developing long-term neurodevelopmental impairment and might be considered candidates for neuroprotective interventions. This article explores some of these high-risk groups, relevant mechanisms of brain injury, and specific mechanisms of cellular injury and death. The potential of erythropoietin (Epo) to act as a neuroprotective agent for neonatal brain injury is discussed. Clinical trials of Epo neuroprotection in preterm and term infants are updated.

> The various blood cell counts of neonates must be interpreted in accordance with high-quality reference intervals based on gestational and postnatal age. Using very large sample sizes, we generated neonatal reference intervals for each element of the complete blood count (CBC). Knowledge of whether a patient has CBC values that are too high (above the upper reference interval) or too low (below the lower reference interval) provides important insights into the specific disorder involved and in many instances suggests a treatment plan.

> Blood component transfusions are important to the care of preterm neonates; however, their use in clinical practice often is not based on high levels of evidence. Five major questions for neonates are discussed: (1) What is the optimal red blood cell (RBC) transfusion threshold? (2) What is the optimal platelet transfusion threshold? (3) Does the storage age of an RBC unit affect outcomes? (4) Does RBC transfusion contribute to the pathogenesis of necrotizing enterocolitis? and (5) Which new practices should be used to prevent transfusion-transmitted infections? Although definitive answers to these questions do not exist, future research should help answer them.

A shortened erythrocyte life span, because of hemolytic disorders, is a common cause of extreme neonatal hyperbilirubinemia. Clinical and laboratory examinations can frequently identify the underlying cause of extreme neonatal hyperbilirubinemia. In this article, several tests, techniques, and approaches have been reviewed, including red blood cell morphology assessment, end-tidal carbon monoxide quantification, eosin-5-maleimide flow cytometry, as well as next-generation DNA sequencing using neonatal jaundice panels.

Perinatal encephalopathy is a leading cause of lifelong disability. Increasing evidence indicates that the pathogenesis of perinatal brain damage is much more complex than originally thought, with multiple pathways involved. An important role of oxidative stress (OS) in the pathogenesis of brain injury is recognized for preterm and term infants. This article examines potential reliable and specific OS biomarkers that can be used in premature and term infants for the early detection and follow-up of the most common neonatal brain injuries, such as hypoxic-ischemic encephalopathy, intraventricular hemorrhage, and periventricular leukomalacia. The next step will be to explore the correlation between brain-specific OS biomarkers and functional brain outcomes.

Umbilical cord blood is a resource that is available to all neonates. Immediately after delivery of the fetus, cord blood can be used for the direct benefit of the premature infant. Delayed cord clamping and milking of the umbilical cord are 2 methods of transfusing additional fetal blood into the neonate after vaginal or cesarean delivery. Additionally, umbilical cord blood can be utilized for neonatal admission laboratory testing rather than direct neonatal phlebotomy. Together these strategies both increase initial neonatal total blood volume and limit immediate loss through phlebotomy.

Erythropoiesis-stimulating agents (ESAs) such as erythropoietin have been studied as red cell growth factors in preterm and term infants for more than 20 years. Recent studies have evaluated darbepoetin (Darbe, a long-acting ESA) for both erythropoietic effects and potential neuroprotection. We review clinical trials of Darbe in term and preterm infants, which have reported significant erythropoietic uses and neuroprotective effects. ESAs show great promise in decreasing or eliminating transfusions, and in preventing and treating brain injury in term and preterm infants.

Neonates receiving fresh frozen plasma (FFP) should do so according to evidence-based guidelines so as to reduce inappropriate use of this life-saving and costly blood product and to minimize associated adverse effects. The consensus-based uses of FFP in neonatology involve neonates with active bleeding and associated coagulopathy. However, because of limited and poor-quality evidence, considerable FFP utilization occurs outside these recommendations. In this review, we describe what we conclude are currently the best practices for the use of FFP in neonates, including interpreting neonatal coagulation tests and strategies for reducing unnecessary FFP transfusions.

Neonates have the highest risk for pathologic thrombosis among pediatric patients. A combination of genetic and acquired risk factors significantly contributes to this risk, with the most important risk factor being the use of central venous catheters. Proper imaging is critical for confirming the diagnosis. Despite a significant number of these events being life- and limb-threatening, there is limited evidence on what the appropriate management strategy should be. Evaluation and treatment of any neonate with a clinically significant thrombosis should occur at a tertiary referral center that has proper support.

PROGRAM OBJECTIVE
The goal of *Clinics in Perinatology* is to keep practicing perinatologists, neonatologists, obstetricians, practicing physicians and residents up to date with current clinical practice in perinatology by providing timely articles reviewing the state of the art in patient care.

TARGET AUDIENCE
Perinatologists, neonatologists, obstetricians, practicing physicians, residents and healthcare professionals who provide patient care utilizing findings from *Clinics in Perinatology*.

LEARNING OBJECTIVES
Upon completion of this activity, participants will be able to:
1. Review new and ongoing research in neonatal transfusion medicine.
2. Discuss the potential uses for stem cells in the treatment of perinatal injury.
3. Recognize how the administration of plasma and umbilical cord blood can be used in various NICU treatments to improve outcomes in the neonate.

ACCREDITATION
The Elsevier Office of Continuing Medical Education (EOCME) is accredited by the Accreditation Council for Continuing Medical Education (ACCME) to provide continuing medical education for physicians.

The EOCME designates this enduring material for a maximum of 15 *AMA PRA Category 1 Credit*(s)™. Physicians should claim only the credit commensurate with the extent of their participation in the activity.

All other health care professionals requesting continuing education credit for this enduring material will be issued a certificate of participation.

DISCLOSURE OF CONFLICTS OF INTEREST
The EOCME assesses conflict of interest with its instructors, faculty, planners, and other individuals who are in a position to control the content of CME activities. All relevant conflicts of interest that are identified are thoroughly vetted by EOCME for fair balance, scientific objectivity, and patient care recommendations. EOCME is committed to providing its learners with CME activities that promote improvements or quality in healthcare and not a specific proprietary business or a commercial interest.

The planning committee, staff, authors and editors listed below have identified no financial relationships or relationships to products or devices they or their spouse/life partner have with commercial interest related to the content of this CME activity:
Giuseppe Buonocore, MD; Patrick D. Carroll, MD, MPH; Gaetano Chirico, MD; Robert D. Christensen, MD; Antonio Del Vecchio, MD; Emoke Deschmann, MD; Anjali Fortna; Erick Henry, MPH; Kerry Holland; Lucky Jain, MD, MBA; Sandra E. Juul, MD, PhD; Joyce M. Koenig, MD; Akhil Maheshwari, MD; Paolo Manzoni, MD, PhD; Marlo Motta, MD; Palani Murugesan; Robert Sheppard Nickel, MD, MSc; Robin K. Ohls, MD; Shrena Patel, MD; Serafina Perrone, MD, PhD; Gillian C. Pet, MD, MS; Costantino Romagnoli, MD; Matthew A. Saxonhouse, MD; Katherine Sparger, MD; Megan Suermann; Maria Luisa Tataranno, MD; Hassan M. Yaish, MD; Momoko Yoshimoto, MD, PhD.

The planning committee, staff, authors and editors listed below have identified financial relationships or relationships to products or devices they or their spouse/life partner have with commercial interest related to the content of this CME activity:
Cassandra D. Josephson, MD is a consultant/advisor for Biomet, Inc.; Immucor, Inc.; and Octapharma AG. **Martha Sola-Visner, MD** is on the speakers' bureau for Sysmex Corporation.

UNAPPROVED/OFF-LABEL USE DISCLOSURE
The EOCME requires CME faculty to disclose to the participants:
1. When products or procedures being discussed are off-label, unlabelled, experimental, and/or investigational (not US Food and Drug Administration [FDA] approved); and
2. Any limitations on the information presented, such as data that are preliminary or that represent ongoing research, interim analyses, and/or unsupported opinions. Faculty may discuss information about pharmaceutical agents that is outside of FDA-approved labelling. This information is intended solely for CME and is not intended to promote off-label use of these medications. If you have any questions, contact the medical affairs department of the manufacturer for the most recent prescribing information.

TO ENROLL

To enroll in the *Clinics in Perinatology* Continuing Medical Education program, call customer service at 1-800-654-2452 or sign up online at http://www.theclinics.com/home/cme. The CME program is available to subscribers for an additional annual fee of $235 USD.

METHOD OF PARTICIPATION

In order to claim credit, participants must complete the following:

1. Complete enrolment as indicated above.
2. Read the activity.
3. Complete the CME Test and Evaluation. Participants must achieve a score of 70% on the test. All CME Tests and Evaluations must be completed online.

CME INQUIRIES/SPECIAL NEEDS

For all CME inquiries or special needs, please contact elsevierCME@elsevier.com.

CLINICS IN PERINATOLOGY

Foreword

Neonatal Hematology and Transfusion Medicine: What We Can Learn from Pediatric Oncology Groups

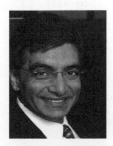

Lucky Jain, MD, MBA
Consulting Editor

A picture is worth a thousand words! One only needs to glance at the survival graph (**Fig. 1**) for children with acute leukemia to see how outcomes have changed in the past 50 years.[1] This is in sharp contrast to survival statistics for similar malignant disorders in adults, and many other chronic diseases in children. What is even more fascinating is that survival statistics look remarkably similar from different regions of the world separated by thousands of miles (**Table 1**).[2]

Many attribute this unprecedented success to uniform protocols and standardization of care in pediatric oncology that began decades ago and continues to date.[3] Where availability of resources is not a constraint, every child diagnosed with a malignancy receives standardized treatment based on one of several well-studied protocols. Outcomes, adverse effects, and details of protocol deviations are recorded at a centralized location. Protocols go through continuous PDSA (plan-do-study-act) cycles. Not surprisingly, similar standardization of care is also being implemented for pediatric hematologic disorders, albeit to a lesser extent.

A quick review of neonatal hematologic disorders and transfusion practices reveals a different story altogether.[4] Different thresholds exist from coast to coast for diagnostic approaches and transfusion practices. Transfusion volumes for packed red cells vary considerably from 10 to 20 mL/kg, transfused over anywhere from 1 to 4 hours. Some neonatologists hold feeds; others don't. Practices for placental transfusion and cord clamping similarly vary considerably, ranging from immediate cord clamping

Clin Perinatol 42 (2015) xv–xvii
http://dx.doi.org/10.1016/j.clp.2015.05.003
0095-5108/15/$ – see front matter © 2015 Published by Elsevier Inc.

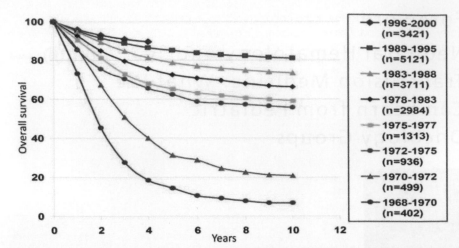

Fig. 1. Improved survival in childhood acute lymphoblastic leukemia. (*Adapted from* Hunger SP, Winick NJ, Sather HN, et al. Therapy of low-risk subsets of childhood acute lymphoblastic leukemia: when do we say enough? Pediatr Blood Cancer 2005;45:876–80; with permission.)

to a 120-second delay with or without cord milking.[5] The result is a huge variation in clinical practices that limits our inability to pin down best practices and eliminate those that cause harm.

Under the leadership of Drs Christensen, Juul, and Del Vecchio, contributing authors to this issue of *Clinics in Perinatology* have done a remarkable job in putting together a more consistent approach to management of neonatal hematologic disorders. Practitioners everywhere are encouraged to embrace these uniform care paths and consistently record outcomes. It is only through standardization of care and comparative effectiveness research that we will reduce morbidity and undesirable outcomes.

Table 1
Outcomes for newly diagnosed childhood acute lymphoblastic leukemia

Cooperative Group	Study	Years	Patients	5-y EFS (%)
Berlin-Frankfurt-Munster	ALL-BFM-95	1995–2000	2169	79.6[a]
Children's Oncology Group	Multiple	2000–2005	7153	90.4
Dana Farber Cancer Institute Consortium	DFCI 95-01	1996–2001	491	82.0
Nordic Society of Pediatric Hematology and Oncology	NOPHO	2002–2007	1023	79.0
St Jude Children's Research Hospital	TOTXV	2000–2007	498	85.6
United Kingdom Acute Lymphoblastic Leukaemia	UKALL 2003	2003–2011	3126	87.2

Abbreviation: EFS, event-free survival.
[a] Six-year EFS used in ALL-BFM-95.
Adapted from Cooper SL, Brown PA. Treatment of pediatric acute lymphoblastic leukemia. Pediatr Clin North Am 2015;62:16; with permission.

As always, I want to thank the editors, authors, and the publishing team at Elsevier (Kerry Holland and Casey Jackson) for another superb issue of the *Clinics in Perinatology*.

Lucky Jain, MD, MBA
Department of Pediatrics
Emory University School of Medicine and
Children's Healthcare of Atlanta
2015 Uppergate Drive
Atlanta, GA 30322, USA

E-mail address:
ljain@emory.edu

REFERENCES

1. Hunger SP, Winick NJ, Sather HN, et al. Therapy of low-risk subsets of childhood acute lymphoblastic leukemia: when do we say enough? Pediatr Blood Cancer 2005;45:876–80.
2. Cooper SL, Brown PA. Treatment of pediatric acute lymphoblastic leukemia. Pediatr Clin North Am 2015;62:1–16.
3. Pui CH, Evans WE. A 50-year journey to cure childhood acute lymphoblastic leukemia. Semin Hematol 2013;50:185–96.
4. Von Lindern JS, Lopriore E. Management and prevention of neonatal anemia: current evidence and guidelines. Expert Rev Hematol 2014;7:195–202.
5. Bhatt S, Polglase GR, Wallace EM, et al. Ventilation before umbilical cord clamping improves the physiological transition at birth. Front Pediatr 2014;2:1–8.

Preface

The Expanding Evidence Base to Guide Neonatal Hematology and Transfusion Medicine Practice

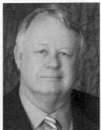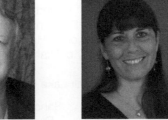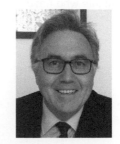

Robert D. Christensen, MD   Sandra E. Juul, MD, PhD   Antonio Del Vecchio, MD
Editors

Hematological problems occur every day in every NICU. Neonatologists, pediatricians, nurse practitioners, and bedside neonatal caregivers cannot work even one shift in a NICU without encountering issues related to cytopenias, hyperbilirubinemia, bleeding or clotting problems, or transfusion decisions. The information needed to provide the best-known solutions for these problems is ever-growing, changing, and increasing in complexity. Keeping up-to-date in clinical neonatal hematology and transfusion medicine is a formidable challenge, but is facilitated by an occasional comprehensive review like the one we have endeavored to produce for this issue of *Clinics in Perinatology*.

Each article of this issue was authored by a neonatal hematologist who has contributed consistently and thematically to the specific areas they volunteered to review. The issue is organized into four sections, dealing with (1) laboratory and blood-banking issues, (2) erythrocytes, (3) leukocytes, and (4) platelets and plasma. Each section contains several highly focused and clinically relevant articles.

The first section deals with pleiotropic effects of hematopoietic growth factors, reference intervals for the elements of a neonate's complete blood count, and the current major issues in neonatal transfusion medicine. The second section focuses on erythrocytes and includes articles on preventing early RBC transfusions by delayed cord clamping/milking and drawing the initial laboratory blood tests from the cord, Darbepoetin use in the NICU, causes of severe neonatal hyperbilirubinemia, and the problem of oxidative stress on neonatal erythrocytes. The third section focuses on leukocytes and includes articles on hematologic and immunologic aspects of necrotizing enterocolitis, hematologic aspects of early- and late-onset sepsis, and the prospects of stem cells as fetal/neonatal therapy. The final section, dealing with platelets, plasma,

http://dx.doi.org/10.1016/j.clp.2015.05.002
0095-5108/15/$ – see front matter © 2015 Published by Elsevier Inc.
perinatology.theclinics.com

thrombosis, and hemostasis, includes four articles authored by neonatal hematologists who have contributed much of what is known about these important clinical issues.

We express our deep appreciation to each article author, and to their teams of co-authors, for assembling the most up-to-date and clinically useful information available on these topics. We sincerely hope that this issue of *Clinics in Perinatology* will be a helpful reference for all NICU clinicians, providing at least some of the answers, and defining several consistent management approaches, thereby improving care of neonatal patients who have hematological and transfusion-related problems.

Robert D. Christensen, MD
Division of Neonatology and
Division of Hematology/Oncology
University of Utah School of Medicine
295 Chipeta Way
Salt Lake City, UT 84108, USA

Sandra E. Juul, MD, PhD
Division of Neonatology
University of Washington School of Medicine
Box 356320
Seattle, WA 98195-6320, USA

Antonio Del Vecchio, MD
Department of Women's and Children's Health
Neonatal Intensive Care Unit
Di Venere Hospital
Bari 70012, Italy

E-mail addresses:
Robert.Christensen@hsc.utah.edu (R.D. Christensen)
sjuul@uw.edu (S.E. Juul)
a.delvecchio@asl.bari.it (A. Del Vecchio)

Erythropoietin and Neonatal Neuroprotection

Sandra E. Juul, MD, PhD*, Gillian C. Pet, MD, MS

KEYWORDS

- Erythropoietin • Brain injury • Extreme prematurity
- Hypoxic ischemic encephalopathy • Apoptosis • Necrosis • Autophagy

KEY POINTS

- Neonates at known high risk of brain injury may be considered candidates for neuroprotective strategies.
- High-risk neonates develop brain injury that is specific to developmental age and mechanism of injury.
- Mechanisms of cell death include apoptosis, necrosis, and autophagy, and these pathways share molecular signals.
- Erythropoietin (Epo) may provide neuroprotection for multiple different pathways of brain injury.

INFANTS AT RISK FOR NEURODEVELOPMENTAL IMPAIRMENT

Neonatology is a new field of medical practice, having come into its own in the 1960s. As the practice has evolved, infants who were previously destined to die now survive, yet their outcomes are frequently burdened by significant neurodevelopmental challenges. Our mandate as neonatologists is to ensure that survivors of these previously fatal conditions can lead fully functional lives without impairment. Examples of infants who previously had little or no hope for survival include those born extremely prematurely (less than 28 weeks of gestation) and term infants with cyanotic heart disease such as hypoplastic left heart syndrome. Survivors of both these conditions have up to 50% neurodevelopmental impairment (NDI).[1–4] Infants who have survived neonatal hypoxic-ischemic encephalopathy (HIE), those with persistent pulmonary hypertension, and those who have undergone ECMO (extra corporeal membrane oxygenation) or neonatal stroke also face significant risks and might be considered candidates for neuroprotective treatments.[5] Common neonatal disorders that might benefit from neuroprotection and their current outcomes are listed in **Box 1**. Mechanisms of injury for 2 of these disorders are discussed.

Disclosures: None.
Division of Neonatology, Department of Pediatrics, University of Washington, 1959 Northeast Pacific Street, Box 356320, Seattle, WA 98195-6320, USA
* Corresponding author.
E-mail address: sjuul@uw.edu

Box 1
Neonatal conditions that may lend themselves to neuroprotection

Extreme prematurity (≤28 weeks gestation)

  7 of 1000 live births[6]

  About 80% survival with up to 50% moderate to severe NDI[1,2]

Hypoxic-ischemic encephalopathy

  1.7 per 1000 live births[7–9]

  About 24% to 33% survival with 27% to 38% moderate to severe NDI[10]

Persistent pulmonary hypertension

  1.5 per 1000 live births

  About 90% survival with up to 25% NDI, particularly hearing loss[11–14]

Cyanotic heart disease

  1.4 per 1000 live births

  Up to 50% moderate to severe NDI[4,15–17]

Stroke

  1 per 4000 live births estimated[18–20]

  Greater than 95% survival with up to 60% NDI[18,21]

Trauma

Preterm Brain Injury

Poor outcomes in premature infants may result from an interruption of normal development or from injury to existing tissues. The vulnerability of the developing brain changes as specific cell populations and structures mature. In the second trimester, neuronal production and migration occurs and synaptogenesis begins. Astrocyte and oligodendrocyte development follows, mediated by bone morphogenetic proteins, wnt, Shh, and Olig 1 and 2. The fetal brain rapidly increases in size, shape, and complexity during the third trimester.[22–24] This period is characterized by maturation of glutamatergic receptor subunits, in particular the K^+-Cl^- cotransporter KCC2, maturation of the neurovascular unit, and neuronal pruning.[25,26] There is concurrent maturation of antioxidant mechanisms systemically. During the period from 24 to 32 weeks of gestation, there is exquisite vulnerability of preoligodendrocytes and subplate neurons to oxidative injury, hypoxia, and excitotoxicity.[27–30] There are also structurally determined susceptibilities due to the developing germinal matrix and vulnerability of the watershed areas, as described by Volpe[31] in his 2009 review. Although the transition from fetal to early postnatal life is the period of greatest vulnerability to brain injury, preterm infants remain at risk for brain injury throughout the period of oligodendrocyte development.[32] This fact is highlighted by the finding that, although the incidence of both severe intracranial hemorrhage and cystic periventricular leukomalacia have diminished significantly over the last decades, neurodevelopmental outcomes for extremely preterm infants have remained largely unchanged.[33,34] It is increasingly appreciated that acute and chronic inflammation play an important role in preterm brain injury.[35,36] Although preterm infants have classically been thought to be at highest risk for white matter injury resulting from oligodendrocyte vulnerability, new findings show that dendritogenesis is also impaired, resulting in loss of both white and gray matter volumes.[37–39]

Hypoxic-Ischemic Encephalopathy

HIE results when there is disruption of both cerebral perfusion and tissue oxygenation. Animal models of acute brain injury show the injury and recovery process occurs in phases. The initial phase occurs during the period of decreased oxygen delivery. The body switches to anaerobic metabolism, which generates less ATP. This loss of cellular energy leads to dysfunction of Na$^+$, K$^+$, and Ca^{++} membrane pumps, accumulation of sodium and calcium in cells, cytotoxic edema, release of excitatory neurotransmitters (in particular, glutamate), and accumulation of free fatty acids. The second phase consists of secondary energy failure that occurs between 6 and 48 hours after the original injury and involves inflammation, cytotoxic edema, nitric oxide synthesis, mitochondrial dysfunction, and further accumulation of excitotoxins.[40] Cell death results from this secondary inflammatory response. Patterns of injury include injury to the deep gray matter (basal ganglia and thalami) in term infants who experience an acute hypoxic-ischemic event and multicystic encephalopathy in term infants who experience an acute event superimposed on more chronic mild to moderate hypoxia.

MECHANISMS OF CELL DEATH

There are 3 known mechanisms of cell death: apoptosis, necrosis, and autophagy. These cell death programs are complex and interrelated and involve signaling pathways that can potentially be inhibited, interrupted, or modified, allowing for targeted neuroprotective strategies (**Fig. 1**). Apoptosis is a form of programmed cell death characterized by immunologically silent cell shrinkage with nuclear pyknosis and intact plasma membranes. It can be activated by intrinsic or extrinsic pathways. The intrinsic, or mitochondrial, pathway depends on the balance of antiapoptotic proteins (such as Bcl-2 and Bcl-xL) and proapoptotic proteins (such as bax and bak). Apoptosis can also be triggered by external signals such as Fas ligand and tumor necrosis factor-alpha activation of proapoptotic receptors on the cell surface, which

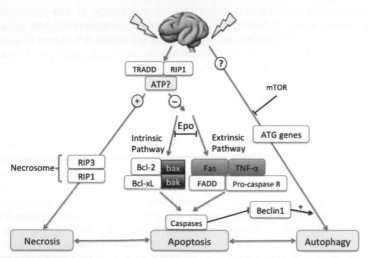

Fig. 1. Hypoxic-ischemic brain injury. FADD, Fas-associated protein with death domain; mTOR, mammalian target of rapamycin; RIP, receptor interacting protein; TNF-α, tumor necrosis factor-alpha; TRADD, tumor necrosis factor receptor–associated death domain.

is known as the extrinsic pathway. Activation leads to a death-inducing signaling complex containing Fas-associated protein with death domain and pro-caspase 8, which then adopts the same effector caspase pathways as the intrinsic pathway. Proapoptotic proteins cause permeabilization of the mitochondrial membrane, allowing factors including caspase to be released into the cytosol leading to apoptosis. Neuronal death following hypoxic-ischemic injury is initially mediated through necrotic pathways and later through apoptotic pathways, suggesting potential pathways for neuroprotection.[41]

Necrotic cell death occurs early after an acute injury such as hypoxia ischemia. It is characterized by profound swelling of cytoplasmic organelles including mitochondria, endoplasmic reticulum, and the nucleus. Necrotic cell death results in release of heat shock proteins and stimulates macrophage activation and cytokine release. Thus, although necrotic cell death requires less energy than apoptosis or autophagy, it stimulates an acute inflammatory response. Following hypoxia-ischemia, members of the tumor necrosis factor receptor (TNFR) superfamily are activated. A conformational change results, allowing interaction with serine/threonine kinase receptor interacting protein 1 (RIP1) and TNFR-associated death domain (TRADD). In the presence of adequate energy stores, the cell goes down the intrinsic apoptotic pathway. In the absence of adequate ATP, there is interaction between RIP1 and RIP3 to form the necrosome.[42] Neuronal necrosis that occurs in the context of excitotoxicity and hypoxic-ischemic injury is mediated by membrane depolarization caused by glutamate-triggered influx of calcium into the cell. Necrosis occurs predominantly in sites of profound energy deprivation such as the core of an ischemic region and is responsible for much of the immediate cell death during the first phase after injury, but there is a continuum between necrotic and apoptotic cell death.

Autophagy is a homeostatic process by which unwanted proteins and damaged organelles are eliminated from cells.[43] It is a catabolic process involving intracellular degradation of cytosolic proteins and organelles by autophagosomes, which fuse with lysosomes to form autophagolysosomes. Autophagy may decrease apoptosis by removing damaged mitochondria from the cell or may itself be a distinct mechanism of cell death that is interrelated to both necrosis and apoptosis.[44] There are several proposed mechanisms for the role of autophagy in cell death following hypoxic-ischemic injury including as an independent mechanism and as a trigger for apoptotic cell death. There are multiple signaling pathways involved in autophagy. Mammalian target of rapamycin (mTOR) pathways inhibit autophagy, and inhibitors of the mTOR pathway (rapamycin) stimulate autophagy.[45] Beclin1 induces autophagy and is negatively regulated by caspases, so caspase inhibitors also induce autophagy. Autophagic cell death is controlled by a series of ATG genes. Targeting pathways of autophagic cell death is a novel approach to neuroprotection.[46–48]

The predominant response to a hypoxic-ischemic event is influenced by the age and gender of the animal. In neonates, for example, neurons are more prone to apoptosis than in adults because of the ongoing pruning that occurs following neurogenesis in the second trimester. Males and females have different pathways of cell death that predominate.[49] Other factors such as ATP availability are also important in determining the cellular response to injury.[50] Cells may die from hybrids of multiples pathways (such as apoptosis and necrosis or apoptosis and autophagy), as there are significant interconnections between pathways (see **Fig. 1**).[51] If one pathway is inhibited, cell death can proceed down an alternative pathway. Each pathway is important for normal functioning; thus, blocking all pathways completely can have negative effects. As understanding of the complex interactions between mechanisms of cell death and survival improve, neuroprotective strategies may include use of multiple agents that work in a complementary manner, either to target different pathways or to use one drug to extend the therapeutic window of another. To date, most neuroprotective efforts have focused on inhibiting apoptosis, but this may result in the unintended consequence of increasing necrotic cell death and the concomitant inflammation that accompanies such cell death.

ERYTHROPOIETIN AS A NEUROPROTECTIVE AGENT FOR NEONATAL NEUROPROTECTION

Epo is a 30.4-kDa cytokine originally recognized for its role in erythropoiesis. Prenatally it is produced primarily in the liver, whereas postnatally it is produced primarily in the kidney. The switch in production site is thought to occur at approximately term postconceptual age. Epo is also produced in developing brain where it functions as both an important growth factor and neuroprotective agent for the central nervous system.[52–55] Epo is produced in brain by multiple cells types, including astrocytes, oligodendrocytes, neurons, and microglia.[56–61] Epo production is stimulated by hypoxia; in the brain, this is mediated by the transcription factor hypoxia-inducible factor (HIF)-1. HIF-2 has also been found to regulate the production of Epo in response to hypoxia in many tissues, although its precise role is less clear. Upregulation of Epo is part of the body's natural response to tissue hypoxia; however, a prolonged stimulus is required (on the order of hours). Elevated circulating or amniotic fluid Epo concentrations may therefore reflect chronic hypoxia in newborns.[62–65] Brief periods of brain perfusion and oxygenation severe enough to result in brain injury may not stimulate endogenous Epo production.[66] In these situations, and possibly others, high-dose exogenous recombinant Epo may provide an excellent neuroprotective strategy.

MECHANISM OF ACTION

Epo binds to 2 cell surface Epo receptors (EpoR) to form a homodimer, which activates Jak2 kinase to phosphorylate Jak2 and EpoR; this activates multiple signaling cascades, including MAPK (mitogen-activated protein kinase)/ERK (extracellular signal-regulated kinases), PI3K (phosphoinositide 3-kinase)/Akt, Stat5, and nuclear factor kappa B (NFkB). NFkB and Stat5 move into the nucleus and act as transcription factors for Bcl-2 and Bcl-xL, which are antiapoptotic genes. Epo also acts indirectly, by decreasing inflammation and oxidative injury. The common beta receptor-EpoR heterodimer may also be important in Epo neuroprotection[67]; however, this is controversial.

Epo is thought to have neuroprotective effects through multiple mechanisms (**Fig. 2**). In the short term, Epo's effects are antiapoptotic,[68,69] anti-inflammatory, neurotrophic, and antioxidant. Long-term effects that may promote brain development and healing include angiogenesis, neurogenesis, and oligodendrogenesis.[53,70–73] Epo also increases erythropoiesis, which in turn increases iron utilization. This increase has the effect of decreasing circulating, potentially unbound iron, which can produce harmful free radicals.[74]

In Vitro and In Vivo Studies

There have been many in vitro studies of Epo effects on cells exposed to hypoxia-ischemia. These studies have shown that Epo is protective for many cell types in the brain, including neurons,[58,75,76] astrocytes,[61,77,78] and oligodendrocytes.[53,79,80]

The effects of Epo on brain injury have been studied in multiple animal models.[81] Animal models have been used both to query Epo effects on gross and histologic brain

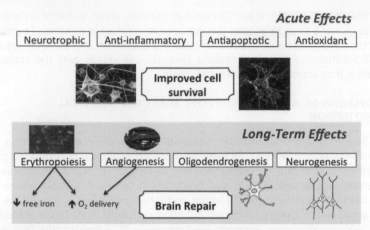

Fig. 2. Neuroprotective effects of Epo: cell and tissue repair.

injury and neurobehavioral outcomes and to elucidate the mechanism of neuroprotection. There is some variability in the results of these studies, likely related to variability in methodology, including duration of hypoxia, timing, dose and frequency of Epo administration, and timing of outcome studied. As hypothermia became standard care for neonates with HIE, it began to be incorporated in animal studies of Epo with variable results depending on the animal model used and other experimental conditions.[66,82,83]

CLINICAL TRIALS OF ERYTHROPOIETIN IN NEONATAL POPULATIONS

In the past 8 years, clinical trials to evaluate the safety and efficacy of Epo in various neonatal conditions have emerged. Neonatal patient populations that have been targeted include preterm infants (**Box 2**)[84–87] and term infants with HIE,[88,89] stroke,[90] and cyanotic heart disease (**Box 3**).[91] Pharmacokinetic and safety studies have shown that Epo dosed from 500 to 3000 U/kg is safe in preterm and term neonates. Two phase I/II studies evaluating the safety[85] and pharmacokinetics[84] of Epo using escalating doses in preterm infants and term infants with HIE[89] being treated with hypothermia showed that a dose of 1000 U/kg produced plasma concentrations similar to those found to be neuroprotective in animals[92,93] and was well tolerated. Follow-up of patients treated with Epo in these phase I/II trials allow for optimism that Epo may be beneficial,[94,95] although the studies were not designed for this purpose. Ohls and colleagues[86] showed that both Epo and darbepoetin had neuroprotective effects (improved cognitive performance assessed by Bayley III) when compared with placebo in preterm infants followed up at 18 to 22 months with preserved benefit at 4 years (Robin Ohls, personal communication, 2015). A preliminary finding of a phase III study of Epo neuroprotection in preterm infants has shown improved white matter integrity at term equivalent age.[87] Long-term neurodevelopmental outcomes of this study, which used 3 doses of 3000 U/kg in the first 3 days of life, are pending. Other phase III studies of Epo neuroprotection for preterm infants are ongoing in the United States (Preterm Epo Neuroprotection [PENUT] trial, NCT01378273) and Europe (Efficacy of Erythropoietin to Improve Survival and Neurologic Outcome in Hypoxic Ischemic Encephalopathy [Neurepo], NCT01732146). Each of these studies is using different dosing strategies and different durations of therapy. The results from these initial trials will inform future studies as to the optimal dose and duration of therapy for individual pathologies.

Box 2
Clinical trials of Epo neuroprotection in preterm neonatal populations

Preterm infants

Phase I/II

- A phase I/II trial of high-dose erythropoietin in extremely low-birth-weight infants: pharmacokinetics and safety[84]

- An approach to using recombinant erythropoietin for neuroprotection in very preterm infants[85]

- Cognitive Outcomes of Preterm Infants Randomized to Darbepoetin, Erythropoietin, or Placebo[86]

- Brain Imaging and Developmental Follow-up of Infants Treated with Erythropoietin (BRITE), NCT01207778

- Darbepoetin Administration to Preterm Infants, NCT00334737

Phase III

- Association between early administration of high-dose erythropoietin in preterm infants and brain MRI abnormality at term-equivalent age[87]

- Does Erythropoietin Improve Outcome in Very Preterm Infants? Swiss EPO Neuroprotection Trial Group Clinical Trial.gov identifier: NCT00413946 Enrollment complete, follow-up pending

- PENUT trial, a multicenter, randomized, placebo-controlled trial of 940 subjects. A National Institute of Neurological Disorders and Stroke–funded project. NCT01378273 Enrollment ongoing

---

SUMMARY OF ANIMAL AND HUMAN STUDIES

Epo has shown significant potential in in vitro and in vivo studies of brain injury.[81,97] It has specific cell receptor-mediated effects that are neuroprotective, as well as effects that are independent of the EpoR,[98] and more general systemic effects (anti-inflammatory, erythropoietic, angiogenic), all of which may be beneficial in the face of brain injury. These basic science studies are now being translated to the bedside. The translation of dose, dosing interval, and duration of treatment from rodent or other animal models to human neonates is tricky. Each of these factors must be individually evaluated in the context of each particular patient population and each injury type, as drug metabolism, drug dose, and duration of therapy may vary widely. For example, brain injury resulting from prematurity is likely chronic, occurring during the vulnerable period of oligodendrocyte maturation and influenced by stress, inflammation, hypoxia, hyperoxia, and necessary medications. In contrast, the injury that results from acute hypoxia-ischemia in the perinatal period of term infants is short lived and likely requires a shorter duration of therapy than prevention or treatment of preterm brain injury. Patients with cyanotic heart disease who undergo hypothermia and bypass surgery may be eligible for pretreatment. Epo neuroprotection must also be evaluated as an adjunct to other therapies. For preterm infants, prenatal steroids, magnesium sulfate, and delayed cord clamping are frequently used before and at birth. Postnatally, caffeine, melatonin, and neuro neonatal intensive care unit care packages are being evaluated to improve outcomes. The role that Epo might play in this emerging environment is unknown. Similarly, for term infants with HIE, therapeutic hypothermia is now standard care. Other adjunctive therapies including Epo, melatonin, and xenon must be evaluated for safety and efficacy in the context of cooling.

Box 3
Clinical trials of Epo neuroprotection in term neonatal populations

Hypoxic-ischemic encephalopathy

Phase I/II

- Neurologic outcome after erythropoietin treatment of neonatal encephalopathy, NCT00808704[88]

- NEAT trial: Erythropoietin for neuroprotection in neonatal encephalopathy: safety and pharmacokinetics, NCT00719407[89]

- NEAT trial follow-up: Erythropoietin and hypothermia for hypoxic-ischemic encephalopathy, NCT00719407[94]

- Erythropoietin in Infants with Hypoxic-Ischemic Encephalopathy, NCT00945789[96]

- Darbe Administration in Newborns Undergoing Cooling for Encephalopathy (DANCE), NCT01471015. Enrollment completed

- NEAT-O trial: Neonatal Epo and therapeutic hypothermia; short-term outcome study, NCT01913340. Enrollment complete, follow-up is ongoing

- Efficacy of Erythropoietin to Improve Survival and Neurological Outcome in Hypoxic Ischemic Encephalopathy (Neurepo), NCT01732146. Enrollment is ongoing

- Neuroprotective role of erythropoietin in perinatal asphyxia, NCT02002039. Enrollment is ongoing

Phase III

- Preventing Adverse Outcomes of Neonatal Encephalopathy with Erythropoietin (PAEAN) study. Enrollment pending

Stroke

Phase I/II

- Feasibility and safety of erythropoietin for neuroprotection after perinatal arterial ischemic stroke[90]

Cyanotic heart disease

Phase I/II

- Erythropoietin neuroprotection in neonatal cardiac surgery: a phase I/II safety and efficacy trial[91]

REFERENCES

1. Stoll BJ, Hansen NI, Bell EF, et al. Neonatal outcomes of extremely preterm infants from the NICHD Neonatal Research Network. Pediatrics 2010;126(3):443–56.
2. Gargus RA, Vohr BR, Tyson JE, et al. Unimpaired outcomes for extremely low birth weight infants at 18 to 22 months. Pediatrics 2009;124(1):112–21.
3. McQuillen PS, Miller SP. Congenital heart disease and brain development. Ann N Y Acad Sci 2010;1184:68–86.
4. Miller SP, McQuillen PS, Hamrick S, et al. Abnormal brain development in new-borns with congenital heart disease. N Engl J Med 2007;357(19):1928–38.
5. Edwards AD, Brocklehurst P, Gunn AJ, et al. Neurological outcomes at 18 months of age after moderate hypothermia for perinatal hypoxic ischaemic encephalopathy: synthesis and meta-analysis of trial data. BMJ 2010;340:c363.
6. Hamilton BE, Hoyert DL, Martin JA, et al. Annual summary of vital statistics: 2010-2011. Pediatrics 2013;131(3):548–58.

7. Wu YW, Escobar GJ, Grether JK, et al. Chorioamnionitis and cerebral palsy in term and near-term infants. JAMA 2003;290(20):2677–84.
8. Wu YW, Backstrand KH, Zhao S, et al. Declining diagnosis of birth asphyxia in California: 1991-2000. Pediatrics 2004;114(6):1584–90.
9. Wu YW, Croen LA, Shah SJ, et al. Cerebral palsy in a term population: risk factors and neuroimaging findings. Pediatrics 2006;118(2):690–7.
10. Tagin MA, Woolcott CG, Vincer MJ, et al. Hypothermia for neonatal hypoxic ischemic encephalopathy: an updated systematic review and meta-analysis. Arch Pediatr Adolesc Med 2012;166(6):558–66.
11. Leavitt AM, Watchko JF, Bennett FC, et al. Neurodevelopmental outcome following persistent pulmonary hypertension of the neonate. J Perinatol 1987; 7(4):288–91.
12. Rohana J, Boo NY, Chandran V, et al. Neurodevelopmental outcome of newborns with persistent pulmonary hypertension. Malays J Med Sci 2011;18(4):58–62.
13. Rosenberg AA, Lee NR, Vaver KN, et al. School-age outcomes of newborns treated for persistent pulmonary hypertension. J Perinatol 2010;30(2):127–34.
14. Eriksen V, Nielsen LH, Klokker M, et al. Follow-up of 5- to 11-year-old children treated for persistent pulmonary hypertension of the newborn. Acta Paediatr 2009;98(2):304–9.
15. Miller SP, McQuillen PS, Vigneron DB, et al. Preoperative brain injury in newborns with transposition of the great arteries. Ann Thorac Surg 2004;77(5): 1698–706.
16. McQuillen PS, Barkovich AJ, Hamrick SE, et al. Temporal and anatomic risk profile of brain injury with neonatal repair of congenital heart defects. Stroke 2007; 38(Suppl 2):736–41.
17. Miller SP, McQuillen PS. Neurology of congenital heart disease: insight from brain imaging. Arch Dis Child Fetal Neonatal Ed 2007;92(6):F435–7.
18. Wu YW, Lynch JK, Nelson KB. Perinatal arterial stroke: understanding mechanisms and outcomes. Semin Neurol 2005;25(4):424–34.
19. Nelson KB. Perinatal ischemic stroke. Stroke 2007;38(Suppl 2):742–5.
20. Raju TN, Nelson KB, Ferriero D, et al, NICHD-NINDS Perinatal Stroke Workshop Participants. Ischemic perinatal stroke: summary of a workshop sponsored by the National Institute of Child Health and Human Development and the National Institute of Neurological Disorders and Stroke. Pediatrics 2007;120(3):609–16.
21. Lynch JK, Nelson KB. Epidemiology of perinatal stroke. Curr Opin Pediatr 2001; 13(6):499–505.
22. Rajagopalan V, Scott JA, Habas PA, et al. Local tissue growth patterns underlying normal fetal human brain gyrification quantified in utero. J Neurosci 2011;31(8): 2878–87.
23. Lodygensky GA, Vasung L, Sizonenko SV, et al. Neuroimaging of cortical development and brain connectivity in human newborns and animal models. J Anat 2010;217(4):418–28.
24. Huppi PS. Growth and development of the brain and impact on cognitive outcomes. Nestle Nutr Workshop Ser Pediatr Program 2010;65:137–49 [discussion 149–51].
25. Zhang LL, Fina ME, Vardi N. Regulation of KCC2 and NKCC during development: membrane insertion and differences between cell types. J Comp Neurol 2006; 499(1):132–43.
26. Li H, Khirug S, Cai C, et al. KCC2 interacts with the dendritic cytoskeleton to promote spine development. Neuron 2007;56(6):1019–33.
27. McQuillen PS, Ferriero DM. Selective vulnerability in the developing central nervous system. Pediatr Neurol 2004;30(4):227–35.

28. Volpe JJ. The encephalopathy of prematurity–brain injury and impaired brain development inextricably intertwined. Semin Pediatr Neurol 2009;16(4):167–78.
29. Back SA, Riddle A, McClure MM. Maturation-dependent vulnerability of perinatal white matter in premature birth. Stroke 2007;38(Suppl 2):724–30.
30. Back SA, Gan X, Li Y, et al. Maturation-dependent vulnerability of oligodendrocytes to oxidative stress-induced death caused by glutathione depletion. J Neurosci 1998;18(16):6241–53.
31. Volpe JJ. Brain injury in premature infants: a complex amalgam of destructive and developmental disturbances. Lancet Neurol 2009;8(1):110–24.
32. Ment LR, Bada HS, Barnes P, et al. Practice parameter: neuroimaging of the neonate: report of the Quality Standards Subcommittee of the American Academy of Neurology and the Practice Committee of the Child Neurology Society. Neurology 2002;58(12):1726–38.
33. Buser JR, Maire J, Riddle A, et al. Arrested preoligodendrocyte maturation contributes to myelination failure in premature infants. Ann Neurol 2012;71(1):93–109.
34. Riddle A, Dean J, Buser JR, et al. Histopathological correlates of magnetic resonance imaging-defined chronic perinatal white matter injury. Ann Neurol 2011;70(3):493–507.
35. Mallard C, Davidson JO, Tan S, et al. Astrocytes and microglia in acute cerebral injury underlying cerebral palsy associated with preterm birth. Pediatr Res 2014;75(1–2):234–40.
36. Hintz SR, Kendrick DE, Stoll BJ, et al. Neurodevelopmental and growth outcomes of extremely low birth weight infants after necrotizing enterocolitis. Pediatrics 2005;115(3):696–703.
37. Back SA. Cerebral white and gray matter injury in newborns: new insights into pathophysiology and management. Clin Perinatol 2014;41(1):1–24.
38. Kidokoro H, Neil JJ, Inder TE. New MR imaging assessment tool to define brain abnormalities in very preterm infants at term. AJNR Am J Neuroradiol 2013;34(11):2208–14.
39. Strunk T, Inder T, Wang X, et al. Infection-induced inflammation and cerebral injury in preterm infants. Lancet Infect Dis 2014;14(8):751–62.
40. Robertson NJ, Tan S, Groenendaal F, et al. Which neuroprotective agents are ready for bench to bedside translation in the newborn infant? J Pediatr 2012;160(4):544–52.e4.
41. Northington FJ, Ferriero DM, Graham EM, et al. Early neurodegeneration after hypoxia-ischemia in neonatal rat is necrosis while delayed neuronal death is apoptosis. Neurobiol Dis 2001;8(2):207–19.
42. Chavez-Valdez R, Martin LJ, Northington FJ. Programmed necrosis: a prominent mechanism of cell death following neonatal brain injury. Neurol Res Int 2012;2012:257563.
43. Boland B, Nixon RA. Neuronal macroautophagy: from development to degeneration. Mol Aspects Med 2006;27(5–6):503–19.
44. Chaabane W, User SD, El-Gazzah M, et al. Autophagy, apoptosis, mitoptosis and necrosis: interdependence between those pathways and effects on cancer. Arch Immunol Ther Exp (Warsz) 2013;61(1):43–58.
45. Lakhani R, Vogel KR, Till A, et al. Defects in GABA metabolism affect selective autophagy pathways and are alleviated by mTOR inhibition. EMBO Mol Med 2014;6(4):551–66.
46. Bendix I, Schulze C, Haefen C, et al. Erythropoietin modulates autophagy signaling in the developing rat brain in an in vivo model of oxygen-toxicity. Int J Mol Sci 2012;13(10):12939–51.

47. Zheng Y, Hou J, Liu J, et al. Inhibition of autophagy contributes to melatonin-mediated neuroprotection against transient focal cerebral ischemia in rats. J Pharmacol Sci 2014;124(3):354–64.

48. Jiang T, Yu JT, Zhu XC, et al. Ischemic preconditioning provides neuroprotection by induction of AMP-activated protein kinase-dependent autophagy in a rat model of ischemic stroke. Mol Neurobiol 2015;51:220–9.

49. Zhu C, Xu F, Wang X, et al. Different apoptotic mechanisms are activated in male and female brains after neonatal hypoxia-ischaemia. J Neurochem 2006;96(4): 1016–27.

50. Eguchi Y, Shimizu S, Tsujimoto Y. Intracellular ATP levels determine cell death fate by apoptosis or necrosis. Cancer Res 1997;57(10):1835–40.

51. Tsujimoto Y, Shimizu S, Eguchi Y, et al. Bcl-2 and Bcl-xL block apoptosis as well as necrosis: possible involvement of common mediators in apoptotic and necrotic signal transduction pathways. Leukemia 1997;11(Suppl 3): 380–2.

52. Yu X, Shacka JJ, Eells JB, et al. Erythropoietin receptor signalling is required for normal brain development. Development 2002;129(2):505–16.

53. Jantzie LL, Miller RH, Robinson S. Erythropoietin signaling promotes oligodendro-cyte development following prenatal systemic hypoxic-ischemic brain injury. Pediatr Res 2013;74(6):658–67.

54. Juul SE, Yachnis AT, Rojiani AM, et al. Immunohistochemical localization of erythropoietin and its receptor in the developing human brain. Pediatr Dev Pathol 1999;2(2):148–58.

55. Chen ZY, Warin R, Noguchi CT. Erythropoietin and normal brain development: receptor expression determines multi-tissue response. Neurodegener Dis 2006; 3(1–2):68–75.

56. Chen ZY, Asavaritikrai P, Prchal JT, et al. Endogenous erythropoietin signaling is required for normal neural progenitor cell proliferation. J Biol Chem 2007;282(35): 25875–83.

57. Sakanaka M, Wen TC, Matsuda S, et al. In vivo evidence that erythropoietin protects neurons from ischemic damage. Proc Natl Acad Sci U S A 1998;95(8): 4635–40.

58. Juul SE, Anderson DK, Li Y, et al. Erythropoietin and erythropoietin receptor in the developing human central nervous system. Pediatr Res 1998;43(1):40–9.

59. Masuda S, Nagao M, Sasaki R. Erythropoietic, neurotrophic, and angiogenic functions of erythropoietin and regulation of erythropoietin production. Int J Hematol 1999;70(1):1–6.

60. Masuda S, Okano M, Yamagishi K, et al. A novel site of erythropoietin production. Oxygen-dependent production in cultured rat astrocytes. J Biol Chem 1994; 269(30):19488–93.

61. Sugawa M, Sakurai Y, Ishikawa-Ieda Y, et al. Effects of erythropoietin on glial cell development; oligodendrocyte maturation and astrocyte proliferation. Neurosci Res 2002;44(4):391–403.

62. Teramo KA, Widness JA, Clemons GK, et al. Amniotic fluid erythropoietin correlates with umbilical plasma erythropoietin in normal and abnormal pregnancy. Obstet Gynecol 1987;69(5):710–6.

63. Buescher U, Hertwig K, Wolf C, et al. Erythropoietin in amniotic fluid as a marker of chronic fetal hypoxia. Int J Gynaecol Obstet 1998;60(3):257–63.

64. Teramo KA, Widness JA. Increased fetal plasma and amniotic fluid erythropoietin concentrations: markers of intrauterine hypoxia. Neonatology 2009;95(2): 105–16.

65. Mikovic Z, Mandic V, Parovic V, et al. Erythropoietin in amniotic fluid as a potential marker in distinction between growth restricted and constitutionally small fetuses. J Matern Fetal Neonatal Med 2014;27(11):1134–7.
66. Traudt CM, McPherson RJ, Bauer LA, et al. Concurrent erythropoietin and hypothermia treatment improve outcomes in a term nonhuman primate model of perinatal asphyxia. Dev Neurosci 2013;35(6):491–503.
67. Brines M, Grasso G, Fiordaliso F, et al. Erythropoietin mediates tissue protection through an erythropoietin and common beta-subunit heteroreceptor. Proc Natl Acad Sci U S A 2004;101(41):14907–12.
68. Juul SE, Beyer RP, Bammler TK, et al. Microarray analysis of high-dose recombinant erythropoietin treatment of unilateral brain injury in neonatal mouse hippocampus. Pediatr Res 2009;65(5):485–92.
69. Rangarajan V, Juul SE. Erythropoietin: emerging role of erythropoietin in neonatal neuroprotection. Pediatr Neurol 2014;51(4):481–8.
70. Shingo T, Sorokan ST, Shimazaki T, et al. Erythropoietin regulates the in vitro and in vivo production of neuronal progenitors by mammalian forebrain neural stem cells. J Neurosci 2001;21(24):9733–43.
71. Tsai PT, Ohab JJ, Kertesz N, et al. A critical role of erythropoietin receptor in neurogenesis and post-stroke recovery. J Neurosci 2006;26(4):1269–74.
72. Wang L, Zhang Z, Wang Y, et al. Treatment of stroke with erythropoietin enhances neurogenesis and angiogenesis and improves neurological function in rats. Stroke 2004;35(7):1732–7.
73. Jantzie LL, Corbett CJ, Firl DJ, et al. Postnatal erythropoietin mitigates impaired cerebral cortical development following subplate loss from prenatal hypoxia-ischemia. Cereb Cortex 2014. http://dx.doi.org/10.1093/cercor/bhu066.
74. Juul SE, Ferriero DM. Pharmacologic neuroprotective strategies in neonatal brain injury. Clin Perinatol 2014;41(1):119–31.
75. Digicaylioglu M, Lipton SA. Erythropoietin-mediated neuroprotection involves cross-talk between Jak2 and NF-kappaB signalling cascades. Nature 2001; 412(6847):641–7.
76. Masuda S, Kada E, Nagao M, et al. In vitro neuroprotective action of recombinant rat erythropoietin produced by astrocyte cell lines and comparative studies with erythropoietin produced by Chinese hamster ovary cells. Cytotechnology 1999; 29(3):207–13.
77. Gunnarson E, Song Y, Kowalewski JM, et al. Erythropoietin modulation of astrocyte water permeability as a component of neuroprotection. Proc Natl Acad Sci U S A 2009;106(5):1602–7.
78. Sinor AD, Greenberg DA. Erythropoietin protects cultured cortical neurons, but not astroglia, from hypoxia and AMPA toxicity. Neurosci Lett 2000;290(3):213–5.
79. Cho YK, Kim G, Park S, et al. Erythropoietin promotes oligodendrogenesis and myelin repair following lysolecithin-induced injury in spinal cord slice culture. Biochem Biophys Res Commun 2012;417(2):753–9.
80. Iwai M, Stetler RA, Xing J, et al. Enhanced oligodendrogenesis and recovery of neurological function by erythropoietin after neonatal hypoxic/ischemic brain injury. Stroke 2010;41(5):1032–7.
81. van der Kooij MA, Groenendaal F, Kavelaars A, et al. Neuroprotective properties and mechanisms of erythropoietin in in vitro and in vivo experimental models for hypoxia/ischemia. Brain Res Rev 2008;59(1):22–33.
82. Fan X, van Bel F, van der Kooij MA, et al. Hypothermia and erythropoietin for neuroprotection after neonatal brain damage. Pediatr Res 2013;73(1):18–23.

83. Fang AY, Gonzalez FF, Sheldon RA, et al. Effects of combination therapy using hypothermia and erythropoietin in a rat model of neonatal hypoxia-ischemia. Pediatr Res 2013;73(1):12–7.
84. Juul SE, McPherson RJ, Bauer LA, et al. A phase I/II trial of high-dose erythropoietin in extremely low birth weight infants: pharmacokinetics and safety. Pediatrics 2008;122(2):383–91.
85. Fauchere JC, Dame C, Vonthein R, et al. An approach to using recombinant erythropoietin for neuroprotection in very preterm infants. Pediatrics 2008; 122(2):375–82.
86. Ohls RK, Kamath-Rayne BD, Christensen RD, et al. Cognitive outcomes of preterm infants randomized to darbepoetin. Pediatrics 2014. http://dx.doi.org/10. 1542/peds.2013-4307.
87. Leuchter RH, Gui L, Poncet A, et al. Association between early administration of high-dose erythropoietin in preterm infants and brain MRI abnormality at term-equivalent age. JAMA 2014;312(8):817–24.
88. Zhu C, Kang W, Xu F, et al. Erythropoietin improved neurologic outcomes in newborns with hypoxic-ischemic encephalopathy. Pediatrics 2009;124(2): e218–26.
89. Wu YW, Bauer LA, Ballard RA, et al. Erythropoietin for neuroprotection in neonatal encephalopathy: safety and pharmacokinetics. Pediatrics 2012; 130(4):683–91.
90. Benders MJ, van der Aa NE, Roks M, et al. Feasibility and safety of erythropoietin for neuroprotection after perinatal arterial ischemic stroke. J Pediatr 2014;164(3): 481–6.e1–2.
91. Andropoulos DB, Brady K, Easley RB, et al. Erythropoietin neuroprotection in neonatal cardiac surgery: a phase I/II safety and efficacy trial. J Thorac Cardiovasc Surg 2013;146(1):124–31.
92. Kellert BA, McPherson RJ, Juul SE. A comparison of high-dose recombinant erythropoietin treatment regimens in brain-injured neonatal rats. Pediatr Res 2007;61(4):451–5.
93. Statler PA, McPherson RJ, Bauer LA, et al. Pharmacokinetics of high-dose recombinant erythropoietin in plasma and brain of neonatal rats. Pediatr Res 2007; 61(6):671–5.
94. Rogers EE, Bonifacio SL, Glass HC, et al. Erythropoietin and hypothermia for hypoxic-ischemic encephalopathy. Pediatr Neurol 2014;51(5):657–62.
95. McAdams RM, McPherson RJ, Mayock DE, et al. Outcomes of extremely low birth weight infants given early high-dose erythropoietin. J Perinatol 2013;33(3): 226–30.
96. Elmahdy H, El-Mashad AR, El-Bahrawy H, et al. Human recombinant erythropoietin in asphyxia neonatorum: pilot trial. Pediatrics 2010;125(5):e1135–42.
97. Pett GC, Juul SE. The potential of erythropoietin to treat asphyxia in newborns. Res Rep Neonatol 2014;4:195–207.
98. Xiong Y, Mahmood A, Qu C, et al. Erythropoietin improves histological and functional outcomes after traumatic brain injury in mice in the absence of the neural erythropoietin receptor. J Neurotrauma 2010;27(1):205–15.

Reference Intervals in Neonatal Hematology

Erick Henry, MPH[a,b,*], Robert D. Christensen, MD[a,c,d]

KEYWORDS

- Complete blood count • CBC • Hemoglobin • Anemia • Erythrocyte indices
- Platelets • Leukocytes

KEY POINTS

- The various blood cell counts of neonates must be interpreted in accordance with high-quality reference intervals based on gestational and postnatal age.
- Using very large sample sizes, we generated neonatal reference intervals for each element of the complete blood count (CBC).
- Knowledge of whether a patient has CBC values that are too high (above the upper reference interval) or too low (below the lower reference interval) provides important insights into the specific disorder involved and in many instances suggests a treatment plan.

REFERENCE INTERVALS

In adult medicine, the elements of the complete blood count (CBC) can be recognized as normal or abnormal by comparing the patient's values with normal ranges established by drawing blood on large numbers of healthy adult volunteers. Normal ranges are not available for neonates, because of justified ethical concerns about drawing blood from healthy neonates for research purposes only. Consequently another approach is used, a concept termed reference intervals. These consist of 5th to 95th percentile values compiled from laboratory tests performed on selected neonates from whom a CBC was drawn for a clinical purpose. The process for selecting the data to be included in the reference range involves retrospectively identifying CBCs from

Disclosures: None.
[a] Women and Newborn's Program, Intermountain Healthcare, 36 S. State Street, Salt Lake City, UT 84111, USA; [b] The Institute for Healthcare Delivery Research, 36 S. State Street Salt Lake City, UT 84111, USA; [c] Division of Neonatology, Department of Pediatrics, University of Utah School of Medicine, 295 Chipeta Way, Salt Lake City, UT, 84108 USA; [d] Division of Hematology/Oncology, Department of Pediatrics, University of Utah School of Medicine, 295 Chipeta Way, Salt Lake City, UT, 84108 USA
* Corresponding author. Women and Newborn's Program, Intermountain Healthcare, Key Bank Building, 36 S. State Street Salt Lake City, UT 84111.
E-mail address: Erick.henry@imail.org

neonates thought to have minimal disorders relevant to the laboratory test, or with disorders unlikely to significantly affect the test results.

To allow for reference ranges not being obtained on healthy volunteers, but on patients, the convention for the range used is different than for normal ranges. Normal ranges include 95% of the measured values, excluding the lowest and the highest 2.5%. In contrast, for reference ranges, 90% of values are included and the lowest and highest 5% are excluded, thus reference ranges are those between the 5th and the 95th percentile values.

Once the relevant database is set, the values within it are displayed in both of 2 ways: (1) data on the day of birth are shown according to gestational age, which is helpful when values at birth vary with gestational age, as is the case for many of the CBC parameters; (2) data on subsequent days are shown, thus illustrating the expected changes over the first weeks or months. These 2 data displays, focused on the 5th percentile value (lower range) and the 95th percentile (upper range) constitute reference intervals for neonates.

Over the past 7 years, we have published 15 reference interval studies focused on individual aspects of the CBC, all based on the Intermountain Healthcare datamarts.[1-15] Intermountain Healthcare is a not-for-profit company that owns and operates hospitals in Utah and Idaho. The present article brings together these individual reports into a single source. It is our hope that practitioners, rather than looking up the various individual publications, will consult this 1 source as a convenient and clinically useful resource.

METHODOLOGY

All reference intervals in this article were derived by identifying every CBC result performed on neonates in the Intermountain Healthcare system between 2005 and 2014. More than 350,000 individual test values were obtained on about 100,000 neonates. The number of values included in each reference interval varied by panel, ranging from a low of 3922 values for neutrophil counts of neonates of 22 to 28 weeks' gestation to a high of 216,869 values for platelet counts in the first 90 days of life. Patients who had an ICD9 (International Classification of Diseases, 9th Revision) code for a chromosomal abnormality were excluded. The neonate's record was matched to delivery information to ascertain the age of the baby in hours and days at the time of the test. Neonates who had received a red blood cell transfusion before their laboratory test for hematocrit, hemoglobin, mean corpuscular volume (MCV), mean corpuscular hemoglobin (MCH), or MCH concentration (MCHC) were excluded from the analysis. The average, 5th, and 95th percentiles were calculated (Statit, Corvallis, OR) and displayed by statistical trend lines.

INDIVIDUAL REFERENCE INTERVALS

Figs. 1–23 show the different neonatal CBC reference intervals. Each figure is constructed to show either the day of birth, giving reference intervals according to gestational age at birth, or postnatal age, giving reference intervals according to hours or days after birth. Where the CBC values for postnatal age vary significantly according to gestational age at birth, separate figures, based on gestational age, are provided. In each figure the 5th percentile is the lower reference interval and the 95th percentile is the upper reference interval. Both of these are shown by dotted lines. The average values are shown by solid lines.

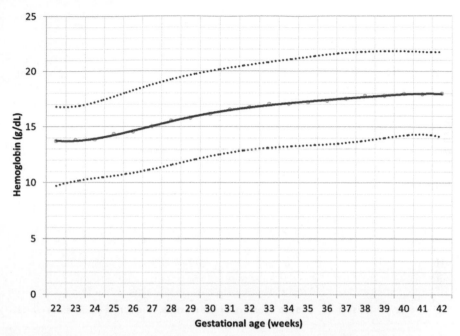

Fig. 1. Blood hemoglobin concentration on the day of birth, according to gestational age.

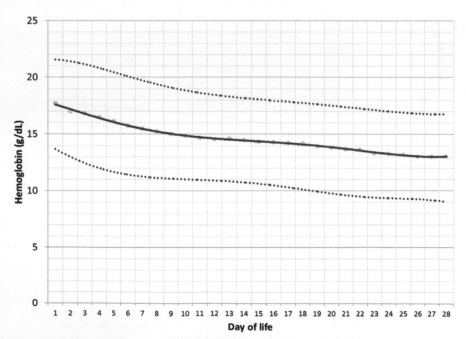

Fig. 2. Blood hemoglobin concentration over the first 28 days of life for neonates born at 35 to 42 weeks' gestation.

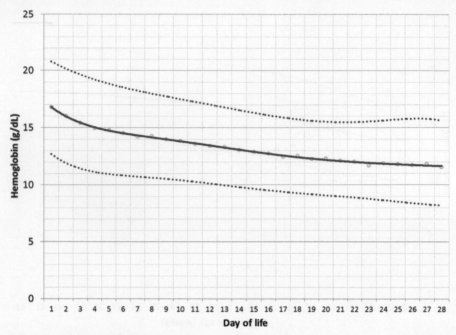

Fig. 3. Blood hemoglobin concentration over the first 28 days of life for neonates born at 29 to 34 weeks' gestation.

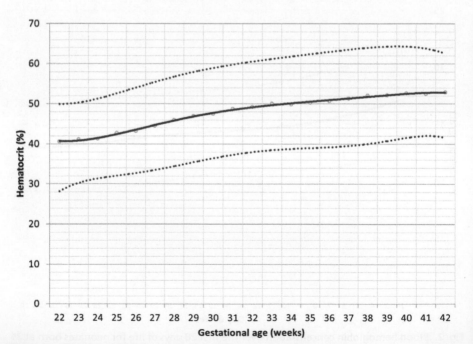

Fig. 4. Hematocrit on the day of birth, according to gestational age.

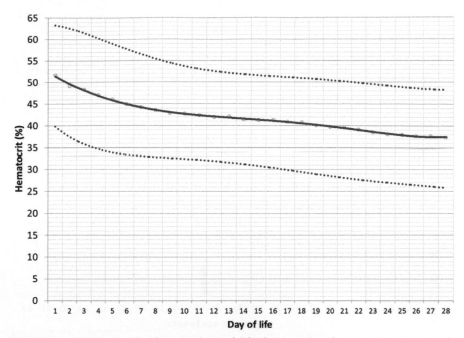

Fig. 5. Hematocrit over the first 28 days of life for neonates born at 35 to 42 weeks' gestation.

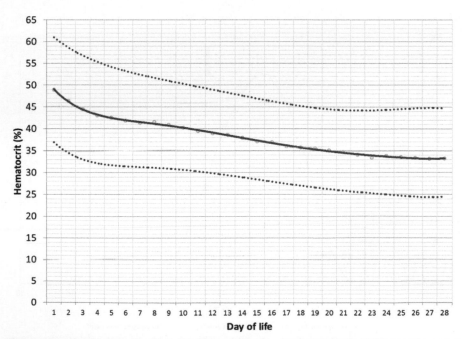

Fig. 6. Hematocrit over the first 28 days of life for neonates born at 29 to 34 weeks' gestation.

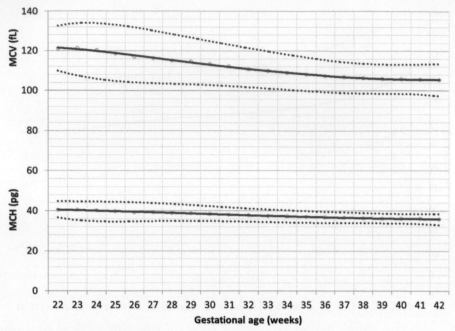

Fig. 7. MCV and MCH on the day of birth, according to gestational age.

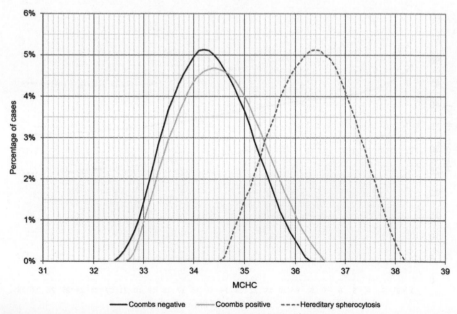

Fig. 8. MCHC of 3 groups of neonates: healthy Coombs negative, ABO hemolytic disease, and hereditary spherocytosis.

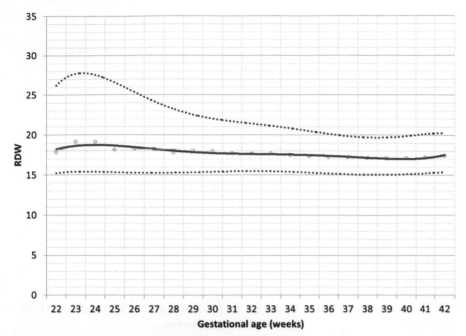

Fig. 9. Red cell distribution width (RDW) on the day of birth, according to gestational age.

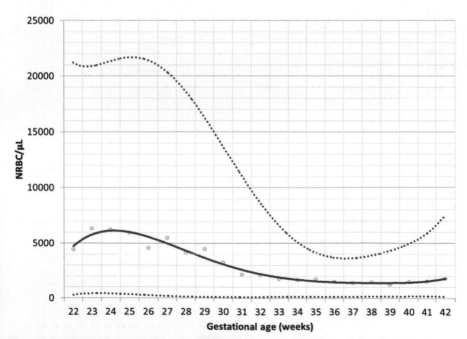

Fig. 10. Nucleated red blood cell (NRBC) levels on the day of birth, according to gestational age.

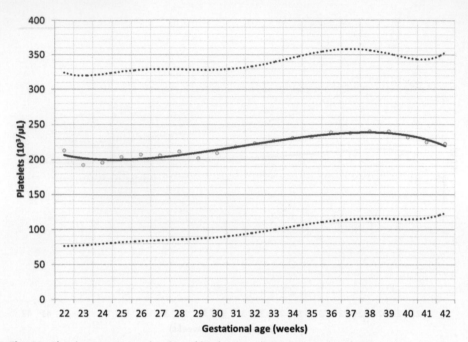

Fig. 11. Platelet counts on the day of birth, according to gestational age.

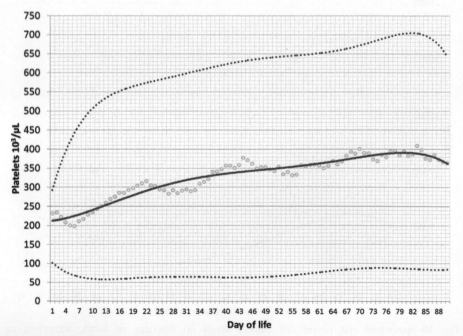

Fig. 12. Platelet counts during the first 90 days of life.

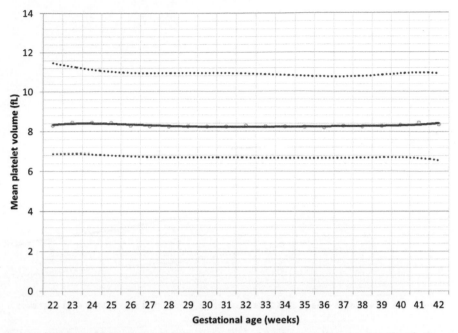

Fig. 13. Mean platelet volume (MPV) on the day of birth, according to gestational age.

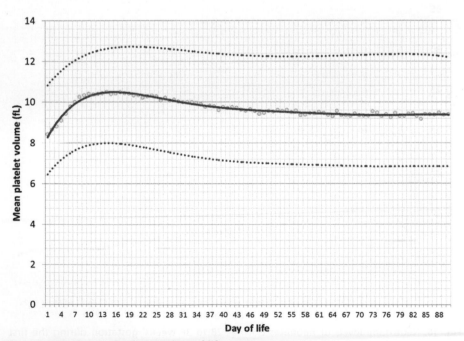

Fig. 14. MPV during the first 90 days of life.

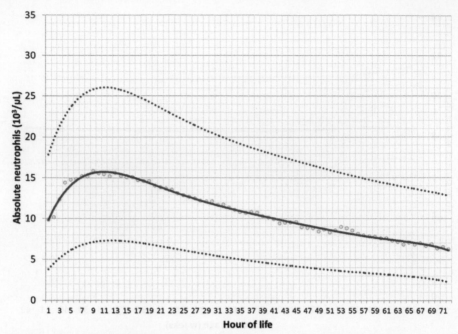

Fig. 15. Neutrophil levels of neonates born at greater than or equal to 36 weeks' gestation during the first 72 hours after birth.

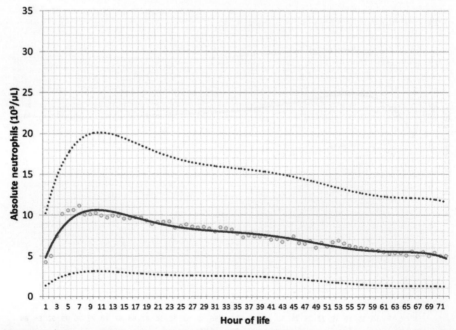

Fig. 16. Neutrophil levels of neonates born at 28 to 36 weeks' gestation during the first 72 hours after birth.

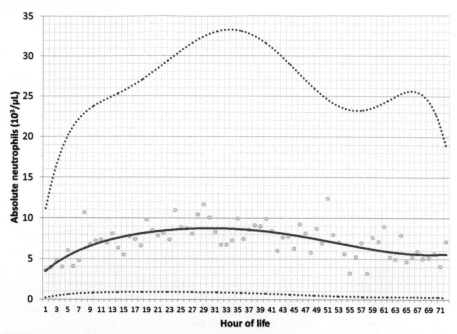

Fig. 17. Neutrophil levels of neonates born at less than 28 weeks' gestation during the first 72 hours of life.

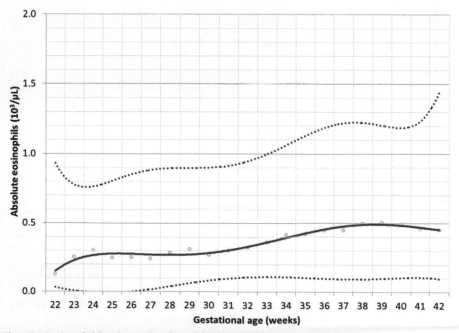

Fig. 18. Eosinophil levels on the day of birth, according to gestational age.

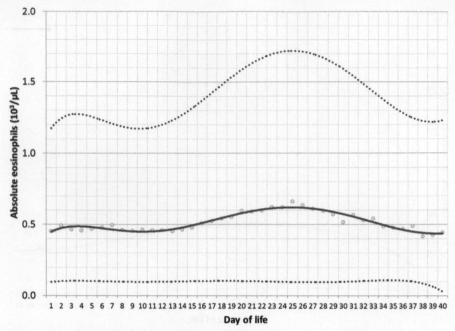

Fig. 19. Eosinophil levels during the first 40 days of life.

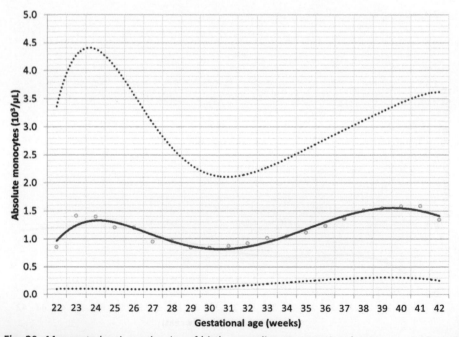

Fig. 20. Monocyte levels on the day of birth, according to gestational age.

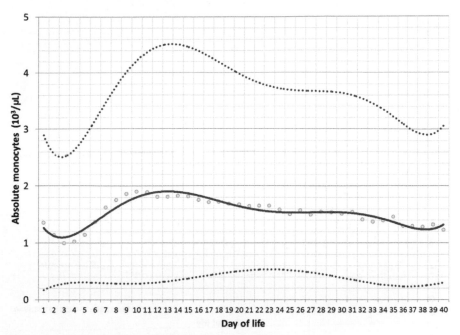

Fig. 21. Monocyte levels during the first 40 days of life.

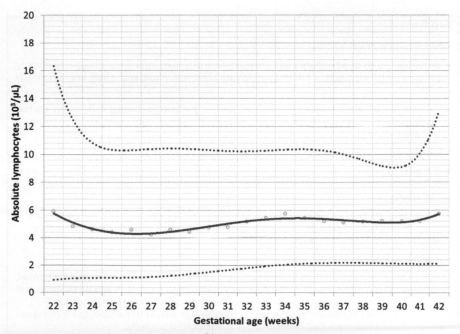

Fig. 22. Lymphocyte levels on the day of birth, according to gestational age.

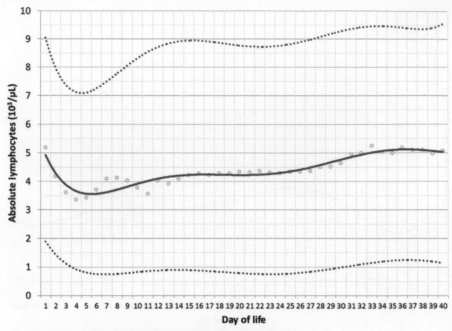

Fig. 23. Lymphocyte levels during the first 40 days of life.

Best Practices

What is current practice?

- When the results of a neonate's CBC are examined, clinicians sometimes struggle to identify precisely which elements are normal, which are abnormally low, and which are abnormally high.

- Patterns of CBC abnormalities can suggest specific pathologic entities but, unless normal ranges (references intervals) are known and available, uncertainty exists about potential CBC abnormalities.

What changes in current practice are likely to improve outcomes?

- Bringing together, into 1 article, multiple neonatal intensive care unit reference ranges publications, covering most aspects of the CBC, can facilitate accurate interpretation of CBC results.

- Future projects that provide neonatal CBC reference intervals in real time, embedded in smart programs to aid diagnosis and treatment, could reduce clinical variability, reduce costs of care, and improve outcomes.

Summary Statement

Making a judgment about whether a hematological value (such as hematocrit level) is normal, low, or high frequently depends on the neonate's gestational age at birth and on the postnatal age when the blood was drawn. Only by consulting data-derived reference intervals, generated from many thousands of neonates like those shown in this article, can a clinician have confidence that each CBC element is being interpreted properly.

REFERENCES

1. Henry E, Walker D, Wiedmeier SE, et al. Hematological abnormalities during the first week of life among neonates with Down syndrome: data from a multihospital healthcare system. Am J Med Genet A 2007;143A(1):42–50.
2. Christensen RD, Jopling J, Henry E, et al. The erythrocyte indices of neonates, defined using data from over 12,000 patients in a multihospital health care system. J Perinatol 2008;28(1):24–8.
3. Schmutz N, Henry E, Jopling J, et al. Expected ranges for blood neutrophil concentrations of neonates: the Manroe and Mouzinho charts revisited. J Perinatol 2008;28(4):275–81.
4. Wiedmeier SE, Henry E, Christensen RD. Hematological abnormalities during the first week of life among neonates with trisomy 18 and trisomy 13: data from a multi-hospital healthcare system. Am J Med Genet A 2008;146A(3):312–20.
5. Del Vecchio A, Latini G, Henry E, et al. Template bleeding times of 240 neonates born at 24 to 41 weeks gestation. J Perinatol 2008;28(6):427–31.
6. Wiedmeier SE, Henry E, Sola-Visner MC, et al. Platelet reference ranges for neonates, defined using data from over 47,000 patients in a multihospital healthcare system. J Perinatol 2009;29(2):130–6.
7. Jopling J, Henry E, Wiedmeier SE, et al. Reference ranges for hematocrit and blood hemoglobin concentration during the neonatal period: data from a multihospital health care system. Pediatrics 2009;123(2):e333–7.
8. Wiedmeier SE, Henry E, Burnett J, et al. Thrombocytosis in neonates and young infants: a report of 25 patients with platelet counts of ≥1,000,000/μL. J Perinatol 2010;30(3):222–6.
9. Baer VL, Lambert DK, Henry E, et al. Severe thrombocytopenia in the NICU. Pediatrics 2009;124(6):e1095–100.
10. Baer VL, Lambert DK, Henry E, et al. Reference ranges for blood concentrations of eosinophils and monocytes during the neonatal period defined from over 63 000 records in a multihospital health-care system. J Perinatol 2010;30(8):540–5.
11. Christensen RD, Henry E, Andres RL, et al. Reference ranges for blood concentrations of nucleated red blood cells in neonates. Neonatology 2011;99(4):289–94.
12. Jensen JD, Wiedmeier SE, Henry E, et al. Linking maternal platelet counts with neonatal platelet counts and outcomes using the data repositories of a multihospital health care system. Am J Perinatol 2011;28(8):597–604.
13. Christensen RD, Baer VL, Gordon PV, et al. Reference ranges for lymphocyte counts of neonates: associations between abnormal counts and outcomes. Pediatrics 2012;129(5):e1165–72.
14. Christensen RD, Baer VL, Lambert DK, et al. Reference intervals for common coagulation tests of preterm infants. Transfusion 2014;54(3):627–32.
15. Christensen RD, Yaish HM, Henry E, et al. Red blood cell distribution width: reference intervals for neonates. J Matern Fetal Neonatal Med 2014;17:1–6.

Neonatal Transfusion Medicine

Five Major Unanswered Research Questions for the Twenty-First Century

Robert Sheppard Nickel, MD, MSc[a], Cassandra D. Josephson, MD[b],*

KEYWORDS

- Neonatal transfusion • Transfusion threshold • Storage age
- Transfusion-associated NEC • Transfusion-transmitted infection

KEY POINTS

- Current studies are seeking to determine the optimal red blood cell (RBC) and platelet transfusion thresholds for neonates.
- Although the use of fresh RBC units does not seem to improve neonatal outcomes, unresolved issues related to product storage age exist.
- Transfusion-associated necrotizing enterocolitis (NEC) likely represents a real clinical entity; however, its exact pathogenesis and methods to prevent it are unclear.
- Leukoreduced, cytomegalovirus (CMV)-seronegative blood products minimize the risk of transfusion-transmitted CMV (TT-CMV), but other infection prevention transfusion practices should be studied in neonates.

INTRODUCTION

Transfusions of RBCs, platelets, and plasma are critical therapies for preterm neonates. A majority of extremely low-birth-weight infants require at least 1 transfusion and many receive multiple transfusions.[1] Historically, evidence-based neonatal transfusion guidelines have been lacking and transfusion practices have varied considerably at different neonatal intensive care units (NICUs).[2–5] Fortunately, a growing body of research has begun to focus on issues related to neonatal transfusion. This review focuses on 5 significant neonatal transfusion medicine research questions,

Disclosures: None.
[a] Department of Pediatrics, Children's National Health System, The George Washington University School of Medicine and Health Sciences, 111 Michigan Avenue North West, Washington, DC 20010, USA; [b] Department of Pathology and Laboratory Medicine, Center for Transfusion and Cellular Therapies, Children's Healthcare of Atlanta, Emory University, 1405 Clifton Road North East, Atlanta, GA 30322, USA
* Corresponding author.
E-mail address: cjoseph@emory.edu

some of which have been previously identified by leading transfusion medicine specialists and the National, Heart, Lung, and Blood Institute (NHLBI).[6–8] Existing literature on these topics is summarized, and directions for current ongoing and future potential work are highlighted.

What Is the Optimal Red Blood Cell Transfusion Threshold for Neonates?

RBC transfusion is a key therapy for improving oxygen delivery in anemic patients. RBC transfusions, however, may also induce adverse immunologic responses, transmit infections, cause volume overload, deliver dangerous amounts of iron, and increase medical costs. Considering the benefits and risks of RBC transfusion, it is imperative to determine when transfusion is indicated. Large, prospective, randomized trials have investigated RBC transfusion thresholds in adults.[9–11] These studies demonstrated that restrictive transfusion (RBC transfusion given at a lower hemoglobin level) was safe and in some cases resulted in superior clinical outcomes[9,11] compared with liberal transfusion (RBC transfusion given at a higher hemoglobin level). Although these results have led to important clinical guidelines[12,13] that advise transfusing RBCs at lower hemoglobin thresholds for most adult clinical populations, they cannot be extrapolated to neonates—especially critically ill premature infants who are at high risk for neurologic damage.

Two prior randomized controlled trials have studied RBC transfusion thresholds in very-low-birth-weight infants (**Table 1**).[14,15] Bell and colleagues[14] enrolled 100 infants weighing 500 to 1300 g to receive either liberal or restrictive transfusions based on hematocrit thresholds that varied depending on 3 phases of respiratory support (assisted mechanical ventilation, nasal continuous positive pressure or supplemental oxygen, and no support). Although many clinical outcomes were not different between the 2 groups, infants in the restrictive-transfusion group were significantly more likely to have grade 4 intraventricular hemorrhage (IVH) or periventricular leukomalacia (PVL) as well as more apnea episodes. In contrast to these results, which favor a liberal transfusion strategy, long-term follow-up of these patients surprisingly showed that patients in the liberal-transfusion group had worse neurocognitive scores[16] and

Table 1
Neonatal studies on liberal versus restrictive red blood cell transfusion

	Study Design	Short-Term Outcomes	Longer-Term Outcomes
University of Iowa trial[14]	RCT of 100 preterm infants (BW 500–1300 g)	Favored liberal-transfusion group. Restrictive-transfusion group had more IVH/PVL and apnea.	Favored restrictive-transfusion group. Liberal-transfusion group had worse neurocognitive scores[16] and smaller brain volumes[17] at age 12 y.
The Premature Infants in Need of Transfusion trial[15]	RCT of 451 preterm infants (BW <1000 g)	No significant differences between the groups.	Favored liberal-transfusion group. Restrictive-transfusion group had more cognitive delay at corrected age 18–21 mo.[19]

Abbreviations: BW, birth weight; RCT, randomized controlled trial.

smaller brain volumes.[17] The investigators hypothesized that these negative long-term neurologic outcomes may have been due to decreased endogenous erythropoietin production (that may be neuroprotective)[18] in the liberal-transfusion group.

In the other neonatal RBC transfusion threshold trial, Kirpalani and colleagues[15] randomized 451 infants weighing less than 1000 g to high or low hemoglobin transfusion thresholds based on patient age (1–7 days, 8–14 days, or ≥15 days) and respiratory support (any respiratory support or no respiratory support). The liberal- and restrictive-transfusion groups had no significant differences in the primary composite clinical outcome, which included death or survival with severe retinopathy, bronchopulmonary dysplasia, or brain injury on cranial ultrasound. A neurodevelopmental evaluation of these patients at 18 to 21 months' corrected age found, however, in a post hoc analysis, that more patients in the restrictive-transfusion group had cognitive delay.[19]

Given the conflicting results and limitations[20–25] of these trials, experts agree that additional research is needed to determine the optimal RBC transfusion threshold for neonates.[6,7,26–28] The National Institute of Child Health and Human Development–sponsored Transfusion Of Prematures (TOP) trial (NCT01702805) seeks to help answer the question of which neonatal RBC transfusion threshold should be adopted. This multicenter trial plans to enroll 1824 infants less than 1000 g and between 22 to 29 weeks' gestational age. Infants are randomized to receive RBC transfusions at a high or low hemoglobin threshold that varies depending on patient age and respiratory support (**Table 2**). The study was designed to detect a 7% absolute difference between the 2 groups in the proportion of patients who died or had serious neurodevelopmental impairment at 22 to 26 months. The study began in 2012 and is estimated to complete enrollment in 2017.

Another multicenter study, Effects of Transfusion Thresholds on Neurocognitive Outcome of Extremely Low Birth-Weight Infants (ETTNO), is also currently active in Germany (NCT01393496). In ETTNO, a planned 920 extremely low-birth-weight infants are randomized to a liberal or restrictive transfusion protocol similar to the TOP trial.[28] Although the TOP and ETTNO trials will provide critical information to assist in devising neonatal RBC transfusion thresholds based on hemoglobin/hematocrit values, future research may further explore the use of other laboratory tests (plasma vascular endothelial growth factor levels) or clinical measurements (near-infrared spectroscopy [NIRS]) to guide RBC transfusion for neonates.[29–31]

What Is the Optimal Platelet Transfusion Threshold for Neonates?

Similar to RBC transfusions, the benefits and risks of platelet transfusions, which have a significantly higher risk of transfusion-transmitted bacterial infection,[32]

Table 2
Transfusion of Prematures trial hemoglobin transfusion thresholds

Time Period	High-Threshold (Liberal) Group		Low-Threshold (Restrictive) Group	
	Respiratory Support	No Support	Respiratory Support	No Support
Week 1	13.0	12.0	11.0	10.0
Week 2	12.5	11.0	10.0	8.5
Weeks ≥3	11.0	10.0	8.5	7.0

Hemoglobin values shown are g/dL. Respiratory support defined as mechanical ventilation, continuous positive airway pressure, fraction of inspired oxygen in excess of 0.35, or oxygen by nasal cannula in excess of 1 L/min.

must also be considered, specifically for neonates. Neonates have unique platelet and coagulation physiology[33–38] and are at especially high risk for IVH. Although platelet transfusions are a critical therapy for bleeding thrombocytopenic infants, the role of prophylactic platelet transfusions to prevent serious bleeding is less clear and significant variability exists in platelet transfusion practices by neonatologists.[3–5]

In an important early study of prophylactic platelet transfusions thresholds, Andrew and colleagues[39] randomized 152 thrombocytopenic neonates less than 33 weeks' gestation age and weighing 500 to 1500 g to receive platelet transfusions to maintain the platelet count either greater than 150×10^9/L or greater than 50×10^9/L for the first week of life. The proportion of infants in the 2 groups who suffered new or worsening IVH was similar, establishing that a liberal 150×10^9/L platelet transfusion threshold does not protect against IVH. This study, however, excluded neonates with an initial platelet count less than 50×10^9/L. To study this population, Murray and colleagues[40] conducted a retrospective observational cohort study of their NICU, which had a variable platelet transfusion practice. None of the preterm infants with platelet counts less than 50×10^9/L in whom platelet transfusions were withheld suffered serious hemorrhage, suggesting that lower platelet count thresholds may be safe for stable infants. von Lindern and colleagues[41] also retrospectively compared 2 similar NICUs with different platelet transfusion guidelines. The liberal platelet transfusion NICU routinely transfused prophylactic platelets, whereas the restrictive NICU transfused platelets only if the platelet count was less than 50×10^9/L and the patient had bleeding symptoms or need for a procedure. The incidence of IVH in these 2 units was not significantly different. Similarly, another recent retrospective study found that infants transfused in a single institution after implementation of a more restrictive platelet transfusion protocol did not have an increased risk of IVH and were less likely to be transfused platelets.[42]

Although these studies offer some important information to help guide neonatal platelet transfusion, the optimal platelet count to trigger transfusion for these patients remains unknown. Experts at a 2009 NHLBI State of the Science Symposium proposed a randomized trial of very-low-birth-weight neonates to liberal versus restrictive platelet transfusion thresholds based on postnatal age and bleeding risk assessment.[6,7] It was estimated that such a trial would require 2252 patients to detect a 3% bleeding rate difference between the groups. This proposed trial has not begun or been funded. In 2011, however, a multicenter European trial was initiated to evaluate the effect of 2 different platelet transfusion thresholds, the Platelets for Neonatal Transfusion—Study 2.[43] This study plans to randomize 660 infants born less than 34 weeks' gestational age to either receive prophylactic platelet transfusions if the platelet count is less than 50×10^9/L or less than 25×10^9/L to detect an 8% difference in mortality and incidence of new major bleeds.

Measures other than platelet count, such as platelet mass (platelet number × platelet volume), may be more helpful than platelet count alone in determining the need for platelet transfusion. Gerday and colleagues[44] found that at 2 NICUs after a change from platelet count–based transfusion guidelines to platelet mass–based guidelines, the proportion of infants receiving platelet transfusions decreased but bleeding rates remained similar. To further explore the use of platelet mass thresholds to reduce unnecessary transfusion, a subsequent feasibility study randomized 30 neonates to receive transfusions based on platelet count or platelet mass.[45] This study, however, did not find that the platelet mass group received fewer transfusions, leading the investigators to conclude that a definitive comparative effectiveness trial on this topic needs to be large.

Does the Storage Age of a Red Blood Cell Unit Affect Clinical Outcomes for Neonates?

It is well established that properties of an RBC unit change over time with storage before the unit expiration date. These storage changes include biochemical (increased supernatant potassium/lactate/iron, decreased 2,3-diphosphoglycerate)[46] and structural (less RBC deformability)[47,48] alterations that may affect transfused erythrocytes ability to effectively deliver oxygen.[49,50] Despite much research characterizing this RBC storage lesion,[51,52] it is not clear if these changes that occur with RBC unit storage actually cause deleterious clinical effects. Although a retrospective study in adult cardiac patients found that transfusion of older stored RBC units was significantly associated with mortality,[53] this finding has not been replicated in any prospective trial.

The issue of RBC storage age is particularly relevant to premature infants who receive multiple transfusions when considering a dedicated donor policy. Such a policy designates that aliquots from a specific RBC unit should be used exclusively to transfuse an infant during hospitalization until the unit expires.[54] This practice has been demonstrated in neonates to successfully decrease blood donor exposures and reduce blood waste and seems safe[55–61]; however, concerns have remained about transfusing older (especially >14 days)[62] stored aliquots.

The Age of Red Blood Cells in Premature Infants (ARIPI) trial sought to address the question of whether older stored RBCs are harmful to neonates. In this multicenter trial, 377 premature infants with a birth weight less than 1250 g were randomized to receive RBCs stored less than or equal to 7 days or standard-issue RBCs (storage time up to 42 days).[63] Patients in both groups received a median of 4 transfusions, with the fresh RBC group having a mean RBC storage age of 5.1 days and the standard-issue RBC group having a mean storage age of 14.6 days. The primary outcome, a composite measure of death and major neonatal morbidities (NEC, retinopathy of prematurity, bronchopulmonary dysplasia, and IVH) and secondary analysis on infections were not different between the 2 groups.

Although the ARIPI trial provides sound evidence that the use of fresh RBCs does not improve outcomes in premature in neonates, it does not resolve all concerns about the use of older stored RBCs.[64] Because few patients in the ARIPI trial received transfusions primarily from RBC units stored longer than 14 days, the study may have failed to detect adverse events related to RBCs stored for greater than 14 days. Fergusson and colleagues[63] acknowledged "a mean RBC storage time of 2 weeks in the standard RBC group may not have been sufficient to detect biological effects attributed to storage or clinically significant storage lesions occurring toward the end of the accepted RBC shelf life." In addition, the findings of the ARIPI trial may have been strongly influenced by patients in the trial having been transfused per a more liberal transfusion strategy. It is possible that adverse events from older RBCs occur only when patients develop severe anemia, something that occurs more commonly using a restrictive transfusion practice.[65] Finally, the RBC storage lesion may be strongly influenced by its preparation and storage in a specific anticoagulant solution or product irradiation practices; the ARIPI trial was not designed to analyze the potential clinical effect of these variables. Although multiple large trials in different adult populations (one of which was recently reported and found that storage age did not affect clinical outcomes)[66] may help determine the clinical significance of RBC storage age, further studies in neonates are still needed.

Does Red Blood Cell Transfusion Contribute to the Pathogenesis of Necrotizing Enterocolitis?

NEC is a serious complication in preterm infants that is characterized by bowel necrosis and multisystem organ failure. Patel and colleagues[67] recently found a significant increase in NEC-related deaths among extremely premature infants in the United States, from 23 per 1000 live births in 2000 to 2003 to 30 per 1000 live births in 2008 to 2011, highlighting the urgent need to better understand and prevent this potentially fatal condition. Multiple studies,[65,68–75] including a meta-analysis,[76] have demonstrated an association between the onset of NEC and RBC transfusion in the prior 48 hours and have coined the terms, *transfusion-associated NEC* and *transfusion-related acute gut injury*.[71] Supporting the idea that transfusion can directly contribute to the pathogenesis of NEC, cases of transfusion-associated NEC have been reported to occur in older, clinically stable neonates without other NEC risk factors.[69,70] Nonetheless, the observed association between transfusion and NEC does not prove causation. The existing literature on this subject is limited to retrospective studies that cannot fully control for all possible confounding variables. In addition, one recent cohort study found that RBC transfusion was actually associated with a decreased risk of NEC for certain groups of infants.[77]

Several theories have been proposed to explain the mechanism of transfusion-associated NEC. Transfusion may trigger an immunologic reaction in the gut, possibly even similar to transfusion-related acute lung injury (TRALI).[71] Transfusion may also affect mesenteric blood flow or tissue oxygenation in a manner that potentiates NEC.[78] In particular, enteral feedings during RBC transfusion have been implicated in intestinal perfusion changes that lead to tissue ischemia.[79] Supporting a link between enteral feeding during RBC transfusion and NEC, El-Dib and colleagues[73] found that after an institutional policy to withhold feeds during RBC transfusion, the incidence of NEC significantly fell (5.3% to 1.3%). Derienzo and colleagues[80] also found a decreased incidence of NEC after the implementation of an institutional policy to stop feeds around transfusion; however, the incidence specifically of transfusion-associated NEC did not significantly change. No randomized controlled trials have been completed to confirm that withholding feeds during RBC transfusion decreases the risk of NEC.

Given the lack of high-quality evidence to guide feeding and transfusion practices, further research investigating this issue is needed. As part of the TOP trial, discussed previously, a subset of enrolled infants will receive NIRS to monitor cerebral and splanchnic tissue oxygen levels. This secondary study aims include evaluating how different NIRS measurements are associated with RBC transfusion and NEC development. In addition, an online registry (www.tragiregistry.com) is currently active that aims to collect clinical information on NEC cases from a diverse group of institutions.[81] Although subject to the problem of reporter bias, this registry nonetheless may provide important data to guide future, more definitive trials on transfusion-associated NEC prevention.

Which New Practices Should Be Used to Prevent Transfusion-Transmitted Infections in Neonates?

Although the risk of infection from transfusion has decreased due to multiple interventions,[82] transfusions still transmit various infections. Prevention of transfusion-transmitted infections is especially important for neonates because any gain in transfusion safety for this population results in more disease-free years of life compared with adults. And, certain transfusion-transmitted infections are of special concern for immunoincompetent patients, such as preterm neonates. CMV is one such transfusion-transmitted infection that can cause serious morbidity and mortality in neonates, especially preterm neonates born to CMV-seronegative mothers.[83,84]

The use of blood products from CMV-seronegative donors effectively decreases the risk of TT-CMV[84]; however, TT-CMV can still occur with this approach because of false-negative serology results[85] and the window period in which a

CMV-seronegative donor has been acutely infected.[86,87] Because latently infected monocytes in the donor blood product are the primary vector of TT-CMV, leukocyte reduction of blood products also effectively decreases the risk of TT-CMV.[88,89] Although some studies in hematopoietic stem cell transplant patients have suggested that unscreened leukoreduced blood products are as safe as CMV-seronegative blood products,[90,91] other studies have concluded that CMV-seronegative blood products are slightly more efficacious in preventing TT-CMV.[92,93] Fortunately, using both these practices (CMV-seronegative donors and leukoreduction), the risk of TT-CMV is extremely low. In a recent prospective study of 539 very-low-birth-weight infants who received a total of 2061 leukoreduced transfusions from CMV-seronegative donors, no cases of TT-CMV occurred.[94] Yet this practice is not ideal because a reliance on CMV-seronegative donors severely limits the donor pool, especially in regions of the United States, like the Southeast, that has a seroprevalence of CMV of approximately 75%[94] and countries where CMV is endemic with seroprevalence rates greater than 95%.[95–97] Future research should consider other less restrictive donor testing, like CMV nucleic acid testing, to further improve the safety of leukoreduced blood products.[98]

An alternative approach to preventing TT-CMV is the use of pathogen inactivation technology (**Table 3**).[99] Pathogen inactivation technology can decrease the risk of a broad range of infections, including many different viruses, protozoa, and bacteria. It is especially attractive because it could also help prevent transmission of unknown, emerging new infectious pathogens. Various pathogen inactivation technologies are at varying stages of development, testing, and clinical implementation.[100] One of the first Food and Drug Administration (FDA)-approved technologies is the INTERCEPT Blood System (Concord, CA) for plasma and platelets.

The INTERCEPT Blood System uses amotosalen HCl, a synthetic psoralen compound that intercalates with nucleic acid and, on activation by UV light, causes cross-linking that inhibits replication of pathogens and white blood cells. This technology has been shown safe in a large, randomized controlled trial of mostly adults,[101–103] but it has not been rigorously tested in neonates. In addition, INTERCEPT is currently

Table 3
Strategies to decrease transfusion-transmitted infections

Strategy	Additional Benefits of This Strategy	Problems with This Strategy
Use of CMV-seronegative donors	None	Only decreases CMV risk, limits pool of donors
Leukocyte reduction	Decreases febrile nonhemolytic transfusion reactions, HLA alloimmunization	Only decreases CMV risk
Photochemical treatment (INTERCEPT)	Decreases risk of transfusion-associated graft-versus-host disease	Only platelets and plasma, not effective against nonenveloped viruses/spores, not well studied in neonates
Solvent/detergent treatment (Octaplas)	Decreases risk of TRALI	Only plasma, not effective against nonenveloped viruses, not well studied in neonates

Abbreviation: HLA, human leukocyte antigen.

contraindicated for neonates treated with phototherapy devices that emit wavelengths less than 425 nm due to the potential for erythema resulting from interaction between UV light and amotosalen. Although hemovigilance monitoring at 2 European blood centers that use this technology reported no serious adverse events in 188 infants who received INTERCEPT-treated plasma,[104] further research in neonates is needed for this and other photochemical treatments.

Another recently FDA-approved product that decreases the risk of infection from plasma transfusion is Octaplas (Octapharma, Hoboken, NJ). Octaplas is a filtered pooled plasma product that undergoes solvent/detergent treatment to inactivate lipid-enveloped viruses. In addition to minimizing pathogen transmission, use of Octaplas is believed to prevent TRALI,[105,106] a potentially fatal transfusion reaction that is likely under-recognized in neonates.[107–109] Although multiple studies have demonstrated that Octaplas is safe and effective in adults,[110–114] the pediatric experience[104,105] is more limited and merits further study especially in neonates. Such research is necessary because the citrate and decreased amount of protein S in Octaplas could possibly cause harm that is unique to neonates.

SUMMARY

The 5 research questions, discussed previously, by no means encompass all the important areas of investigation in neonatal transfusion medicine. Significant work remains related to defining the proper use of plasma product transfusions and recombinant erythropoietin in neonates. Research further describing the immunology of hemolytic disease of the newborn and neonatal alloimmune thrombocytopenia with a goal of devising treatments to better prevent these conditions is also clearly needed. And, as new transfusion technologies and therapies emerge, it remains important to specifically study them in neonates.

ACKNOWLEDGMENTS

The authors would like to thank Dr R. Patel for his helpful comments on this article.

Best Practices

What is the current practice?

1. Neonates receive RBC and platelet transfusions at varying hemoglobin values and platelet counts, depending on gestational age, clinical status, and individual centers' practices.

2. Although a randomized controlled study has demonstrated that RBC units stored for less than 7 days are not superior, neonates are still routinely transfused with fresher RBC units given concerns about RBC storage.

3. Given that understanding of the link between RBC transfusion and NEC is still evolving, centers have varying feeding and transfusion policies.

4. The use of leukoreduced blood products obtained from CMV-seronegative donors is effective in preventing TT-CMV; however, other infectious concerns remain for neonates.

Which changes in current practice are likely to improve outcomes?

1. Active clinical research is seeking to better define optimal RBC and platelet count transfusion thresholds for neonates to develop evidence-based practice recommendations that specifically seek to optimize neurocognitive outcomes.

2. Future research accounting for variables, including transfusion threshold and product manipulation, should further clarify the safety and efficacy of transfusing older stored RBC units.

3. Better understanding of the pathogenesis of transfusion-associated NEC should inform feeding recommendations to prevent this potentially fatal complication.

4. Additional research using FDA-approved pathogen inactivation technology (INTERCEPT) and treated pooled products (Octaplas) for neonates will likely help further prevent existing and emerging transfusion-transmitted infections in neonates.

Summary Statement

Neonatal transfusion medicine has many unanswered questions. Research seeking to answer these questions will lead not only to improved use of the blood product resource but also to improved clinical outcomes for neonates.

REFERENCES

1. Maier RF, Sonntag J, Walka MM, et al. Changing practices of red blood cell transfusions in infants with birth weights less than 1000 g. J Pediatr 2000;136(2):220–4.
2. Bednarek FJ, Weisberger S, Richardson DK, et al. Variations in blood transfusions among newborn intensive care units. SNAP II Study Group. J Pediatr 1998;133(5):601–7.
3. Kahn DJ, Richardson DK, Billett HH. Inter-NICU variation in rates and management of thrombocytopenia among very low birth-weight infants. J Perinatol 2003; 23(4):312–6.
4. Josephson CD, Su LL, Christensen RD, et al. Platelet transfusion practices among neonatologists in the United States and Canada: results of a survey. Pediatrics 2009;123(1):278–85.
5. Cremer M, Sola-Visner M, Roll S, et al. Platelet transfusions in neonates: practices in the United States vary significantly from those in Austria, Germany, and Switzerland. Transfusion 2011;51(12):2634–41.
6. Blajchman MA, Glynn SA, Josephson CD, et al. Clinical trial opportunities in transfusion medicine: proceedings of a national heart, lung, and blood institute state-of-the-science symposium. Transfus Med Rev 2010;24(4):259–85.
7. Josephson CD, Glynn SA, Kleinman SH, et al. A multidisciplinary "think tank": the top 10 clinical trial opportunities in transfusion medicine from the National Heart, Lung, and Blood Institute-sponsored 2009 state-of-the-science symposium. Transfusion 2011;51(4):828–41.
8. Josephson CD, Mondoro TH, Ambruso DR, et al. One size will never fit all: the future of research in pediatric transfusion medicine. Pediatr Res 2014;76(5):425–31.
9. Hebert PC, Wells G, Blajchman MA, et al. A multicenter, randomized, controlled clinical trial of transfusion requirements in critical care. Transfusion Requirements in Critical Care Investigators, Canadian Critical Care Trials Group. N Engl J Med 1999;340(6):409–17.
10. Carson JL, Terrin ML, Noveck H, et al. Liberal or restrictive transfusion in high-risk patients after hip surgery. N Engl J Med 2011;365(26):2453–62.
11. Villanueva C, Colomo A, Bosch A, et al. Transfusion strategies for acute upper gastrointestinal bleeding. N Engl J Med 2013;368(1):11–21.
12. Carson JL, Grossman BJ, Kleinman S, et al. Red blood cell transfusion: a clinical practice guideline from the AABB. Ann Intern Med 2012;157(1):49–58.
13. Hicks LK, Bering H, Carson KR, et al. The ASH Choosing Wisely(R) campaign: five hematologic tests and treatments to question. Blood 2013;122(24):3879–83.
14. Bell EF, Strauss RG, Widness JA, et al. Randomized trial of liberal versus restrictive guidelines for red blood cell transfusion in preterm infants. Pediatrics 2005; 115(6):1685–91.

15. Kirpalani H, Whyte RK, Andersen C, et al. The Premature Infants in Need of Transfusion (PINT) study: a randomized, controlled trial of a restrictive (low) versus liberal (high) transfusion threshold for extremely low birth weight infants. J Pediatr 2006;149(3):301–7.
16. McCoy TE, Conrad AL, Richman LC, et al. Neurocognitive profiles of preterm infants randomly assigned to lower or higher hematocrit thresholds for transfusion. Child Neuropsychol 2011;17(4):347–67.
17. Nopoulos PC, Conrad AL, Bell EF, et al. Long-term outcome of brain structure in premature infants: effects of liberal vs restricted red blood cell transfusions. Arch Pediatr Adolesc Med 2011;165(5):443–50.
18. Juul S. Neuroprotective role of erythropoietin in neonates. J Matern Fetal Neonatal Med 2012;25(Suppl 4):105–7.
19. Whyte RK, Kirpalani H, Asztalos EV, et al. Neurodevelopmental outcome of extremely low birth weight infants randomly assigned to restrictive or liberal hemoglobin thresholds for blood transfusion. Pediatrics 2009;123(1):207–13.
20. Boedy RF, Mathew OP. Randomized trial of liberal versus restrictive guidelines for red blood cell transfusion in preterm infants. Pediatrics 2005;116(4): 1048–9 [author reply: 1049–50].
21. Murray N, Roberts I, Stanworth S. Red blood cell transfusion in neonates. Pediatrics 2005;116(6):1609 [author reply: 1609–10].
22. Swamy RS, Embleton ND. Red blood cell transfusions in preterm infants: is there a difference between restrictive and liberal criteria? Pediatrics 2006;117(1): 257–8 [author reply: 258–9].
23. Meyer MP. Transfusion thresholds for preterm infants. J Pediatr 2007;150(6): e90–1.
24. Bell EF. Transfusion thresholds for preterm infants: how low should we go? J Pediatr 2006;149(3):287–9.
25. Alkalay AL, Simmons CF. Transfusion threshold in anemic premature infants. J Pediatr 2007;151(3):e10 [author reply: e10].
26. Crowley M, Kirpalani H. A rational approach to red blood cell transfusion in the neonatal ICU. Curr Opin Pediatr 2010;22(2):151–7.
27. Whyte RK. Neurodevelopmental outcome of extremely low-birth-weight infants randomly assigned to restrictive or liberal hemoglobin thresholds for blood transfusion. Semin Perinatol 2012;36(4):290–3.
28. ETTNO Investigators. The 'Effects of transfusion thresholds on neurocognitive outcome of extremely low birth-weight infants (ETTNO)' study: background, aims, and study protocol. Neonatology 2012;101(4):301–5.
29. Tschirch E, Weber B, Koehne P, et al. Vascular endothelial growth factor as marker for tissue hypoxia and transfusion need in anemic infants: a prospective clinical study. Pediatrics 2009;123(3):784–90.
30. Wardle SP, Garr R, Yoxall CW, et al. A pilot randomised controlled trial of peripheral fractional oxygen extraction to guide blood transfusions in preterm infants. Arch Dis Child Fetal Neonatal Ed 2002;86(1):F22–7.
31. Banerjee J, Aladangady N. Biomarkers to decide red blood cell transfusion in newborn infants. Transfusion 2014;54(10):2574–82.
32. Lafeuillade B, Eb F, Ounnoughene N, et al. Residual risk and retrospective analysis of transfusion-transmitted bacterial infection reported by the French National Hemovigilance Network from 2000 to 2008. Transfusion 2015;55(3): 636–46.
33. Israels SJ, Odaibo FS, Robertson C, et al. Deficient thromboxane synthesis and response in platelets from premature infants. Pediatr Res 1997;41(2):218–23.

34. Israels SJ, Daniels M, McMillan EM. Deficient collagen-induced activation in the newborn platelet. Pediatr Res 1990;27(4 Pt 1):337–43.
35. Gelman B, Setty BN, Chen D, et al. Impaired mobilization of intracellular calcium in neonatal platelets. Pediatr Res 1996;39(4 Pt 1):692–6.
36. Andrew M, Paes B, Johnston M. Development of the hemostatic system in the neonate and young infant. Am J Pediatr Hematol Oncol 1990;12(1):95–104.
37. Ferrer-Marin F, Chavda C, Lampa M, et al. Effects of in vitro adult platelet transfusions on neonatal hemostasis. J Thromb Haemost 2011;9(5):1020–8.
38. Ferrer-Marin F, Stanworth S, Josephson C, et al. Distinct differences in platelet production and function between neonates and adults: implications for platelet transfusion practice. Transfusion 2013;53(11):2814–21 [quiz: 2813].
39. Andrew M, Vegh P, Caco C, et al. A randomized, controlled trial of platelet transfusions in thrombocytopenic premature infants. J Pediatr 1993;123(2):285–91.
40. Murray NA, Howarth LJ, McCloy MP, et al. Platelet transfusion in the management of severe thrombocytopenia in neonatal intensive care unit patients. Transfus Med 2002;12(1):35–41.
41. von Lindern JS, Hulzebos CV, Bos AF, et al. Thrombocytopaenia and intraventricular haemorrhage in very premature infants: a tale of two cities. Arch Dis Child Fetal Neonatal Ed 2012;97(5):F348–52.
42. Borges JP, dos Santos AM, da Cunha DH, et al. Restrictive guideline reduces platelet count thresholds for transfusions in very low birth weight preterm infants. Vox Sang 2013;104(3):207–13.
43. Curley A, Venkatesh V, Stanworth S, et al. Platelets for neonatal transfusion - study 2: a randomised controlled trial to compare two different platelet count thresholds for prophylactic platelet transfusion to preterm neonates. Neonatology 2014;106(2):102–6.
44. Gerday E, Baer VL, Lambert DK, et al. Testing platelet mass versus platelet count to guide platelet transfusions in the neonatal intensive care unit. Transfusion 2009;49(10):2034–9.
45. Zisk JL, Mackley A, Clearly G, et al. Transfusing neonates based on platelet count vs. platelet mass: a randomized feasibility-pilot study. Platelets 2014;25(7):513–6.
46. Karam O, Tucci M, Toledano BJ, et al. Length of storage and in vitro immunomodulation induced by prestorage leukoreduced red blood cells. Transfusion 2009;49(11):2326–34.
47. Relevy H, Koshkaryev A, Manny N, et al. Blood banking-induced alteration of red blood cell flow properties. Transfusion 2008;48(1):136–46.
48. Frank SM, Abazyan B, Ono M, et al. Decreased erythrocyte deformability after transfusion and the effects of erythrocyte storage duration. Anesth Analg 2013;116(5):975–81.
49. Marik PE, Sibbald WJ. Effect of stored-blood transfusion on oxygen delivery in patients with sepsis. JAMA 1993;269(23):3024–9.
50. Tsai AG, Cabrales P, Intaglietta M. Microvascular perfusion upon exchange transfusion with stored red blood cells in normovolemic anemic conditions. Transfusion 2004;44(11):1626–34.
51. Zimring JC. Fresh versus old blood: are there differences and do they matter? Hematology Am Soc Hematol Educ Program 2013;2013:651–5.
52. Hess JR. Measures of stored red blood cell quality. Vox Sang 2014;107(1):1–9.
53. Koch CG, Li L, Sessler DI, et al. Duration of red-cell storage and complications after cardiac surgery. N Engl J Med 2008;358(12):1229–39.

54. Meyer EK, Josephson CD. Neonatal and pediatric transfusion practice. In: Fung M, editor. Technical manual. 18th edition. Bethesda (MD): AABB Press; 2014. p. 571–92.
55. Strauss RG, Burmeister LF, Johnson K, et al. AS-1 red cells for neonatal transfusions: a randomized trial assessing donor exposure and safety. Transfusion 1996;36(10):873–8.
56. Strauss RG, Burmeister LF, Johnson K, et al. Feasibility and safety of AS-3 red blood cells for neonatal transfusions. J Pediatr 2000;136(2):215–9.
57. Liu EA, Mannino FL, Lane TA. Prospective, randomized trial of the safety and efficacy of a limited donor exposure transfusion program for premature neonates. J Pediatr 1994;125(1):92–6.
58. Lee DA, Slagle TA, Jackson TM, et al. Reducing blood donor exposures in low birth weight infants by the use of older, unwashed packed red blood cells. J Pediatr 1995;126(2):280–6.
59. Cook S, Gunter J, Wissel M. Effective use of a strategy using assigned red cell units to limit donor exposure for neonatal patients. Transfusion 1993;33(5):379–83.
60. Wood A, Wilson N, Skacel P, et al. Reducing donor exposure in preterm infants requiring multiple blood transfusions. Arch Dis Child Fetal Neonatal Ed 1995; 72(1):F29–33.
61. Fernandes da Cunha DH, Nunes Dos Santos AM, Kopelman BI, et al. Transfusions of CPDA-1 red blood cells stored for up to 28 days decrease donor exposures in very low-birth-weight premature infants. Transfus Med 2005;15(6): 467–73.
62. Collard KJ. Transfusion related morbidity in premature babies: possible mechanisms and implications for practice. World J Clin Pediatr 2014;3(3):19–29.
63. Fergusson DA, Hebert P, Hogan DL, et al. Effect of fresh red blood cell transfusions on clinical outcomes in premature, very low-birth-weight infants: the ARIPI randomized trial. JAMA 2012;308(14):1443–51.
64. Patel RM, Josephson CD. Storage age of red blood cells for transfusion of premature infants. JAMA 2013;309(6):544–5.
65. Singh R, Visintainer PF, Frantz ID 3rd, et al. Association of necrotizing enterocolitis with anemia and packed red blood cell transfusions in preterm infants. J Perinatol 2011;31(3):176–82.
66. Steiner ME, Triulzi DJ, Assmann SF, et al. Randomized trial results: red cell storage are is not associated with a significant difference in multiple-organ dysfunction score or mortality in transfused cardiac surgery patients. Transfusion 2014; 54(Suppl):15A.
67. Patel RM, Kandefer S, Walsh MC, et al. Causes and timing of death in extremely premature infants from 2000 through 2011. N Engl J Med 2015;372(4):331–40.
68. McGrady GA, Rettig PJ, Istre GR, et al. An outbreak of necrotizing enterocolitis. Association with transfusions of packed red blood cells. Am J Epidemiol 1987; 126(6):1165–72.
69. Christensen RD, Lambert DK, Henry E, et al. Is "transfusion-associated necrotizing enterocolitis" an authentic pathogenic entity? Transfusion 2010;50(5): 1106–12.
70. Mally P, Golombek SG, Mishra R, et al. Association of necrotizing enterocolitis with elective packed red blood cell transfusions in stable, growing, premature neonates. Am J Perinatol 2006;23(8):451–8.
71. Blau J, Calo JM, Dozor D, et al. Transfusion-related acute gut injury: necrotizing enterocolitis in very low birth weight neonates after packed red blood cell transfusion. J Pediatr 2011;158(3):403–9.

72. Josephson CD, Wesolowski A, Bao G, et al. Do red cell transfusions increase the risk of necrotizing enterocolitis in premature infants? J Pediatr 2010;157(6): 972–8.e1–3.
73. El-Dib M, Narang S, Lee E, et al. Red blood cell transfusion, feeding and necrotizing enterocolitis in preterm infants. J Perinatol 2011;31(3):183–7.
74. Carter BM, Holditch-Davis D, Tanaka D, et al. Relationship of neonatal treatments with the development of necrotizing enterocolitis in preterm infants. Nurs Res 2012;61(2):96–102.
75. Paul DA, Mackley A, Novitsky A, et al. Increased odds of necrotizing enterocolitis after transfusion of red blood cells in premature infants. Pediatrics 2011; 127(4):635–41.
76. Mohamed A, Shah PS. Transfusion associated necrotizing enterocolitis: a meta-analysis of observational data. Pediatrics 2012;129(3):529–40.
77. Elabiad MT, Harsono M, Talati AJ, et al. Effect of birth weight on the association between necrotising enterocolitis and red blood cell transfusions in <=1500 g infants. BMJ Open 2013;3(11):e003823.
78. Krimmel GA, Baker R, Yanowitz TD. Blood transfusion alters the superior mesenteric artery blood flow velocity response to feeding in premature infants. Am J Perinatol 2009;26(2):99–105.
79. Marin T, Josephson CD, Kosmetatos N, et al. Feeding preterm infants during red blood cell transfusion is associated with a decline in postprandial mesenteric oxygenation. J Pediatr 2014;165(3):464–71.e1.
80. Derienzo C, Smith PB, Tanaka D, et al. Feeding practices and other risk factors for developing transfusion-associated necrotizing enterocolitis. Early Hum Dev 2014;90(5):237–40.
81. La Gamma EF, Blau J. Transfusion-related acute gut injury: feeding, flora, flow, and barrier defense. Semin Perinatol 2012;36(4):294–305.
82. Luban NL. Transfusion safety: where are we today? Ann N Y Acad Sci 2005; 1054:325–41.
83. Adler SP, Chandrika T, Lawrence L, et al. Cytomegalovirus infections in neonates acquired by blood transfusions. Pediatr Infect Dis 1983;2(2):114–8.
84. Yeager AS, Grumet FC, Hafleigh EB, et al. Prevention of transfusion-acquired cytomegalovirus infections in newborn infants. J Pediatr 1981;98(2):281–7.
85. Zhu J, Shearer GM, Marincola FM, et al. Discordant cellular and humoral immune responses to cytomegalovirus infection in healthy blood donors: existence of a Th1-type dominant response. Int Immunol 2001;13(6):785–90.
86. Zanghellini F, Boppana SB, Emery VC, et al. Asymptomatic primary cytomegalovirus infection: virologic and immunologic features. J Infect Dis 1999;180(3): 702–7.
87. Revello MG, Zavattoni M, Sarasini A, et al. Human cytomegalovirus in blood of immunocompetent persons during primary infection: prognostic implications for pregnancy. J Infect Dis 1998;177(5):1170–5.
88. Gilbert GL, Hayes K, Hudson IL, et al. Prevention of transfusion-acquired cytomegalovirus infection in infants by blood filtration to remove leucocytes. Neonatal Cytomegalovirus Infection Study Group. Lancet 1989;1(8649): 1228–31.
89. Eisenfeld L, Silver H, McLaughlin J, et al. Prevention of transfusion-associated cytomegalovirus infection in neonatal patients by the removal of white cells from blood. Transfusion 1992;32(3):205–9.
90. Bowden RA, Slichter SJ, Sayers M, et al. A comparison of filtered leukocyte-reduced and cytomegalovirus (CMV) seronegative blood products for the

prevention of transfusion-associated CMV infection after marrow transplant. Blood 1995;86(9):3598–603.

91. Thiele T, Kruger W, Zimmermann K, et al. Transmission of cytomegalovirus (CMV) infection by leukoreduced blood products not tested for CMV antibodies: a single-center prospective study in high-risk patients undergoing allogeneic hematopoietic stem cell transplantation (CME). Transfusion 2011;51(12):2620–6.

92. Nichols WG, Price TH, Gooley T, et al. Transfusion-transmitted cytomegalovirus infection after receipt of leukoreduced blood products. Blood 2003;101(10): 4195–200.

93. Vamvakas EC. Is white blood cell reduction equivalent to antibody screening in preventing transmission of cytomegalovirus by transfusion? A review of the literature and meta-analysis. Transfus Med Rev 2005;19(3):181–99.

94. Josephson CD, Caliendo AM, Easley KA, et al. Blood transfusion and breast milk transmission of cytomegalovirus in very low-birth-weight infants: a prospective cohort study. JAMA Pediatr 2014;168(11):1054–62.

95. Gargouri J, Elleuch H, Karray H, et al. Prevalence of anti-CMV antibodies in blood donors in the Sfax region (value in blood transfusion). Tunis Med 2000; 78(8–9):512–7 [in French].

96. Das B, Kaur G, Basu S. Seroprevalence of cytomegalovirus antibodies among blood donors and multitransfused recipients–a study from north India. Transfus Apher Sci 2014;50(3):438–42.

97. Souza MA, Passos AM, Treitinger A, et al. Seroprevalence of cytomegalovirus antibodies in blood donors in southern, Brazil. Rev Soc Bras Med Trop 2010; 43(4):359–61.

98. Roback JD, Josephson CD. New insights for preventing transfusion-transmitted cytomegalovirus and other white blood cell-associated viral infections. Transfusion 2013;53(10):2112–6.

99. Roback JD, Conlan M, Drew WL, et al. The role of photochemical treatment with amotosalen and UV-A light in the prevention of transfusion-transmitted cytomegalovirus infections. Transfus Med Rev 2006;20(1):45–56.

100. Schlenke P. Pathogen inactivation technologies for cellular blood components: an update. Transfus Med Hemother 2014;41(4):309–25.

101. McCullough J, Vesole DH, Benjamin RJ, et al. Therapeutic efficacy and safety of platelets treated with a photochemical process for pathogen inactivation: the SPRINT Trial. Blood 2004;104(5):1534–41.

102. Snyder E, McCullough J, Slichter SJ, et al. Clinical safety of platelets photochemically treated with amotosalen HCl and ultraviolet A light for pathogen inactivation: the SPRINT trial. Transfusion 2005;45(12):1864–75.

103. Murphy S, Snyder E, Cable R, et al. Platelet dose consistency and its effect on the number of platelet transfusions for support of thrombocytopenia: an analysis of the SPRINT trial of platelets photochemically treated with amotosalen HCl and ultraviolet A light. Transfusion 2006;46(1):24–33.

104. Cazenave JP, Waller C, Kientz D, et al. An active hemovigilance program characterizing the safety profile of 7483 transfusions with plasma components prepared with amotosalen and UVA photochemical treatment. Transfusion 2010; 50(6):1210–9.

105. Sinnott P, Bodger S, Gupta A, et al. Presence of HLA antibodies in single-donor-derived fresh frozen plasma compared with pooled, solvent detergent-treated plasma (Octaplas). Eur J Immunogenet 2004;31(6):271–4.

106. Sachs UJ, Kauschat D, Bein G. White blood cell-reactive antibodies are undetectable in solvent/detergent plasma. Transfusion 2005;45(10):1628–31.

107. Wu TJ, Teng RJ, Tsou Yau KI. Transfusion-related acute lung injury treated with surfactant in a neonate. Eur J Pediatr 1996;155(7):589–91.
108. Lieberman L, Petraszko T, Yi QL, et al. Transfusion-related lung injury in children: a case series and review of the literature. Transfusion 2014;54(1):57–64.
109. Joshi VH, Joshi PV, Webert K, et al. Does transfusion-related acute lung injury occur in newborns. Paediatr Child Health 2006;11(Suppl B) [CAP abstract: 042].
110. Haubelt H, Blome M, Kiessling AH, et al. Effects of solvent/detergent-treated plasma and fresh-frozen plasma on haemostasis and fibrinolysis in complex coagulopathy following open-heart surgery. Vox Sang 2002;82(1):9–14.
111. Jilma-Stohlawetz P, Kursten FW, Horvath M, et al. Recovery, safety, and tolerability of a solvent/detergent-treated and prion-safeguarded transfusion plasma in a randomized, crossover, clinical trial in healthy volunteers. Transfusion 2013;53(9):1906–17.
112. Edel E, Al-Ali HK, Seeger S, et al. Efficacy and safety profile of solvent/detergent plasma in the treatment of acute thrombotic thrombocytopenic purpura: a single-center experience. Transfus Med Hemother 2010;37(1):13–9.
113. Williamson LM, Llewelyn CA, Fisher NC, et al. A randomized trial of solvent/detergent-treated and standard fresh-frozen plasma in the coagulopathy of liver disease and liver transplantation. Transfusion 1999;39(11–12):1227–34.
114. Scully M, Longair I, Flynn M, et al. Cryosupernatant and solvent detergent fresh-frozen plasma (Octaplas) usage at a single centre in acute thrombotic thrombocytopenic purpura. Vox Sang 2007;93(2):154–8.

Hemolytic Disorders Causing Severe Neonatal Hyperbilirubinemia

Robert D. Christensen, MD[a,b],*, Hassan M. Yaish, MD[b]

KEYWORDS

- Bilirubin • Hemoglobin • Anemia • Jaundice • Next-generation DNA sequencing
- Kernicterus • BIND • End-tidal carbon monoxide

KEY POINTS

- A shortened erythrocyte life span, because of hemolytic disorders, is a common cause of extreme neonatal hyperbilirubinemia.
- Clinical and laboratory examinations can frequently identify the underlying cause of extreme neonatal hyperbilirubinemia.
- Newer diagnostic tests include end-tidal carbon monoxide to identify hemolytic jaundice, eosin-5-maleimide (EMA) flow cytometry to identify red blood cell (RBC) membrane defects such as hereditary spherocytosis (HS), and next-generation sequencing (NGS) of relevant genes to look for mutations and polymorphisms.

NEONATAL HEMOLYTIC DISORDERS

After RBCs are released from the marrow into the blood, they circulate for about 120 days before they are culled by the reticuloendothelial system and their constituents recycled.[1] It is widely accepted that the circulating life span of RBCs in neonates is significantly shorter than 120 days, perhaps approximating 80 days.[2–5] When a neonate's RBC life span is significantly shorter than 80 days, because of intrinsic or extrinsic factors, erythropoiesis increases in an attempt to compensate, as evidenced by a rise in reticulocyte count. However, when RBC production cannot increase sufficiently to keep pace with the increased loss of RBCs because of their short life

Disclosures: Dr R.D. Christensen is a noncompensated advisor to Capnia Inc, Palo Alto, CA.
[a] Women and Newborn's Program, Division of Neonatology, Department of Pediatrics, Intermountain Healthcare, University of Utah School of Medicine, 295 Chipeta Way, Salt Lake City, UT 84108, USA; [b] Division of Hematology/Oncology, Department of Pediatrics, University of Utah School of Medicine, Salt Lake City, UT, USA
* Corresponding author. Department of Pediatrics, University of Utah, 295 Chipeta Way, Salt Lake City, UT 84108.
E-mail address: Robert.christensen@hsc.utah.edu

Clin Perinatol 42 (2015) 515–527
http://dx.doi.org/10.1016/j.clp.2015.04.007

span, the hematocrit and amount of hemoglobin decrease, defining the condition as hemolytic anemia.

During the first days and weeks after birth, the major adverse consequence of a short RBC life span is hyperbilirubinemia,[6,7] which is because each molecule of heme liberated from RBC by hemolysis is metabolized to 1 molecule of bilirubin.[6–10] High levels of bilirubin in the serum can lead to transient or permanent neurologic impairment.[11–13]

A week or so after birth, the bilirubin-metabolizing system has generally matured sufficiently to conjugate and excrete the bilirubin load imposed by a moderately fore-shortened RBC life span. Thus, in neonates with a shortened RBC life span, jaundice is the primary problem during the first days, and then anemia becomes the more significant issue in the weeks that follow. In some instances, a relatively slow insidious drop in hemoglobin culminates in a clinical deterioration, with pallor, poor feeding, tachypnea, and tachycardia, a clinical picture that somewhat resembles that of an infectious process. Such neonates may present to emergency departments with significant unanticipated anemia requiring emergent transfusion.[13]

The most common causes of neonatal hemolytic jaundice and anemia are listed in **Table 1**. The laboratory tests required to confirm hemolysis are listed in **Table 2**; these tests are divided into 2 categories, the first being those that indicate accelerated hemoglobin metabolism and the second being those that confirm accelerated erythropoiesis to compensate for hemolysis. At the onset of a hemolytic episode, the tests indicating hemolysis usually yield positive result, whereas those indicating accelerated erythropoiesis in response to the hemolysis may require several days before they give positive result.

HEMOLYTIC DISORDERS ARE FREQUENTLY RESPONSIBLE FOR EXTREME NEONATAL HYPERBILIRUBINEMIA

Intermountain Healthcare is a not-for-profit health care system in the western United States that owns and manages 18 hospitals with labor and delivery services. A review of 10 years of data from the Intermountain Healthcare system revealed

Table 1 Causes of neonatal hemolytic jaundice	
Varieties	**Examples**
Alloimmune	ABO hemolytic disease
	Rh hemolytic disease
	Hemolytic disease involving RBC antigens (Kell, Kidd, Duffy)
Mutations in RBC structural proteins	HS
	Hereditary elliptocytosis
	Pyropoikilocytosis
Mutations in RBC enzymes	G6PD deficiency
	Pyruvate kinase deficiency
	Others
Unstable hemoglobins	F Poole
	Hasharon
	Others
Microangiopathic hemolytic disorders	DIC
	Infection without DIC
	T-activation
	Infantile pyknocytosis

Abbreviations: DIC, disseminated intravascular coagulation; G6PD, glucose-6-phosphate dehydrogenase.

Table 2
Laboratory evidence of neonatal hemolytic disease

	Laboratory Test	Neonatal Reference Range
Tests for excessive hemoglobin degradation	Elevated end-tidal carbon monoxide	First 10–14 d after birth 1.4–1.7 ppm (5th to 95th percentile reference range) After day 14 should be <1 ppm[14]
	Elevated levels of carboxyhemoglobin	Value >1.5%–2% by co-oximetry
	Hemoglobinuria, in the absence of RBC, in the urine	There is normally no hemoglobin reported on the urine analysis, in the absence of RBC in the urine. Even trace hemoglobinura suggests hemolysis
	Low levels of serum haptoglobin	Absent haptoglobin (a value below the lower limit of assay detection) may be a reasonable good marker of hemolysis. See Ref.[15]
	Elevated levels of serum unconjugated (indirect) bilirubin	Compare patient value with hour-specific bilirubin nomogram
Tests for a compensatory increase in erythropoiesis	Elevated reticulocyte count	The reticulocyte count, typically 4%–7% at birth, generally falls to <2–3% after 24 h
	Elevated immature reticulocyte fraction	Not adequately defined in newborn infants.
	Elevated NRBC (nucleated red blood cell) count	Upper reference range limit among late-preterm and term infants is 3000/μL. For detailed reference ranges, see Ref.[16]

that 76% (85/112) of neonates with a serum bilirubin level exceeding 30 mg/dL had no explanation identified for their jaundice.[13] It was also found that 65% of neonates with total serum bilirubin level greater than 30 mg/dL had no explanation identified. The authors' findings were consistent with figures reported nationally. For instance, among 125 neonates listed in the voluntary USA kernicterus Registry from 1992 to 2004, 55% had no specific diagnosis identified to explain their hyperbilirubinemia and were termed cases of idiopathic jaundice.[17]

Many cases of extreme neonatal jaundice in which no cause for the hyperbilirubinemia is obvious are the result of hemolysis.[18] Some of these cases are the result of genetically based hemolytic conditions that only cause hyperbilirubinemia during the neonatal period, and will be compensated for adequately thereafter because of maturation of mechanisms involved in bilirubin metabolism.[7]

IDENTIFYING HEMOLYTIC CAUSES OF NEONATAL JAUNDICE

Five diagnostic tests that prove useful in diagnosing hemolytic jaundice are reviewed. These tests can assist physicians caring for jaundiced neonates to reach an accurate underlying diagnosis. The authors propose that making a precise diagnosis can be satisfying for both the physician and the family, enabling anticipatory guidance when chronic hemolytic conditions are identified. Such guidance can involve anticipating anemia during childhood with or without early bilirubin cholelithiasis. The 5 diagnostic tests or approaches are (1) erythrocyte morphology, (2) end-tidal carbon monoxide (ETCO) measurement, (3) EMA flow cytometry as a test for HS and other membrane defects, (4) NGS of relevant genes, and (5) an algorithm to assist in the judicious use of the standard tests and the selective use of the newer confirmatory tests.

RBC Morphology

Fig. 1 and **Table 3** demonstrate 5 of the more common morphologic abnormalities in RBC that frequently lead to neonatal jaundice,[19] namely, (1) microspherocytes, (2) elliptocytes, (3) blister/bite cells, (4) echinocytes, (5) and schistocytes.

Spherocytes are identified by the lack of a central pallor zone that is characteristic of normal erythrocytes. Spherocytes have lost part of the cell membrane and thus have a low mean corpuscular volume (MCV), maintaining the same hemoglobin content in a smaller cell volume, leading to an elevated mean corpuscular hemoglobin concentration (MCHC).[20–25] When abundant spherocytes are observed on the blood smear of a

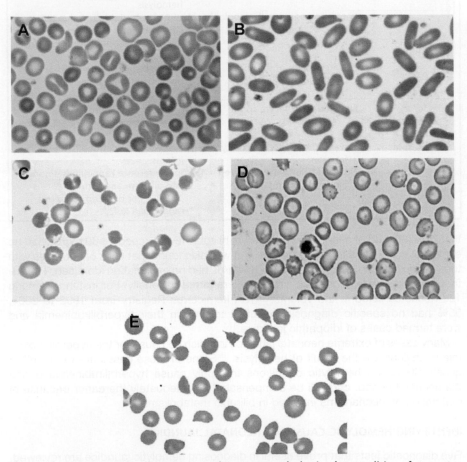

Fig. 1. Photomicrographs illustrating erythrocyte morphologic abnormalities of neonates with hemolytic jaundice (Wrights stain, 1000× magnification). (*A*) HS. Notice microspherocytes, lacking zone of central pallor, and large polychromatophilic erythrocytes. (*B*) Hereditary elliptocytosis. Notice many elliptical erythrocytes. (*C*) G6PD deficiency in a neonate with hemolysis after an oxidative exposure. Notice several erythrocytes with blisters, some spherocytes, and rare schistocytes. (*D*) Pyruvate kinase deficiency. Notice echinocytes and one orthochromatic normoblast. (*E*) Microangiopathic hemolytic anemia. Notice triangular and other abnormally shaped erythrocytes. Notice 2 polychromatophilic erythrocytes.

Table 3
Morphologic abnormalities of erythrocytes from neonates with jaundice

Abnormal Erythrocyte Morphology	Most Likely Causes	Suggested Laboratory Testing/Findings	Other Features
Microspherocytes	HS	• DAT (−) • EMA flow (+) • Persistent spherocytosis • Reticulocytosis	MCHC/MCV elevated (>36, likely >40)[18]
	ABO hemolytic disease	• DAT (+) • Transient spherocytosis • Reticulocytosis	MCHC/MCV normal (<36, likely <34)
Elliptocytes	Hereditary elliptocytosis	DAT (−)	MCHC normal MCV normal
Bite & blister cells	G6PD deficiency Unstable hemoglobin	G6PD enzyme activity Heinz body preparation	• Typically affects males but rarely females are also affected • Ethnicity of equatorial origin
Echinocytes	PK deficiency Other glycolytic enzyme deficiency	PK enzyme activity Quantify activity of other glycolytic enzymes	Autosomal recessive, likely to have no family history
Schistocytes	• DIC and/or perinatal asphyxia • Heinz body HA	• Low levels of FV and FVIII, elevated levels of D-dimers • Positive result of Heinz body preparation	• Low or falling platelet count • Normal to high IPF • Normal to high MPV DIC, perinatal asphyxia
	ADAMTS13 deficiency (TTP)	Severely decreased ADAMTS13 activity (<0.1 U/mL) high levels of LDH	• ADAMTS13 deficiency, early neonatal HUS, and giant hemangiomas all involve platelet consumption from endothelial injury and all have a similar neonatal presentation
	Neonatal hemolytic uremic syndrome	Acute renal failure	
	Homozygous protein C deficiency	Severely decreased functional protein C activity (<1%)	
	Giant hemangioma	May be internal or external	

Abbreviations: DAT, direct antiglobulin test; DIC, disseminated intravascular coagulation; FV, factor V; FVIII, factor VIII; G6PD, glucose-6-phosphate dehydrogenase; HA, hemolytic anemia; HUS, hemolytic uremic syndrome; IPF, immature platelet fraction; LDH, lactic dehydrogenase; MCHC, mean corpuscular hemoglobin concentration; MCV, mean corpuscular volume; MPV, mean platelet volume; PK, pyruvate kinase; TTP, thrombotic thrombocytopenic purpura.

neonate with jaundice, 2 main entities should be considered: ABO hemolytic disease and HS. Although the direct antiglobulin test (DAT) generally gives positive result in the former and negative result in the latter, there may rarely be a jaundiced neonate with ABO hemolytic disease with a negative result of DAT because of a low-titer maternal antibody, insufficient to render the test result positive but still sufficient to cause some degree of hemolysis. Also, the DAT sometimes gives negative result, whereas the indirect Coombs test gives positive result.

Elliptocytes are oval or elliptical. Elliptocytosis generally occurs as an autosomal dominantly inherited condition, with a variety of genotypes and with phenotypes ranging from completely asymptomatic to moderately severe hemolytic anemia.[19] Most neonates with hereditary elliptocytosis (HE) do not have significant jaundice or anemia and the condition commonly goes undetected in the neonatal period. However, an important exception, often resulting in severe neonatal jaundice, occurs when a neonate inherits an HE mutation from one parent, and also inherits a different RBC membrane defect from the other parent, similar to an autosomal recessive condition. The authors have recently reported such a neonate in detail with a condition termed pyropoikilocytosis.[26]

Blister cells and bite cells have lost a small portion of the hemoglobin content as a result of oxidative stress leading to denaturation of the hemoglobin, which is usually picked by the spleen leading to an empty space covered by a thin outer membrane (blister), which later becomes a bite cell after losing its thin membrane.[19] When these cells are observed in a jaundiced neonate, it usually suggests that the hemolytic process is precipitated by an episode of oxidative stress because of challenged unstable hemoglobin or glucose-6-phosphate dehydrogenase (G6PD)-deficient RBCs.[27]

Echinocytes are contracted and dehydrated cells with numerous rather uniform spicules. In the authors' experience, pyruvate kinase (PK) deficiency is the most common condition in jaundiced neonates giving rise to these cells.[28]

Schistocytes are fragments of erythrocytes and are usually encountered when mechanical destruction of red cells within the vasculature occurs or in the aftermath of oxidative stress such as seen in acute schistocytic (Heinz body) hemolytic anemia. The authors recommend that if greater than 1% of erythrocytes on a blood film of full-term neonates are schistocytes, or if more than 5% schistocytes are found in a premature baby, the term schistocytosis is appropriate. Other specific causes of schistocytic jaundice and anemia in neonates are reviewed elsewhere.[19]

End-Tidal Carbon Monoxide

Tidmarsh and colleagues[29] recently emphasized the clinical relevance of determining ETCO levels in jaundiced neonates. Carbon monoxide is generated stoichiometrically as heme is metabolized to bilirubin.[6,7] Thus, measuring the ETCO (minus the ambient CO) in jaundiced neonates may not only confirm hemolysis as a cause of the hyperbilirubinemia but also quantify the rate of hemolysis. **Fig. 2** shows an ETCO measurement taking place in a neonate who had an elevated serum bilirubin level. The upper reference range level of ETCO during the first week after birth is 1.7 ppm, and the authors generally use a level exceeding 2.0 ppm to confirm neonatal hemolysis.[14] It is feasible to quantify ETCO of jaundiced neonates during their birth hospitalization. When hemolytic jaundice is identified, physicians and parents typically comply with the American Academy of Pediatrics follow-up guidelines to have serum bilirubin levels measured within 24 hours after discharge from the birth hospital.[30]

EMA Flow Cytometry

When the diagnosis of HS is to be made, EMA binding can be a helpful test (**Fig. 3**).[31] EMA binding is a flow-cytometry-based test measuring the relative amount of fluorescently labeled EMA dye bound to band 3 and Rh-related proteins in the erythrocyte membrane. In HS, the reduction in band 3 and other membrane proteins leads to decreased fluorescence intensity. In the authors' hematology clinic at Primary Children's Hospital, EMA flow has outperformed other diagnostic tests for HS in newborn infants and has replaced osmotic fragility testing.

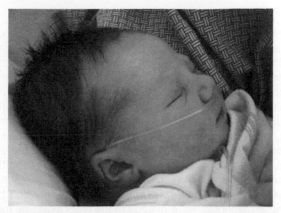

Fig. 2. Screening for hemolytic jaundice using end-tidal carbon monoxide quantification. A neonate with jaundice (serum bilirubin in the high-intermediate-risk zone) where ETCO is measured by a single-nare cannula attached to the CoSense monitor.

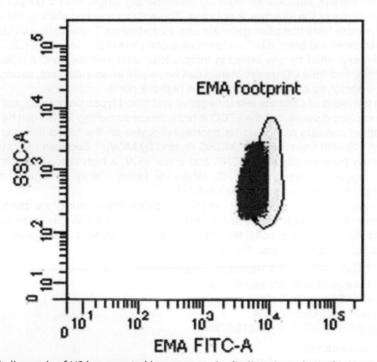

Fig. 3. A diagnosis of HS is supported in a neonate by finding that a large fraction of erythrocytes display reduced EMA binding. Fewer than normal EMA-tagged erythrocytes are indicated by a leftward displacement of events compared with the normal range (footprint). FITC-A, fluorescein isothiocyanate; SSC-A, side scatter.

Next-Generation Sequencing

Laboratory techniques collectively termed next-generation sequencing, developed only a few years ago, are currently being adopted by clinical reference laboratories as diagnostic tests for mutations or polymorphisms causing human genetically based disorders. Because multiple candidate genes from a patient can be sequenced in parallel in a single run, the cost of the procedure can be several orders of magnitude less than previous methods in which mutations are sought by sequencing candidate genes one at a time. Moreover, using the barcoding technique to identify which DNA fragments belong to which patients, the DNA of multiple patients can be sequenced in a single run, further reducing costs as a clinical test. The test usually reports the exact mutation and not only the gene involved. When novel mutations or genetically complex conditions are present, involving mutations in several genes, NGS can identify the situation, while previous techniques frequently do not. The quality of patient data generated by NGS, and the usefulness to clinical diagnosis, have already made NGS available for diagnosing the cause of congenital hemolytic jaundice and also for congenital bone marrow failure disorders. Attempts are underway to generate NGS like the one illustrated in **Table 4** to identify the underlying genetic causes of neonatal jaundice. Limited availability to date, and limited reports, are generating useful information.[18,23–26,32]

Algorithm

Fig. 4 illustrates a method that the authors advocate for evaluating the cause of problematic cases of neonatal jaundice. For the purpose of this algorithm, the authors define problematic jaundice as requiring phototherapy longer than a couple of days when the cause of the jaundice is not clear. The authors suggest starting the evaluation with simple tests that often generate useful information. These tests include blood typing of mother and baby, (DAT or Coombs), a complete blood cell count (CBC) with a blood film examined by one skilled in morphologic interpretation, and a reticulocyte count. Also, end-tidal CO determination can be helpful as an initial test, strongly suggesting a hemolytic disorder if the ETCO is high (>2 ppm).

When the result of Coombs test is negative and blood types do not suggest alloimmune hemolytic disease, but the ETCO is high, simple screening for HS can be useful. This method consists of looking for microspherocytes on the blood film and calculating the HS ratio from the CBC (MCHC divided by MCV).[20] Because neonates with HS typically have an elevated MCHC and a low MCV, a high ratio, exceeding 0.36 or 0.37 suggests a diagnosis of HS. When the family history is negative for HS, EMA flow cytometric testing can be useful.[31]

Enzymatic testing for G6PD deficiency or PK deficiency is usually inexpensive and rapid. When the pathogenesis is still unclear after these rather simple tests, hematology consultation with additional testing is sometimes needed. Laboratories in which such testing is offered include the following:

Blood Disease Reference Hematology Laboratory
http://www.yalebloodddiseaselab.org/
310 Cedar Street, CB 541a
New Haven, CT 06520, USA
Tel. (203)737-1349, Fax (203)785-3896.

ARUP Laboratories
http://www.aruplab.com/testing.
500 Chipeta Way
Salt Lake City, UT 84108, USA
Tel. (800)522-2787, Fax (800)522-2706.

Table 4
The genes sequenced in the problematic neonatal jaundice NGS panel

Gene Symbol	Gene Description	OMIM ID	Associated Hematological Disorder
SPTA1	Spectrin alpha	182860	Elliptocytosis, spherocytosis, pyropoikilocytosis
SPTB	Spectrin beta	182870	Elliptocytosis, spherocytosis
ANK1	Ankyrin 1	612641	Spherocytosis
SLC4A1	Solute carrier family 4, anion exchanger, member 1 (erythrocyte membrane protein band 3)	109270	Spherocytosis, stomatocytosis, acanthocytosis, ovalocytosis
EPB41	Erythrocyte membrane protein band 4.1	130500	Elliptocytosis
EPB42	Erythrocyte membrane protein band 4.2	177070	Spherocytosis
PIEZO1	Piezo-type mechanosensitive ion channel component 1	611184	Xerocytosis
CYB5R3	Cytochrome b reductase 3	613213	Methemoglobinemia type 1 and 2
G6PD	Glucose-6-phosphate dehydrogenase	305900	G6PD deficiency
GPI	Glucose phosphate isomerase	172400	GPI deficiency
GSR	Glutathione reductase	138300	GSR deficiency
HK1	Hexokinase 1	142600	Hemolytic anemia
NT5C3	Pyrimidine 5′-nucleotidase	606224	Hemolytic anemia
PGK1	Phosphoglycerate kinase 1	311800	PGK1 deficiency
PKLR	Pyruvate kinase (liver and red cell)	609712	PKLR deficiency
PKM	Pyruvate kinase (muscle)	179050	Bloom syndrome
TPI1	Triosephosphate isomerase 1	190450	TPI1 deficiency
GSS	Glutathione synthase	601002	GSS deficiency
ADA	Adenosine deaminase	608958	ADA deficiency
AK1	Adenylate kinase 1	103000	AK1 deficiency
PFKM	Phosphofructokinase (muscle)	610681	PFKM deficiency, glycogen storage disease type 7
PFKL	Phosphofructokinase (liver)	171860	?
UGT1A1	UDP glycosyltransferase 1 family, polypeptide A1	19174	Crigler-Najjar syndrome 1 and 2
UGT1A6	UDP glycosyltransferase 1 family, polypeptide A6	606431	UGT1A6 deficiency
UGT1A7	UDP glycosyltransferase 1 family, polypeptide A7	606432	UGT1A7 deficiency
SLCO1B1	Solute carrier organic anion transporter family, member 1B1	604843	Rotor syndrome
SLCO1B3	Solute carrier organic anion transporter family, member 1B3	605495	Rotor syndrome

Abbreviations: OMIM, Online Mendelian Inheritance in Man; UDP, uridine diphosphate.

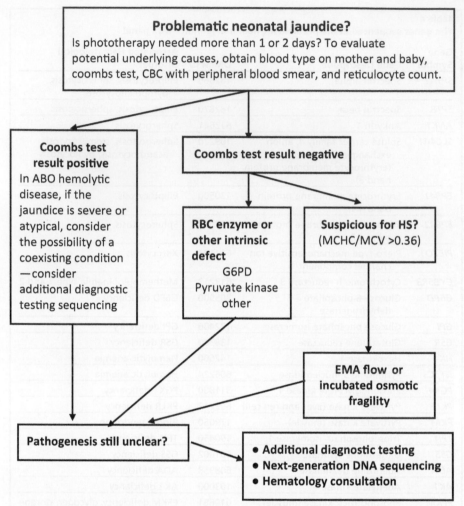

Fig. 4. Algorithm for evaluating the underlying cause in neonates with problematic jaundice. G6PD, glucose-6-phosphate dehydrogenase; MCHC, mean corpuscular hemoglobin concentration; MCV, mean corpuscular volume.

GeneDx
http://www.genedx.com.
207 Perry Parkway Gaithersburg
MD 20877, USA
Tel. (301)519-2100, Fax (301)519-2892.

Mayo Medical Laboratories.
http://www.mayomedicallaboratories.com/
3050 Superior Drive NW
Rochester, MN 55901, USA.
Tel. (800)553-1710, Fax (507)284-1759.

Best Practices

What is current practice?

- Conscientious attempts are made to prevent hazardous neonatal hyperbilirubinemia and thereby avert bilirubin-induced neurologic dysfunction.

- Methods used to reduce the risk of hazardous neonatal hyperbilirubinemia include universal screening of serum or transcutaneous bilirubin levels during the birth hospitalization.

- Neonates who are recognized as having significant jaundice are managed with phototherapy and careful follow-up, to assess bilirubin rebound after stopping phototherapy.

- Despite concerted efforts, kernicterus still occurs.

- The most common cause of rehospitalization during the first week after birth is neonatal jaundice.

What changes in current practice are likely to improve outcomes?

- Rapidly identifying specific hemolytic causes of jaundice can alert clinicians to the need for rigorous inpatient and outpatient bilirubin follow-up.

- Rapid recognition of the most common genetic contributors to hazardous neonatal hemolytic jaundice can facilitate anticipatory guidance of these patients, thereby avoiding adverse outcomes.

Summary Statement

Tests, techniques, and approaches reviewed in this article include assessing RBC morphology, end-tidal carbon monoxide quantification, EMA flow cytometry, next-generation DNA sequencing using neonatal jaundice panels, and the algorithms presented in this article.

REFERENCES

1. Glader G, Allen GA. Neonatal hemolysis. In: deAlarcon PA, Werner EJ, Christensen RD, editors. Neonatal hematology. 2nd edition. Cambridge (United Kingdom): Cambridge University Press; 2014. p. 91.
2. Pearson HA. Life-span of the fetal red blood cell. J Pediatr 1967;70:166–71.
3. Bard H, Widness JA. The life span of erythrocytes transfused to preterm infants. Pediatr Res 1997;42:9–11.
4. Kuruvilla DJ, Nalbant D, Widness JA, et al. Mean remaining life span: a new clinically relevant parameter to assess the quality of transfused red blood cells. Transfusion 2014;54(10 Pt 2):2724–9.
5. Mock DM, Widness JA, Veng-Pedersen P, et al. Measurement of posttransfusion red cell survival with the biotin label. Transfus Med Rev 2014;28(3):114–25.
6. Stevenson DK, Vreman HJ, Wong RJ. Bilirubin production and the risk of bilirubin neurotoxicity. Semin Perinatol 2011;35(3):121–6.
7. Cohen RS, Wong RJ, Stevenson DK. Understanding neonatal jaundice: a perspective on causation. Pediatr Neonatol 2010;51(3):143–8.
8. Maisels MJ, Pathak A, Nelson NM, et al. Endogenous production of carbon monoxide in normal and erythroblastotic newborn infants. J Clin Invest 1971;50(1):1–8.
9. Maisels MJ, Kring E. The contribution of hemolysis to early jaundice in normal newborns. Pediatrics 2006;118(1):276–9.
10. Kaplan M, Bromiker R, Hammerman C. Hyperbilirubinemia, hemolysis, and increased bilirubin neurotoxicity. Semin Perinatol 2014;38(7):429–37.
11. Johnson L, Bhutani VK. The clinical syndrome of bilirubin-induced neurologic dysfunction. Semin Perinatol 2011;35(3):101–13.

12. Kaplan M, Hammerman C. Understanding severe hyperbilirubinemia and preventing kernicterus: adjuncts in the interpretation of neonatal serum bilirubin. Clin Chim Acta 2005;356(1–2):9–21.
13. Christensen RD, Lambert DK, Henry E, et al. Unexplained extreme hyperbilirubinemia among neonates in a multihospital healthcare system. Blood Cells Mol Dis 2013;50(2):105–9.
14. Christensen RD, Lambert DK, Henry E, et al. End-tidal carbon monoxide as an indicator of the hemolytic rate. Blood Cells Mol Dis 2015;54(3):292–6.
15. Chavez-Bueno S, Beasley JA, Goldbeck JM, et al. Haptoglobin concentrations in preterm and term newborns'. J Perinatol 2011;31(7):500–3.
16. Christensen RD, Henry E, Andres RL, et al. Neonatal reference ranges for blood concentrations of nucleated red blood cells. Neonatology 2010;99:289–94.
17. Johnson L, Bhutani VK, Karp K, et al. Clinical report from the pilot USA Kernicterus Registry (1992 to 2004). J Perinatol 2009;29(Suppl 1):S25–45.
18. Christensen RD, Nussenzveig RH, Yaish HM, et al. Causes of hemolysis in neonates with extreme hyperbilirubinemia. J Perinatol 2014;34(8):616–9.
19. Christensen RD, Yaish HM, Lemons RS. Neonatal hemolytic jaundice: morphologic features of erythrocytes that will help you diagnose the underlying condition. Neonatology 2014;105(4):243–9.
20. Yaish HM, Christensen RD, Henry E, et al. A simple method of screening newborn infants for hereditary spherocytosis. J Appl Hematol 2013;4:27–32.
21. Christensen RD, Henry E. Hereditary spherocytosis in neonates with hyperbilirubinemia. Pediatrics 2010;125(1):120–5.
22. Sheffield MJ, Christensen RD. Evaluating neonatal hyperbilirubinemia in late preterm Hispanic twins led to the diagnosis of hereditary spherocytosis in them, and in their sibling and in their mother. J Perinatol 2011;31(9):625–7.
23. Christensen RD, Yaish HM, Nussenzveig RH, et al. Acute kernicterus in a neonate with O/B blood group incompatibility and a mutation in SLC4A1. Pediatrics 2013; 132(2):e531–4.
24. Yaish HM, Christensen RD, Agarwal A. A neonate with Coombs-negative hemolytic jaundice with spherocytes but normal erythrocyte indices: a rare case of autosomal-recessive hereditary spherocytosis due to alpha-spectrin deficiency. J Perinatol 2013;33(5):404–6.
25. Nussenzveig RH, Christensen RD, Prchal JT, et al. Novel α-spectrin mutation in trans with α-spectrin causing severe neonatal jaundice from hereditary spherocytosis. Neonatology 2014;106(4):355–7.
26. Christensen RD, Nussenzveig RH, Reading NS, et al. Variations in both α-spectrin (SPTA1) and β-spectrin (SPTB) in a neonate with prolonged jaundice in a family where nine individuals had hereditary elliptocytosis. Neonatology 2014;105(1): 1–4.
27. Christensen RD, Yaish HM, Wiedmeier SE, et al. Neonatal death suspected to be from sepsis was found to be kernicterus with G6PD deficiency. Pediatrics 2013; 132(6):e1694–8.
28. Christensen RD, Yaish HM, Johnson CB, et al. Six children with pyruvate kinase deficiency from one small town: molecular characterization of the PK-LR gene. J Pediatr 2011;159(4):695–7.
29. Tidmarsh GF, Wong RJ, Stevenson DK. End-tidal carbon monoxide and hemolysis. J Perinatol 2014;34(8):577–81.
30. Maisels MJ, Bhutani VK, Bogen D, et al. Hyperbilirubinemia in the newborn infant > or =35 weeks' gestation: an update with clarifications. Pediatrics 2009; 124:1193–8.

31. Christensen RD, Agarwal AM, Nussenzveig RH, et al. Evaluating eosin-5-maleimide binding as a diagnostic test for hereditary spherocytosis in newborn infants. J Perinatol 2014. http://dx.doi.org/10.1038/jp.2014.202.
32. Yaish HM, Nussenzveig RH, Agarwal AM, et al. A previously unknown mutation in the pyruvate kinase gene (PKLR) identified from a neonate with severe jaundice. Neonatology 2014;106(2):140–2.

Plasma Biomarkers of Oxidative Stress in Neonatal Brain Injury

Maria Luisa Tataranno, MD, Serafina Perrone, MD, PhD*, Giuseppe Buonocore, MD

KEYWORDS

- Oxidative stress • Newborn infant • Brain damage • Plasma biomarkers
- Lipid peroxidation • Inflammation • Hypoxia-ischemia

KEY POINTS

- Pathogenesis of perinatal encephalopathy is quite complex. An important role for oxidative stress is now recognized.
- Prostanoids and non–protein bound iron represent specific plasma oxidative biomarkers reflecting oxidative stress injury to neuronal cells.
- Sensitive and specific biomarkers of oxidative stress can be used in premature and term infants for the early detection and follow-up of brain injury.

BACKGROUND

The preterm and term brain is particularly vulnerable to the insult of oxidative stress (OS) because rapidly growing tissues are especially sensitive to the harmful effects of free radicals (FRs).[1,2] OS causes endothelial cell damage, hemostatic abnormalities, inflammatory reactions, astrocyte dysfunction, N-methyl-D-aspartate (NMDA) receptor impairment, and synaptosome structural damage.[3–6] According to current knowledge, the pathophysiology of brain injury almost always involves multiple factors including hemodynamic, metabolic, nutritional, toxic, and infectious mechanisms, acting in the antenatal or postnatal period. The combination of these factors often triggers neuronal death processes.[4] Perinatal hypoxia-ischemia[7] and the so-called "encephalopathy of prematurity" encompassing intraventricular hemorrhage (IVH) and periventricular leukomalacia are major contributors to neonatal brain injury. Chronic placental inflammation and acute fetal and neonatal inflammation also increase the risk of brain injury.[8] Complex disturbance on the infant's subsequent brain development also plays an important role.[9]

Disclosure: The authors state that there are no commercial or financial conflicts of interest.
Department of Molecular and Developmental Medicine, University of Siena, Via Banchi di Sotto, 55, 53100 Siena, Italy
* Corresponding author.
E-mail address: saraspv@yahoo.it

The pathogenesis of perinatal brain damage is complex with multiple contributory pathways and mechanisms of injury.[10] Efforts to understand and prevent neonatal brain injury are worthwhile because of the huge number of infants involved and the enormous cost to society.

OS plays a pivotal role in the pathogenesis of brain injury, being the final common pathway for multiple converging events. OS may result from many different pathways including glutamate release and NMDA receptor activation leading to excitotoxic processes; mitochondrial dysfunction; activation of enzymes, such as nitric oxide synthase (NOS); phagocyte activation; arachidonic acid cascade; Fenton reaction driven by the release of non–protein bound iron (NPBI); and deficiency of the antioxidant system of the immature brain.[11,12]

OS occurs at birth in all newborns as a consequence of the hyperoxic challenge that occurs with the transition from the hypoxic intrauterine environment to extrauterine life. It happens when the production of FRs exceeds the capacity of antioxidant defenses and is primarily caused by a disturbance in the delicate balance between the production of FRs and the biologic system's ability to readily detoxify the FRs or to repair the resulting damage.[13] Hypoxia-ischemia is a main event inducing an overproduction of FRs.[14] Chronic placental inflammation, acute fetal inflammation, and neonatal inflammation interact in contributing oxidative risk and/or directly damaging the developing brain.[4] Some FRs can even act as second messengers: at low levels, they are signaling molecules, and at high levels, they can damage organelles, particularly the mitochondria. Oxidative damage and the associated mitochondrial dysfunction may result in energy depletion, accumulation of cytotoxic mediators, and cell death.[15]

The discovery and validation of specific OS biomarkers of neonatal brain injury represents a key step in the evolution of neonatal neuroprotection and is based on the measurement of a single or a panel of biomarkers in biologic fluids and tissues reflecting OS injury to neuronal cells. Clinicians do not currently have access to biomarkers for early diagnosis or intervention in neonates with brain injury. Thus there is a need to develop specific OS biomarkers to enable caregivers to make an early prediction of newborns at high risk, to start preventative neuroprotective strategies, and to monitor the progression of the disease. This article examines potential reliable and specific plasma OS biomarkers that can be used in premature and term infants for the early detection and follow-up of the most common neonatal brain injuries, such as hypoxic-ischemic encephalopathy (HIE), IVH, and periventricular leukomalacia.

PLASMA BIOMARKERS OF OXIDATIVE STRESS

The quantification of OS is based on the measurement of specific biomarkers in biologic fluids and tissues, which reflect induced oxidative damage to lipids, proteins, and DNA or an increased risk for injury to macromolecules. Several biomarkers have been proposed for OS detection, but only a small number of them can be considered truly specific and reliable for brain injury; these include prostanoids and NPBI.[11,16,17] Biomarkers can be considered as indicators of a disease process, but they can also give information about the worsening and progression of the process. A reliable biomarker should be biologically plausible, with a high sensitivity and specificity, and should be measured with a reproducible and standardized methodology.

The measurement of OS level in vivo is known to be difficult because FRs usually have a short half-life. Furthermore, some tests to measure FRs suffer from problems related to low specificity and sensitivity. The discovery of more stable compounds has led to the possibility of more reliable biomarkers of neonatal brain injury.

Isoprostanes

Nonenzymatic in vivo and in vitro peroxidation of polyunsaturated fatty acids leads to the production of prostanoids, which are prostaglandin-like compounds. F2-isoprostanes (IsoPs) are first produced in phospholipids and then they are released into the blood. The mechanism involved in their formation implies that FR insult causes hydrogen abstraction from arachidonic acid and addition of molecular oxygen to form a peroxyl radical.[18] The following intermediates undergo double 5-exo-trig cyclization and addition of second molecular oxygen to form prostaglandin G_2–like compounds, which are rapidly reduced to F2-IsoPs.[19,20] These prostanoids are more stable compared with other peroxidation products, such as aldehydes or peroxyl radicals, thus they can be detected in biologic fluids.[21] Prostanoids can be measured in plasma, tissues, cells, urine, cerebral spinal fluid, bile, and bronchoalveolar lavage fluid[21] for the assessment of in situ oxidative injury. F2-IsoP detection and measurement requires sophisticated and expensive methods, such as gas chromatography/mass spectrometry. From the same family, F3-IsoPs are stable, specific, and reliable markers of lipid peroxidation, more specifically derived from oxidation of eicosapentenoic acid. Consequently, decreased levels could indicate a reduced intake of eicosapentanoic acid.[16] Eicosapentanoic acid is a direct precursor of docosahexaenoic acid (DHA), a primary structural component of the human brain and particularly cerebral cortex. Finally, F2-dihomo-IsoPs are specific and reliable OS markers of cerebral white matter lipid oxidation, because they are directly derived from oxidation of adrenic acid[16] highly concentrated in myelin within the brain white matter of primates.

Isofurans

The prostanoid profile can be affected by oxygen tension. An oxygen insertion step blocks the intermediates from the IsoPs pathway to form different compounds, termed isofurans (IsoFs), which contain a substituted tetrahydrofuran ring. The IsoFs, similar to the IsoPs, are chemically and metabolically stable and are well suited to act as in vivo biomarkers of oxidative damage. The ratio of IsoFs to IsoPs also provides information about the relative oxygen tension where the lipid peroxidation is occurring. This was clearly shown in pigs, in which exposure to high oxygen tension increased IsoFs production and reduced IsoPs levels in the brain.[22,23]

Neuroprostanes

The oxidation in vivo and in vitro of DHA, a major component of neuronal membranes, leads to the formation of IsoP-like compounds termed neuroprostanes.[24] The most studied series is the four-series neuroprostanes, mainly F4-neuroprostane. The neuroprostanes are the only quantitative in vivo biomarker of oxidative damage selective for neurons, thus they are a specific and reliable marker of cerebral gray matter lipid oxidation.

Neurofurans

Similar to IsoFs, in high oxygen tension conditions, an alternative pathway of oxidation of DHA leads to the formation of compounds termed neurofurans. Thus hyperoxic or hypoxic conditions can be detected through quantitative assessment of neurofurans and IsoFs in vivo. Given the abundance of DHA in the brain, analysis of neurofurans may be of particular value in the quantitative assessment of lipid peroxidation in brain damage.[25] IsoFs and neurofurans are new promising markers and their potential is being investigated because they can be good markers of oxidative injury in conditions of high oxygen tension. Little data exist in humans, mostly because of a lack of commercially standard references.[16,26]

Non–Protein Bound Iron

In physiologic conditions, iron is safely sequestered by transport proteins, such as transferrin and lactoferrin, and stored in proteins, such as ferritin and hemosiderin.[27,28] Because iron ions cannot be free in plasma, the term NPBI was introduced to indicate a low-molecular-mass iron form, free from binding to plasma proteins. NPBI levels can be measured using high-performance liquid chromatography.[29] Iron toxicity is inversely proportional to the presence of ferritin, which is able to bind and detoxify ferrous ion, and directly proportional to the quantity of hydrogen peroxide to produce hydroxyl radicals through the Fenton reaction. Furthermore, lipid exposure to high concentration of NPBI leads to formation of IsoPs.[30,31]

OXIDATIVE STRESS AND NEONATAL BRAIN INJURY

In many animals but especially in humans, the neonatal brain undergoes huge and substantial qualitative and quantitative changes during development, including cell division, differentiation and migration, axonal and dendritic proliferation, synaptogenesis, myelination, programmed cell death, and formation of neuronal networks.[32] Many factors, such as the existence of a complex network of signaling molecules, ion channel cerebral expression, receptor maturation, and growth factor synthesis, are important for these sophisticated processes.[33] Energy production is central to life and the brain is particularly sensitive to any disturbances in energy generation, and even a short-term interruption can result in long-lasting, irreversible damage. Many papers underline the role of OS in the pathogenesis of many neurologic neonatal diseases, such as IVH,[34] HIE,[35] and epilepsy.[36] The role of hypoxic-ischemic insult in injury to the developing brain may be related to intrinsic regional metabolic factors, such as the cerebral metabolic rate for glucose and for oxygen, energy consumption, and cerebral blood flow, which are higher than in the mature brain. These changes in metabolism lead to structural and functional modifications to the mitochondrial activity (ie, the number of mitochondria per cell, mitochondrial protein and respiratory enzyme content, and mitochondrial matrix density).[33] A characteristic feature of the fetal brain is the presence of many leptomeningeal anastomoses among major cerebral arteries that leads to the relative sparing of gray matter, whereas the telencephalic white matter, especially in the depths of the sulci, represents a border zone of blood supply between major cerebral arteries. Furthermore, the very high levels of polyunsaturated fatty acids in the neonatal brain predisposes to the generation of FRs and to OS injury. Polyunsaturated fatty acid constituents of membrane lipids in the white matter are highly susceptible to FR damage. FR attacks on immature myelin lead to lipid peroxidation and lipid peroxides are themselves FRs.[37] The relative immaturity of the antioxidant system facilitates the exposure of fetuses and newborns to the damaging effects of OS. Particularly, superoxide dismutase, catalase, and glutathione peroxidase antioxidant enzyme systems are less active and are present in lower concentrations in the immature brain.[38] The presence in the developing brain of a transient increase in density and distribution of glutamate receptors could amplify brain injury caused by hypoxic damage.[39]

Following hypoxic stimulus there is a certain degree of swelling and calcium deposit inside the mitochondria,[40] which leads to chromatin condensation, thus triggering apoptosis. Cerebral apoptosis starts with cytochrome C translocation from mitochondria, followed by caspase-9 activation and then caspase-3 activation. Many apoptosis-related factors are upregulated in the immature brain including caspase-3, Apaf-1, Bcl-2, and Bax.[41] In the developing brain, NMDA receptor activation depresses mitochondrial respiration and induces apoptosis, a phenomenon that is not seen in the adult brain (the so-called NMDA-paradox).[42] Subtype is essential for the antiapoptotic signaling integrity of amino acid receptors of the NMDA. The developing brain is prone to produce FRs from oxygen and nitric oxide (NO); they operate intramitochondrial protein nitrosilation, which triggers cell death and/or apoptosis. It is thus plausible that the intramitochondrial scavenging system in the developing brain fails to detoxify nitrogen and oxygen FRs.[43] It is clear that mitochondria play crucial roles in the activation of apoptotic mechanisms; they are initiators and targets of OS. In a prospective study conducted on 90 newborns (>32 weeks gestational age) with various stages of HIE, Peeters-Scholte and colleagues[44] studied glutathione peroxidase activity in the cerebrospinal fluid in the first 48 hours of life as an index of OS. They also examined the concentration of neuron-specific enolase at 72 hours of life as a marker of brain injury. Neurologic outcome was assessed at 12 months of corrected gestational age using the Denver Developmental screening test. They found a correlation between glutathione peroxidase activity and gestational age, clinical stage of HIE, neuron-specific enolase levels, and neurodevelopmental outcome. It has also been suggested that the broad variation in the final effects of hypoxia-ischemia on the neonatal brain is caused by genetic factors and that there is a gender difference regarding response to hypoxic-ischemic injury, with male newborns being more susceptible to injury than females.[20,45]

The negative effects of OS may start from intrauterine life. It has been demonstrated that OS plays a key role in some pathologic conditions associated with neurologic impairment (ie, cerebral palsy, cognitive and behavioral disorders), such as intrauterine growth retardation.[46] An in vivo and ex vivo rat model of intrauterine growth retardation shows the delay in oligodendrocyte differentiation and myelination, likely caused by bone morphogenetic protein 4 upregulation induced by OS. Normal myelination has been observed when abrogating bone morphogenetic protein signaling.[47] Down syndrome originates from an extra chromosome 21 in the cellular karyotype. The superoxide dismutase gene is localized on chromosome 21. This enzyme dismutates superoxide anion with the participation of catalase and glutathione peroxidase. Increased levels of 8-iso-PGF2 IsoP, a reliable biomarker of OS, were found in the amniotic fluid of pregnancies with a Down syndrome fetus.[48] The immature oligodendroglial cells are glutathione peroxidase and catalase deficient, so overexpression of superoxide dismutase can be dangerous rather than protective. The early occurrence of OS in pregnancies with a trisomy 21 fetus and the subsequent oxidative damage as a major contributing factor in brain aging and cognitive function decline are likely because of the overexpression of superoxide dismutase caused by the supernumerary chromosome. Superoxide dismutase is also overexpressed in the immature brain, especially under stress conditions.

Hypoxia-ischemia, infection, inflammation, and excitotoxicity are all important causes participating in the development of injury.[4,49,50] The sudden or chronic interruption of oxygen availability in the perinatal period determines a radical shift from aerobic metabolism to the less efficient anaerobic metabolism.[6,51] The reoxygenation process, which is a fundamental requisite for survival, can lead to sustained overexpression of alternative metabolic pathways, thus prolonging the energy deficit and/or generating OS.[52,53] Perinatal hypoxia alters mechanisms that regulate cerebral blood flow and can trigger a cascade of biochemical events that begins with a shift from oxidative to anaerobic metabolism leading to oxidative brain damage.[54] By favoring intracellular release of NPBI into plasma, asphyxia and acidosis supply redox-cycling iron, predisposing to OS.[55-57] NPBI leads to the catalysis of O_2-, H_2O_2, and the generation of the damaging OH. In presence of free iron, huge increases in FR generation are possible, with the potential to cause tissue damage. Plasma NPBI may leak into the brain through a damaged blood-brain barrier and can be particularly damaging when taken up directly by cells. When NPBI gains access to the extracellular space, cellular uptake is enhanced by intracellular calcium and paradoxically also by increased levels of intracellular iron. Differentiating oligodendrocytes are particularly vulnerable to FRs damage, being rich in iron that is required for differentiation.[58] Plasma NPBI has been found to be the best early predictive marker of neurodevelopmental outcome in newborns (gestational age, 24–42 weeks) with clinical signs of perinatal hypoxia at birth. This marker showed 100% sensitivity and 100% specificity for good outcome until the second year of age at 0 to 1.16 µmol/L and for poor outcome at greater than 15.2 µmol/L.[11] The role of NO in the pathogenesis of injury is also very important. NO is a weak FR, produced by the actions of NOS isoforms, and has several physiologic roles including the physiologic modulation of cerebral blood flow, the modulation of cellular respiration, and FR production in the mitochondria. Finally, it also has antioxidant properties.[59,60] There are three well-known isoforms of NOS: (1) neuronal NOS (nNOS), (2) endothelial NOS (eNOS), and (3) inducible NOS. The latter is principally produced in macrophages, microglia, endothelial cells, and astrocytes. nNOS is principally produced in neurons, and eNOS in endothelial cells.[61-63] Both nNOS and eNOS are up-regulated following neonatal hypoxia-ischemia.[64] nNOS knockout mice seem to be protected from neonatal hypoxic-ischemic injury.[61] Studies from eNOS knockout mice suggest eNOS may play a protective role against hypoxic-ischemic injury in the adult brain,[65] which may be caused by eNOS influencing neural migration and outgrowth and acting as a downstream regulator of angiogenesis.[66] Finally, polyunsaturated fatty acids are constituents of lipid membrane in white matter and they are highly susceptible to FR attack. The lipid peroxidation that occurs following acute hypoxia in the fetal brain[67] may be caused by the generation of peroxynitrite, following the nonenzymatic combination of NO and superoxide.[68] Lipid peroxidation affects immature oligodendrocytes in particular in the preterm fetal brain,[69] and may be a major factor in the white matter damage that can arise from hypoxia or infection in the developing brain.[38,69-71]

Chronic placental inflammation, acute fetal inflammation, and neonatal inflammation interact in contributing to oxidative risk and/or directly damaging the developing brain.[4] Intrauterine infection may be followed by brain damage caused by the direct effects of bacterial toxins and lipopolysaccharides on glial cells, by astrocyte deregulation, and by the effects of phagocyte activation, particularly on coagulation and endothelium.[71] During a primary systemic immune response, there is a systemic upregulation of proinflammatory cytokines and activation of microglia in the brain.[72] Microglia enhance injury by expressing inflammatory mediators and proinflammatory cytokines.[73] Cytokine-activated cells release toxic substances, including proteolytic enzymes, myeloperoxidase, and reactive oxygen species.[74,75] The superoxide anion, the most abundant radical species, is also the first stage of the bacterial killing reaction, which is followed by the production of other FRs, such as hydrogen peroxide (H_2O_2) by superoxide dismutase, hydroxyl radicals catalyzed by transition metals, and $HOCl^-$ by myeloperoxidase. These substances contribute to bacterial killing but also favor tissue damage. Moreover, these agents determine increased capillary permeability that facilitates the passage of cytokines. Thus, a close relation between inflammation and OS has been established.[76]

SUMMARY

The neonatal brain is particularly vulnerable to OS insult because the rapidly growing tissues are especially sensitive to the harmful effects of FRs. Plasma OS biomarkers have the potential to early identify newborns at high risk for brain damage. Nevertheless there are few publications that validated the role of OS biomarkers of brain injury with more accurate brain damage assessment, such as brain MRI. Furthermore, the correlation between OS biomarkers and functional brain outcomes, such as amplitude-integrated electroencephalogram, near-infrared spectroscopy, and long-term neurodevelopmental follow-up, should be explored. Further studies are urgently needed to explore the diagnostic and predictive value of different OS biomarkers in assessing the severity of brain injury to improve the outcome of the high-risk newborn.

ACKNOWLEDGMENTS

The authors thank the EURAIBI Foundation (Europe Against Infant Brain Injury) for the partial contribution.

Best Practices

What is the current practice?

Perinatal encephalopathy in term and preterm infants is one of the main leading causes of lifelong disability. Increasing evidences on perinatal brain damage indicate a complex pathogenesis. In this context OS plays an important role because cerebral fast-growing tissues are especially sensitive to the harmful effects of FRs. Nowadays clinicians do not routinely use biomarkers for early diagnosis or intervention in neonates with brain injury.

What changes in current practice are likely to improve outcomes?

The discovery and validation of specific plasma OS biomarkers to predict the occurrence and severity of neonatal brain injury represent a key step in the evolution of neonatal neuroprotection based on the measurement of a single or a panel of biomarkers.

Major recommendations

Plasma OS biomarkers have the potentiality to early identify newborns at high risk for brain damage. The correlation between OS biomarkers and structural and functional brain outcomes, such as MRI, amplitude integrated electroencephalogram, near-infrared spectroscopy, and long-term neurodevelopmental follow-up should be explored. Further studies are urgently needed to explore the diagnostic and predictive value of different OS biomarkers in assessing the severity of brain injury to improve the outcome of this high-risk population.

Summary statement

OS plays a fundamental role in the pathogenesis of brain injury in preterm and term infants. The discovery and validation of specific plasma OS biomarkers of neonatal brain injury represents a key step in the evolution of neonatal neuroprotection based on the measurement of a single or a panel of biomarkers.

REFERENCES

1. Goplerud JM, Mishra OP, Delivoria-Papadopoulos M. Brain cell membrane dysfunction following acute asphyxia in newborn piglets. Biol Neonate 1992;61: 33–41.

2. Perrone S, Tataranno LM, Stazzoni G, et al. Brain susceptibility to oxidative stress in the perinatal period. J Matern Fetal Neonatal Med 2013. [Epub ahead of print].

3. Palmer C, Menzies SL, Roberts RL, et al. Changes in iron histochemistry after hypoxic-ischemic brain injury in the neonatal rat. J Neurosci Res 1999;56: 60–71.

4. Korzeniewski SJ, Romero R, Cortez J, et al. A "multi-hit" model of neonatal white matter injury: cumulative contributions of chronic placental inflammation, acute fetal inflammation and postnatal inflammatory events. J Perinat Med 2014;42: 731–4.

5. Buonocore G, Perrone S. Biomarkers of hypoxic brain injury in the neonate. Clin Perinatol 2004;31:107–16.

6. Akhter W, Ashraf QM, Zanelli SA, et al. Effect of graded hypoxia on cerebral cortical genomic DNA fragmentation in newborn piglets. Biol Neonate 2001;79: 187–93.

7. Low JA. Determining the contribution of asphyxia to brain damage in the neonate. J Obstet Gynaecol Res 2004;30:276–86.

8. Ofek-Shlomai N, Berger I. Inflammatory injury to the neonatal brain: what can we do? Front Pediatr 2014;2:30.

9. Douglas-Escobar M, Weiss MD. Biomarkers of brain injury in the premature infant. Front Neurol 2013;22(3):185.

10. Damman O, Ferriero D, Gressen P. Neonatal enchepalophathy or hypoxic-ischemic encepalophathy? Appropriate terminology matter. Pediatr Res 2011; 70:1–2.

11. Buonocore G, Perrone S, Longini M, et al. Non protein bound iron as early predictive marker of neonatal brain damage. Brain 2003;126:1224–30.

12. Piscopo P, Bernardo A, Calamandrei G, et al. Altered expression of cyclooxygenase-2, presenilins and oxygen radical scavenging enzymes in a rat model of global perinatal asphyxia. Exp Neurol 2008;209:192–8.

13. Buonocore G, Perrone S, Tataranno ML. Oxygen toxicity: chemistry and biology of reactive oxygen species. Semin Fetal Neonatal Med 2010;15:186–90.

14. Mishra OP, Delivoria Papadopoulos M. Cellular mechanisms of hypoxic injury in the developing brain. Brain Res Bull 1999;48:233–8.

15. Lee J, Giordano S, Zhang J. Autophagy, mitochondria and oxidative stress: cross-talk and redox signalling. Biochem J 2012;441:523–40.

16. Milne GL, Yin H, Hardy KD, et al. Isoprostane generation and function. Chem Rev 2011;111:5973–96.

17. Tonni G, Leoncini S, Signorini C, et al. Pathology of perinatal brain damage: background and oxidative stress markers. Arch Gynecol Obstet 2014;290: 13–20.

18. Leung KS, Galano JM, Durand T, et al. Current development in non-enzymatic lipid peroxidation products, isoprostanoids and isofuranoids, in novel biological samples. Free Radic Res 2014;1:1–11.

19. Jahn U, Galano JM, Durand T. Beyond prostaglandins: chemistry and biology of cyclic oxygenated metabolites formed by free-radical pathways from polyunsaturated fatty acids. Angew Chem Int Ed Engl 2008;47:5894–955.

20. Galano JM, Mas E, Barden A, et al. Isoprostanes and neuroprostanes: total synthesis, biological activity and biomarkers of oxidative stress in humans. Prostaglandins Other Lipid Mediat 2013;107:95–102.

21. Casetta B, Longini M, Proietti F, et al. Development of a fast and simple LC-MS/MS method for measuring the F2-isoprostanes in newborns. J Matern Fetal Neonatal Med 2012;25(Suppl 1):114–8.

22. Solberg R, Longini M, Proietti F, et al. Resuscitation with supplementary oxygen induces oxidative injury in the cerebral cortex. Free Radic Biol Med 2012;53: 1061–7.
23. de La Torre A, Lee YY, Oger C, et al. Synthesis, discovery, and quantitation of dihomo-isofurans: biomarkers for in vivo adrenic acid peroxidation. Angew Chem Int Ed Engl 2014;53:6249–52.
24. Arneson KO, Roberts LJ 2nd. Measurement of products of docosahexaenoic acid peroxidation, neuroprostanes, and neurofurans. Meth Enzymol 2007;433: 127–43.
25. Balduini W, Carloni S, Perrone S, et al. The use of melatonin in hypoxic-ischemic brain damage: an experimental study. J Matern Fetal Neonatal Med 2012; 25(Suppl 1):119–24.
26. Song WL, Lawson JA, Reilly D, et al. Neurofurans, novel indices of oxidant stress derived from docosahexaenoic acid. J Biol Chem 2008;283:6–16.
27. Perrone S, Tataranno ML, Negro S, et al. Early identification of the risk for free radical-related diseases in preterm newborns. Early Hum Dev 2010;86:241–4.
28. Papanikolaou G, Pantopoulos K. Iron metabolism and toxicity. Toxicol Appl Pharmacol 2005;202:199–211.
29. Paffetti P, Perrone S, Longini M, et al. Non-protein-bound iron detection in small samples of biological fluids and tissues. Biol Trace Elem Res 2006; 112:221–32.
30. Signorini C, Perrone S, Sgherri C, et al. Plasma esterified F2-isoprostanes and oxidative stress in newborns: role of nonprotein-bound iron. Pediatr Res 2008; 63:287–91.
31. Ozawa H, Nishida A, Mito T, et al. Immunohistochemical study of ferritin-positive cells in the cerebellar cortex with subarachnoidal hemorrhage in neonates. Brain Res 1994;651:345–8.
32. Lu PP, Ramanan N. A critical cell-intrinsic role for serum response factor in glial specification in the CNS. J Neurosci 2012;32:8012–23.
33. Erecinska M, Cherian S, Silver IA. Energy metabolism in mammalian brain during development. Prog Neurobiol 2004;73:397–445.
34. Chua CO, Vinukonda G, Hu F, et al. Effect of hyperoxic resuscitation on propensity of germinal matrix haemorrhage and cerebral injury. Neuropathol Appl Neurobiol 2010;36:448–58.
35. Ten VS, Starkov A. Hypoxic-ischemic injury in the developing brain: the role of reactive oxygen species originating in mitochondria. Neurol Res Int 2012;2012: 542976.
36. Waldbaum S, Patel M. Mitochondrial dysfunction and oxidative stress: a contributing link to acquired epilepsy? J Bioenerg Biomembr 2010;42:449–55.
37. Halliwell B. Reactive oxygen species and the central nervous system. J Neurochem 1992;59:1609–23.
38. Baud O, Greene AE, Li J, et al. Glutathione peroxidase-catalase cooperativity is required for resistance to hydrogen peroxide by mature rat oligodendrocytes. J Neurosci 2004;24:1531–40.
39. Jantzie LL, Talos DM, Jackson MC, et al. Developmental expression of n-methyl-d-aspartate (NMDA) receptor subunits in human White and Gray matter: potential mechanism of increased vulnerability in the immature brain. Cereb Cortex 2015; 25:482–95.
40. Puka-Sundvall M, Gajkowska B, Cholewinski M, et al. Subcellular distribution of calcium and ultrastructural changes after cerebral hypoxia-ischemia in immature rats. Brain Res Dev Brain Res 2000;125:31–41.

41. Ota K, Yakovlev AG, Itaya A, et al. Alteration of apoptotic protease-activating factor-1 (APAF-1)-dependent apoptotic pathway during development of rat brain and liver. J Biochem 2002;131:131–5.
42. Ikonomidou C, Bosch F, Miksa M, et al. Blockade of NMDA receptors and apoptotic neurodegeneration in the developing brain. Science 1999;283:70–4.
43. Vasiljevic B, Maglajlic-Djukic S, Gojnic M, et al. New insights into the pathogenesis of perinatal hypoxic-ischemic brain injury. Pediatr Int 2011;53:454–62.
44. Peeters-Scholte C, Koster J, Veldhuis W, et al. Neuroprotection by selective nitric oxide synthase inhibition at 24 hours after perinatal hypoxia–ischemia. Stroke 2002;33:2304–10.
45. Nunez JL, McCarthy MM. Sex differences and hormonal effects in a model of preterm infant brain injury. Ann N Y Acad Sci 2003;1008:281–4.
46. Longini M, Perrone S, Kenanidis A, et al. Isoprostanes in amniotic fluid: a predictive marker for fetal growth restriction in pregnancy. Free Radic Biol Med 2005;38: 1537–41.
47. Reid MV, Murray KA, Marsh ED, et al. Delayed myelination in an intrauterine growth retardation model is mediated by oxidative stress upregulating bone morphogenetic protein 4. J Neuropathol Exp Neurol 2012;71:640–53.
48. Perrone S, Longini M, Bellieni CV, et al. Early oxidative stress in amniotic fluid of pregnancies with Down syndrome. Clin Biochem 2007;40:177–80.
49. Thornton C, Rousset CI, Kichev A, et al. Molecular mechanisms of neonatal brain injury. Neurol Res Int 2012;2012:506320.
50. Haldipur P, Dupuis N, Degos V, et al. HIP/PAP prevents excitotoxic neuronal death and promotes plasticity. Ann Clin Transl Neurol 2014;1:739–54.
51. Herrera-Marschitz M, Morales P, Leyton L, et al. Perinatal asphyxia: current status and approaches towards neuroprotective strategies, with focus on sentinel proteins. Neurotox Res 2011;19:603–27.
52. McCord JM. Oxygen-derived free radicals in postischemic tissue injury. N Engl J Med 1985;312:159–63.
53. Marzocchi B, Ciccoli L, Tani C, et al. Hypoxia-induced post-translational changes in red blood cell protein map of newborns. Pediatr Res 2005;58:660–5.
54. Perrone S, Bracci R, Buonocore G. New biomarkers of fetal-neonatal hypoxic stress. Acta Paediatr Suppl 2002;91:135–8.
55. Buonocore G, Zani S, Perrone S, et al. Intraerythrocyte nonprotein-bound iron and plasma malondialdehyde in the hypoxic newborn. Free Radic Biol Med 1998;25:766–70.
56. Ciccoli L, Rossi V, Leoncini S, et al. Iron release in erythrocytes and plasma non protein-bound iron in hypoxic and non hypoxic newborns. Free Radic Res 2003; 37:51.
57. Comporti M, Signorini C, Buonocore G, et al. Iron release, oxidative stress and erythrocyte ageing. Free Radic Biol Med 2002;32:568–76.
58. Ozawa H, Nishida A, Mito T, et al. Development of ferritin-containing cells in the pons and cerebellum of the human brain. Brain Dev 1994;16:92–5.
59. Beltrán B, Mathur A, Duchen MR, et al. The effect of nitric oxide on cell respiration: a key to understanding its role in cell survival or death. Proc Natl Acad Sci U S A 2000;97:14602–7.
60. Li C, Jackson RM. Reactive species mechanisms of cellular hypoxia-reoxygenation injury. Am J Physiol Cell Physiol 2002;282:C227–41.
61. Ferriero DM, Holtzman DM, Black SM, et al. Neonatal mice lacking neuronal nitric oxide synthase are less vulnerable to hypoxic-ischemic injury. Neurobiol Dis 1996;3:64–71.

62. McLean C, Ferriero D. Mechanisms of hypoxic-ischemic injury in the term infant. Semin Perinatol 2004;28:425–32.
63. Kaur C, Ling EA. Periventricular white matter damage in the hypoxic neonatal brain: role of microglial cells. Prog Neurobiol 2009;87:264–8.
64. van den Tweel ER, Nijboer C, Kavelaars A, et al. Expression of nitric oxide synthase isoforms and nitrotyrosine formation after hypoxia-ischemia in the neonatal rat brain. J Neuroimmunol 2005;167(1–2):64–71.
65. Huang Z, Huang PL, Ma J, et al. Enlarged infarcts in endothelial nitric oxide synthase knockout mice are attenuated by nitro-L-arginine. J Cereb Blood Flow Metab 1996;16:981–7.
66. Chen J, Zacharek A, Zhang C, et al. Endothelial nitric oxide synthase regulates brain-derived neurotrophic factor expression and neurogenesis after stroke in mice. J Neurosci 2005;25:2366–75.
67. Castillo-Meléndez M, Chow JA, Walker DW. Lipid peroxidation, caspase-3 immunoreactivity, and pyknosis in late-gestation fetal sheep brain after umbilical cord occlusion. Pediatr Res 2004;55:864–71.
68. Tan S, Zhou F, Nielsen VG, et al. Sustained hypoxia-ischemia results in reactive nitrogen and oxygen species production and injury in the premature fetal rabbit brain. J Neuropathol Exp Neurol 1998;57:544–53.
69. Back SA, Gan X, Li Y, et al. Maturation-dependent vulnerability of oligodendrocytes to oxidative stress-induced death caused by glutathione depletion. J Neurosci 1998;18:6241–53.
70. Baburamani AA, Ek CJ, Walker DW, et al. Vulnerability of the developing brain to hypoxic-ischemic damage: contribution of the cerebral vasculature to injury and repair? Front Physiol 2012;3:424.
71. Dammann O, Leviton A. Coagulation, inflammation, and the risk of neonatal white matter damage. Pediatr Res 2004;55:541–5.
72. Berger I, Peleg O, Ofek-Shlomai N. Inflammation and early brain injury in term and preterm infants. Isr Med Assoc J 2012;14:318–23.
73. Leviton A, Dammann O, Durum SK. The adaptive immune response in neonatal cerebral white matter damage. Ann Neurol 2005;58:821–8.
74. Okazaki K, Nishida A, Kato M, et al. Elevation of cytokine concentrations in asphyxiated neonates. Biol Neonate 2006;89:183–9.
75. Buonocore G, Gioia D, De Filippo M, et al. Superoxide anion release by polymorphonuclear leukocytes in whole blood of newborns and mothers during the peripartal period. Pediatr Res 1994;36(5):619–22.
76. Eliwan H, Watson R, Aslam S, et al. Neonatal brain injury and systemic inflammation: modulation by activated protein C ex vivo. Clin Exp Immunol 2015;179(3):477–84.

Umbilical Cord Blood—An Untapped Resource

Strategies to Decrease Early Red Blood Cell Transfusions and Improve Neonatal Outcomes

Patrick D. Carroll, MD, MPH[a,b,*]

KEYWORDS

- Delayed cord clamping • Milking • Cord blood • Transfusion
- Intraventricular hemorrhage

KEY POINTS

- Umbilical cord blood is fetal blood still remaining in the umbilical cord/placental circulation at the time of cord clamping.
- Delayed cord clamping (DCC) or milking of the umbilical cord (MUC) has been recommended as the standard of care for premature deliveries and the first step in the resuscitation process.
- In addition to resulting in higher hematocrit, fewer transfusions, and more rapid resuscitation, DCC or MUC leads to decreased intraventricular hemorrhage (IVH) and higher survival in very preterm neonates.
- In premature neonates, umbilical cord blood can be used for essential initial admission laboratory testing, thereby leading to fewer erythrocyte transfusions due to phlebotomy loss.
- Adequate volumes of umbilical cord blood can be obtained for admission laboratory testing even after DCC or MUC.

INTRODUCTION

During the past several decades, ingenious, dramatic life-saving discoveries have led to improved neonatal outcomes. Of particular note are antenatal steroid administration, exogenous surfactant, neonatal specific mechanical ventilators, and more sophisticated incubators. Together these advances have contributed to improved

Disclosures: The authors do not have any commercial or financial conflicts of interest.
[a] Women and Newborn's Program, Intermountain Healthcare, 36 South State Street, Salt Lake City, UT 84111, USA; [b] Neonatal Services, Dixie Regional Medical Center, 544 East 400 South, St George, UT 84770, USA
* NICU, Dixie Regional Medical Center, 544 East 400 South, St George, UT 84770.
E-mail address: Patrick.carroll@imail.org

survival for neonates. The survival rate of extremely low-birth-weight (ELBW) infants weighing 500 to 750 g increased from 44% to 65% in 12 years from 1987–88 to 1999–2000.[1] Despite these advances, preterm infants, particularly ELBW neonates, remain at significant risk for the most frequent life-threatening complications of prematurity such as IVH, necrotizing enterocolitis (NEC), retinopathy of prematurity, and anemia. As the limit of viability has decreased, so too has the weight at birth and by extension, the total circulating blood volume of these infants. Indeed, the smallest infants cared for in the neonatal intensive care unit (NICU) routinely may have birth weights less than 500 g, leading to total circulating blood volumes of less than 40 mL; this leads to the current state in which transfusions have become almost universal among the smallest patients, primarily as a result of the frequent laboratory testing required by these critically ill groups. Efforts to increase the initial total circulating volume and slow its rapid rate of decline as a result of bleeding into the laboratory have been shown to decrease erythrocyte transfusions and improve other outcomes among premature infants. This article reviews the practices and outcomes associated with delayed clamping or MUC and with obtaining blood for essential initial admission laboratory testing from the umbilical cord.

DELAYED CORD CLAMPING OR MILKING OF THE UMBILICAL CORD
Transition During Gestation and from Fetal to Neonatal Circulation

Fetal oxygen delivery is accomplished by transfer of oxygen from maternal blood to fetal blood through the placental trophoblastic membrane (**Fig. 1**). Once placental oxygen is bound to fetal hemoglobin, it enters the fetus through the umbilical vein and is preferentially delivered to the fetal brain. To do so, most of the fetal blood flow first

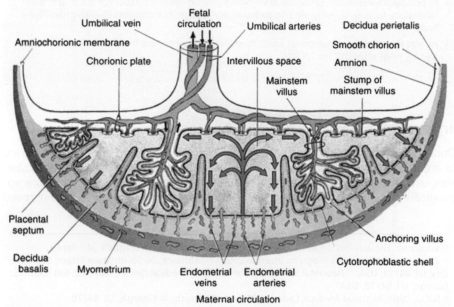

Fig. 1. Placental anatomy demonstrating components of both maternal and fetal circulation. Maternal and fetal circulation are separated by the trophoblastic membrane (cytotrophoblastic shell). (*From* Moore KL. The developing human: clinically oriented embryology. 5th edition. Philadelphia: WB Saunders; 1993. p. 117; with permission.)

passes the fetal liver via the ductus venosus and next bypasses the fetal lungs via the foramen oval and the ductus arteriosus. These bypass shunts result in a small percentage of cardiac output being delivered to the liver and the pulmonary arterial beds. A study using fetal Doppler echocardiography evaluated the cardiac output in the second half of pregnancy. This study demonstrated that 75% to 87% of fetal cardiac output filled systemic circulatory beds through the aorta and 13% to 25% was directed to the fetal pulmonary circulation.[2]

At birth, the circulation of the newly born infant changes as the pressures within the circulation change. With the first breaths of air containing higher levels of oxygen, the pulmonary vascular resistance decreases. At the same time, the absence of a low-pressure placental circuit leads to an increase in systemic vascular resistance. These changes naturally lead to an increased proportion of blood flow to the now oxygen-rich lung at the expense of systemic blood flow. This increase is of particular importance in premature infants for whom cerebral autoregulation is impaired[3] and for whom fluctuations in mean arterial pressure may increase the risk of IVH in the regions in which delicate and fragile capillary networks are found.

Neonatal Blood Volume Following Delayed Cord Clamping/Milking of the Umbilical Cord

Studies more than 40 years ago demonstrated increasing fetal blood volume and decreasing placental blood volume as a result of delaying cord clamping for up to 180 seconds.[4] In term infants, Yao and Lind[5] elegantly demonstrated a correlation between infant blood volume and the duration between birth and clamping of the umbilical cord. Delaying cord clamping by 30, 60, or 180 seconds showed an increase in infant blood volume by 6, 13.6, or 22.5 mL/kg using a radiolabeled iodinated albumin dilution technique (**Fig. 2**). Using gravity by adjusting the position of the infant relative to the mother in both vaginal and cesarean delivery was shown in early studies to increase the volume of fetal blood transfused following DCC.[6] A multicenter trial[7] of term

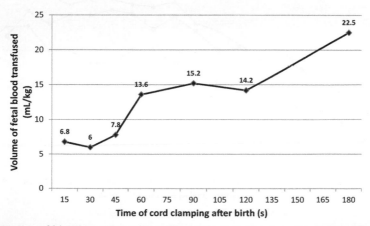

Fig. 2. Amount of blood transfused from the placenta to the neonate during delayed cord clamping at various time intervals compared with early cord clamping at 5 seconds. (*Adapted from* Yao AC, Lind J, Tiisala R, et al. Placental transfusion in the premature infant with observation on clinical course and outcome. Acta Paediatr Scand 1969;58(6):561–6; with permission.)

infants born by vaginal delivery also demonstrated increased neonatal blood volume following DCC using a simple method of periodically weighing the infant to determine the volume of fetal blood transfused from the placenta. In contrast to previous studies, this randomized controlled trial demonstrated a similar volume of fetal blood transferred from the placenta to the infant independent of infant position, suggesting gravity did not have an effect on transfused volume.[7]

It is feasible that once the fetus is born, the umbilical artery contraction[8] could result in only the blood in the umbilical vein being effectively transfused or some of the transfused blood being returned to the placenta via the umbilical arteries.[9] This transfusion could still result in an increase of 5 to 19 mL of circulating blood volume following a single MUC.

MUC is another method of transfusing fetal blood from the placenta into the fetus. This method offers the potential advantage of being completed more quickly than DCC. It may also be more enthusiastically adopted by obstetricians who may feel uncomfortable holding a premature infant during DCC without any perceived intervention. Several studies have sonographically investigated the umbilical vessel sizes at various gestational ages.[10–12] The umbilical vein and umbilical artery diameters were used to estimate in situ the blood volume within the umbilical cord of a fetus (**Fig. 3**). This study suggests that milking a 30-cm segment of umbilical cord may provide an additional 8 to 28 mL of blood to a neonate born at 23 to 34 weeks' gestation.

Hosono and colleagues[13] sought to identify the actual volume of blood that cord milking could deliver. This study demonstrated that a 30-cm segment of umbilical cord among 20 ELBW infants contained a mean volume of 15.5 ± 6.7 mL of residual fetal blood. Although this study may have overestimated the cord blood volume because the proximal and distal ends of the umbilical cord were not clamped

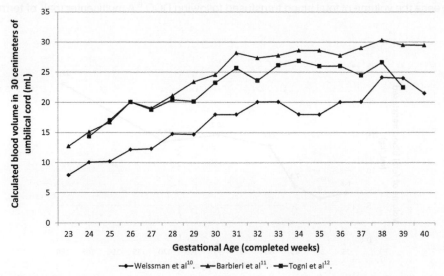

Fig. 3. In utero volume of blood contained within a 30-cm segment of umbilical cord at various gestational ages calculated from sonographically measured umbilical vein and artery diameters reported in the obstetric literature. (*Data from* Refs.[10–12]; and *From* Carroll PD, Christensen RD. Use of cord blood in perinatal care. Matern Health Neonatol Perinatol, in press; with permission.)

simultaneously, it is the first study directly measuring cord blood volume in a specific length of umbilical cord.

Physiologic Changes in Circulation Following Delayed Cord Clamping/Milking of the Umbilical Cord

Premature infant brains are sensitive to fluctuations in blood pressure, particularly hypotension due to poor cerebral autoregulation.[3] Maintaining stable blood pressure may be a factor in limiting IVH.[14] Katheria and colleagues[15] demonstrated improved superior vena cava blood flow and right ventricular output, both markers of systemic blood flow, in preterm infants following MUC compared with immediate cord clamping (ICC). In addition, the diastolic and mean blood pressures within the first 6 hours of life were increased in the MUC group. This finding is consistent with previous studies on MUC.[16,17] Although no studies on SVC (superior vena cava) flow have been done following DCC, blood pressure has been shown to be improved after DCC compared with ICC.[18]

For DCC to effectively transfuse placental blood to the newly delivered neonate, fetal blood in the placenta must continue to transfer into the neonate for a period, that is, potentially until the umbilical cord is clamped or cord pulsations cease. If the opposite results, the neonate would hemorrhage back into the placenta. To study this, the direction of blood flow during DCC was evaluated using Doppler ultrasonography in term infants after vaginal delivery.[9] The duration of flow in the umbilical vein and both umbilical arteries varied among the 30 infants in this study. About 90% had venous flow toward the neonate noted immediately after birth, whereas the remaining 10% demonstrated no blood flow. Venous flow continued until the cord was clamped in 10 of 30 patients. Venous flow was bidirectional, with the direction of flow associated with the respiratory pattern. In some cases, retrograde umbilical cord flow was observed during vigorous crying. It has been postulated that umbilical arterial flow ceases quickly after delivery.[8] However, in this series of term infants, flow continued until the cord was clamped in 13 of 30 patients. In half of the infants, the umbilical arterial and venous flow ceased at the same time, and in 7 of the 30, arterial flow stopped before venous flow. In 8 of the 30, venous flow stopped before cessation of arterial flow.[19] This study did not quantify flow rate or ratios of flow in versus flow from the neonate back to the placenta in cases in which both arterial and venous flow continued. Additional studies are needed to further clarify these blood flow patterns in premature infants after vaginal and cesarean delivery.

Neonatal Outcomes After Delayed Cord Clamping/Milking of the Umbilical Cord

The overall risks and benefits of DCC versus ICC have been assessed in premature infants. Although the definition for DCC varied from 30 to 120 seconds, by 2004, there were at least 7 randomized controlled trials comparing ICC with DCC in preterm infants. A 2012 Cochrane review comparing both DCC up to 180 seconds and MUC randomized controlled trials versus ICC included 15 studies.[18]

Risks of delayed cord clamping/milking of the umbilical cord

Physicians have raised concerns about potential risks of DCC. In particular, obstetricians reported a concern that DCC may delay resuscitation, result in lower Apgar scores, increase rates of hypothermia, or cause IVH.[20,21] Neonatologists and pediatricians have reported concerns of hyperbilirubinemia and polycythemia as potential risks. When these outcomes were investigated,[18] there was no difference in the Apgar scores at 1, 5, or 10 minutes. There was also no difference in rates of hypothermia on admission. The average admission temperature was 0.14°C (95% confidence interval [CI], −0.03 to 0.31) higher in the DCC/MUC group. The peak bilirubin level in the DCC/MUC group was 15.01 µmol/L higher (0.88 mg/dL) than the ICC group. However, there was no difference in the frequency of phototherapy, although there was a trend toward more phototherapy (relative risk [RR], 1.21; 95% CI, 0.94–1.55). Finally, the cord pH between groups was not different.

Effect of delayed cord clamping/milking of the umbilical cord on initial resuscitation
Following MUC, a small randomized group of preterm infants was evaluated and found to have higher oxygen saturations and decreased supplemental oxygen exposure during the first 10 minutes of life. Oxygen saturation was higher in the cord milking group through the first 4 minutes of life.[22] These findings are similar to those found in an observational cohort of term infants undergoing DCC. In this study of uncomplicated term deliveries, the oxygen saturation range was higher with less variability for the first 3 minutes of life in the DCC group.[9] In addition, the heart rate of the infants demonstrated less variability and no refractive tachycardia as was seen in the ICC group at 2 to 4 minutes of life.

Benefits of delayed cord clamping/milking of the umbilical cord
Initial studies demonstrated that DCC was associated with higher hematocrit values, fewer transfusions, and less IVH.[23] Some were studying DCC, whereas others were investigating MUC as a more pragmatic and rapid alternative.[16,17] When these 2 approaches were evaluated for efficacy in a 2012 Cochrane review, the results demonstrated that for the combined DCC and MUC groups, there were 39% fewer transfusions for anemia (7 studies), 41% fewer patients with IVH (12 studies), and 38% fewer patients with NEC (4 studies).[18] Although there was also a 37% decrease in death reported, this finding did not reach statistical significance for all infants (RR, 0.63; 95% CI, 0.31–1.28).

In a separate meta-analysis limited to infants less than 32 completed weeks of gestation who underwent either DCC or MUC, Backes and colleagues[24] demonstrated that mortality was decreased by 58% (8 studies). Thus, with nearly 4 million births annually in the United States,[25] of which 1.93% are born before 32 weeks' gestation,[26] DCC or MUC could result in approximately 4500 lives saved. The finding of decreased mortality was also independently reported in an article describing a quality improvement initiative following the implementation of MUC in all infants less than 30 weeks' gestation.[27] Compared with historical controls, the rate of survival in the MUC group increased from 84% to 94% and 76% to 91% among infants less than 30 and less than 27 weeks' gestation, respectively. Researchers continue to investigate the optimal duration of DCC, and debate persists regarding the efficacy of DCC versus MUC.

Obstetric Acceptance of Delayed Cord Clamping/Milking of the Umbilical Cord

There are insufficient data to assess the frequency of DCC as a broadly accepted standard of care. Nonetheless, Rabe and colleagues[28] reported in their comparison of DCC and MUC that a control group of patients with ICC was not enrolled because this practice was considered outside of the standard of care at the study site. Despite the recent American College of Obstetric and Gynecology committee opinion[29] supporting DCC in preterm infants, the practices of DCC or MUC is not universally practiced (**Table 1**). A 2015 survey assessing practices of obstetricians in the Netherlands reported a low number of practice protocols (6.3%) endorsing DCC as the standard of care, although most practice protocols in this study did not address timing of cord clamping.[21] A related survey in the United States[20] reported that 53% of obstetricians thought the timing of cord clamping was either very or moderately important. In this

Table 1
Results of survey data indicating frequency of delayed cord clamping

Author, Year	Frequency of Delayed Cord Clamping
Ononeze and Hutchon,[46] 2009	9.3% always, 53.4% occasionally
Farrar et al,[47] 2010	44% of preterm vaginal deliveries,[a] 37% of preterm cesarean section
Boere et al,[21] 2015	54% of preterm deliveries,[a] 12% of term cesarean sections

[a] Obstetrician and midwives. Midwives reported higher rates of DCC.

survey, 76% of the obstetricians with any concerns about DCC cited delayed neonatal resuscitation as a reason to clamp the cord immediately. Although 12.6% of these obstetricians were inclined to DCC to prevent IVH, 29.6% were inclined to ICC fearing that DCC may cause IVH despite strong evidence of the protective effects of DCC/MUC on IVH.

USE OF UMBILICAL CORD BLOOD FOR INITIAL LABORATORY TESTING

Some laboratory testing is necessary in the care of critically ill patients in the NICU. These neonates often have the lowest birth weights and gestational ages. Very-low-birth-weight (VLBW) infants consistently experience their greatest phlebotomy blood loss on the first day of life, often surpassing 10 mL/kg, that is, 10% to 15% of these infants' total blood volume.[30] Obtaining admission laboratory studies from the otherwise discarded fetal blood remaining in the umbilical cord or placenta is a justified, well-validated alternative to drawing blood for admission laboratory studies directly from the infant (**Table 2**).[31] As indicated later, following the relevant review of placental anatomy, data are provided on the use of umbilical cord blood for complete blood count, blood culture, blood type, antibody screen, newborn metabolic state screening, and genetic testing. A procedure for drawing umbilical cord blood for neonatal admission laboratory testing and a description of neonatal outcomes resulting from this approach are also provided.

Placental Anatomy

Before delivery, the fetus depends on the placenta for survival. Oxygen and nutrients are delivered to the fetus by passing from maternal to fetal circulation through the trophoblastic membrane, which is composed of the cytotrophoblast and syncytiotrophoblast (see **Fig. 1**). This membrane is a semipermeable membrane separating maternal and fetal circulation while allowing transfer of nutrients and waste products to and from the fetus, respectively. Blood in the umbilical cord therefore is fetal blood and is identical to blood in the fetus. At any given time, a blood cell in the fetoplacental circuit may be in the fetus, umbilical cord, or fetal side of the placenta.

Laboratory Tests Performed on Umbilical Cord Blood

There have been several reports that have investigated the validity of using umbilical cord blood for the initial laboratory testing in neonates following birth. Several studies have directly compared paired samples of neonatal and cord blood, whereas others have compared research data to historical controls (see **Table 2**).

Complete blood count

In paired samples, complete blood count and manual differential counts have been shown to be equivalent in both term and preterm infants.[32–36] In a study comparing

Table 2
List of articles that report or discuss use of umbilical cord blood for neonatal laboratory testing along with brief description of findings

Laboratory Test	Author, Year	Comments
CBC	Hansen et al,[33] 2005	113 term infant paired umbilical cord & neonatal samples. High correlation of WBC, hematocrit, platelets. I:T ratio reported
	Carroll et al,[32] 2012	174 preterm infant umbilical cord & neonatal paired samples. High correlation of WBC, hemoglobin, platelets. False-positive thrombocytopenia on 4 cord samples
	Christensen et al,[35] 2011	10 VLBW infant pilot study. No difference in CBC compared with historical controls
	Beeram et al,[34] 2012	200 term and preterm infant umbilical cord & neonatal paired samples. Similar results between sources. Higher rate of leukopenia in cord samples noted
	Baer et al,[43] 2013	91 VLBW infants. No paired samples. Outcome study
	Rotshenker-Olshinka et al,[36] 2014	305 term and preterm infant umbilical cord & neonatal paired samples. Significant correlation between cord and infant CBC
Blood culture	Polin et al,[38] 1981	200 cord blood cultures with 29 paired infant cultures. Cord sterilized with 2% tincture of iodine. One septic patient had positive cord and infant culture. Similar contamination rate between cord samples (2.5%) and infant samples (3.4%)
	Herson et al,[37] 1998	81 term infants, 35 high-risk umbilical cord & neonatal paired samples. Placental vein sterilized with povidone-iodine. 5-mL blood samples from cord obtained. 20% true positive from cord vs 3% true positive from infant cultures of paired samples
	Hansen et al,[33] 2005	113 term infants. Cord sterilized with alcohol. Zero contaminants or true positive cultures
	Christensen et al,[35] 2011	10 VLBW infant pilot study. No positive cultures from cases or historical controls
	Beeram et al,[34] 2012	200 term and preterm umbilical cord & neonatal paired samples. Cord sterilized with povidone-iodine and then swabbed with alcohol. 2 contaminants from cord blood. One contaminant and one pathogen from infant blood
	Baer et al,[43] 2013	91 VLBW infants. Prospective outcome study with historical controls
	Rotshenker-Olshinka et al,[36] 2014	223 term and preterm infant umbilical cord & neonatal paired samples. Cord sterilized with chlorhexidine before placental delivery. No cases of sepsis. High contamination rate from both cord sample (12.5%) and infant sample (2.5%)

Blood type	American Academy of Pediatrics Subcommittee on Hyperbilirubinemia,[41] 2004	Recommends "direct antibody test, blood type, and Rh (D) type on the infant's (cord) blood"
	Judd,[42] 2001	Practice guideline for immunohematology. Endorses obtaining blood type from cord blood or infant blood
	Christensen et al,[35] 2011	10 VLBW infant pilot prospective outcome study with historical controls
	Baer et al,[43] 2013	91 VLBW infants. Prospective outcome study with historical controls
Antibody screen	Josephson et al,[44] 2011	American Association of Blood Banking technical manual. Recommends antibody testing using plasma or serum from the infant or mother
	Christensen et al,[35] 2011	10 VLBW infant pilot study
	Baer et al,[43] 2013	91 VLBW infants. No paired samples. Outcome study
Newborn metabolic screen	Miller & Tuerck,[45] 2008	CLSI newborn screening guidelines. Recommends first newborn metabolic test be obtained on admission of premature infants
	Christensen et al,[35] 2011	10 VLBW infant pilot study
	Baer et al,[43] 2013	91 VLBW infants. No paired samples. Outcome study

Abbreviations: CBC, complete blood count; CLSI, Clinical and Laboratory Standards Institute; WBC, white blood cell.

From Carroll PD, Christensen RD. Use of cord blood in perinatal care. Matern Health Neonatol Perinatol, in press; with permission.

paired umbilical cord blood and neonatal samples among preterm infants, the correlation coefficient of white blood cells (WBCs), hemoglobin, and platelets was 0.82, 0.72, and 0.76, respectively.[32] A later study replicated these results, with similar correlation coefficients of 0.89, 0.61, and 0.65 of WBCs, hematocrit, and platelets, respectively.[34] The rate of false-positive immature to total granulocyte ratio (I:T ratio), defined as elevated I:T ratio with negative culture from the same source, was 5% from umbilical cord blood and 9% directly from the infant.[33] Together, these studies produce compelling evidence that umbilical cord blood can safely be used in place of direct neonatal blood sampling for a complete blood count with leukocyte differential.

Blood culture

Blood culture results from umbilical cord segments or placental fetal vessels have been investigated in several studies when compared with what can be technically and ethically drawn from infants after birth.[33–38] The former method offers the benefits of increased blood culture volume, thereby increasing the sensitivity of the blood culture[37,39,40] and sparing the neonate from additional phlebotomy loss. Concern is frequently raised regarding contamination rates of umbilical cord blood cultures, particularly because birth takes place through a nonsterile birth canal. It is important, however, to remember that the neonate is delivered through the same environment as the umbilical cord and placenta. Hansen and colleagues[33] obtained paired blood cultures from more than 100 term infants successfully without any contaminated cultures; this differs considerably from a more recent study in which the contamination rate was more than 12% from cord blood cultures and also more than2% from the neonate.[36] Another study of both term and preterm infants had a contamination rate of less than 1% for both cord blood and direct neonatal blood cultures.[34] This variation in contamination underscores the importance of technique in obtaining reliable cord blood cultures.

Blood type and antibody screen

Neonatal blood type is routinely obtained from umbilical cord blood. Both the pediatric[41] and obstetric[42] literature specifically identify cord blood as an appropriate source for identifying infant blood type and Rh (D) status for treatment of hyperbilirubinemia. The authors are unaware of any studies that have specifically endorsed or refuted this practice for purposes of neonatal transfusion. It is the authors' opinion that cord blood can be typed for the purpose of neonatal transfusion[43] provided the sample is obtained from the umbilical cord and not from a vein on the placental surface; this is because, although the blood in the placental vein is fetal blood, obtaining a sample in this manner introduces the possibility of operator error if the needle passes through the fetal vessel and into the maternal chorionic villus space with resultant aspiration of maternal blood. However, the authors are unaware of any reports of this occurring. Antibody screening for the purpose of transfusion of a neonate can also be performed on umbilical cord blood. Although umbilical cord blood is not specifically mentioned, the American Association of Blood Banking states, "initial patient testing must include a screen for unexpected red cell antibodies, using either plasma or serum from the infant or mother."[44]

Newborn metabolic screen

Many states recommend drawing the first newborn metabolic screening test from VLBW infants before any antibiotics are administered, blood products are transfused, or amino acid–containing hyperalimentation solutions are administered. In many cases, this is on admission to the NICU. For premature infants, the Clinical and Laboratory Standards Institute recommends obtaining their first newborn metabolic screen on admission.[45] Obtaining the first newborn screen sample from umbilical cord blood results in similar limitations as an admission sample obtained directly from the infant. Specifically, despite being reliable for hemoglobinopathies, GALT (galactose-1-phosphate uridyl transferase), and biotinidase enzymes, as well as providing baseline testing for amino acids and acylcarnitines, admission testing can result in inaccurate results for thyroid-stimulating hormone and 17-hydroxyprogesterone levels and IRT (immunoreactive trypsinogen) cystic fibrosis screening. In both scenarios, repeat testing is required.

Procedure for Umbilical Cord Blood Sampling

Before initiation of the umbilical cord blood sampling, all of the supplies needed should be gathered (**Box 1**). Next, the following schedule of events is recommended:

- Remind the delivering provider to clamp the distal end of the umbilical cord. Inspect the fetal side of the placenta for signs of umbilical vessel rupture.
- Swab the base of the cord insertion on the placenta and up the umbilical cord 8 to 10 cm 3 times with povidone-iodine.
- Allow for the Betadine to dry. While waiting, use the alcohol pad to wipe the top of the blood culture bottle. Once the povidone-iodine has dried, grasp the umbilical cord and insert the 18-gauge needle, bevel down, into the umbilical vein 6 to 8 cm above the placental insertion site.
- Aspirate 10 mL of blood to fill the syringe or until you can obtain no more. Once the needle is removed, the cord may continue to bleed. Remove the needle from the syringe and attach a sterile blood transfer device. Transfer 1 to 4 mL blood into the blood culture bottle, followed by 1.5 mL into the ethylenediaminetetraacetic acid (EDTA) vacutainer and 3 to 4 mL into the Na-heparin vacutainer.
- Remove the blood transfer device and drip 0.5 mL of blood into an EDTA microtainer for complete blood count with differential.

Box 1
Supplies needed for the proper collection of cord blood for laboratory testing

- Clean gloves
- Betadine sticks
- Alcohol swab
- Eighteen-guage needle
- Ten-milliliter syringe
- Blood transfer devise
- Twenty-five-guage needle
- Blood culture bottle
- EDTA collection tube (for type and screen)
- EDTA microtainer (for CBC/diff)
- Newborn metabolic screen card #1 (may vary by state)
- Optional: Na-heparin collection tube for chromosomes and microarray

Abbreviations: CBC/diff, complete blood count with differential; EDTA, ethylenediaminetetraacetic acid.

- Apply blood spots onto the state newborn metabolic screen filter paper. It may be helpful to use a needle for more control in applying these drops to the filter paper.
- Clearly label all samples at the time of collection, making certain to distinctly label samples from twins or higher-order multiples.

Particular care must be taken in adequately sterilizing the field before obtaining blood cultures just as when obtaining blood cultures from other sites. Multiple methods have been reported to adequately achieve a sterile cord/placenta, including use of alcohol, Betadine, and tincture of iodine. Because the surface of the placenta is often wet and contains depressions between vessels that allow for pooling of fluid, it is advisable to first dry the surface before initiation of sterilization technique to allow adequate drying in a reasonable time. This procedure is not necessary when a cord segment is used for obtaining a cord blood sample. With the existing compelling data endorsing DCC or MUC, there is also evidence that adequate cord blood volumes can be obtained following either DCC or MUC.[43]

Neonatal Outcomes

To date, 1 pilot study[35] and 1 multicenter study[43] have been published reporting neonatal outcomes as a result of using umbilical cord blood for the admission laboratory testing in premature infants. The initial pilot study reported the outcomes of 10 VLBW neonates compared with historical matched controls. The control patients experienced 7.5 ± 5.2 mL/kg of phlebotomy blood loss in the first day of life compared with 1.5 ± 2.3 mL/kg among study patients. In this study, a decrease in red blood cell (RBC) transfusions and in IVH was observed in the intervention group. The larger multicenter trial enrolled 96 patients and successfully obtained umbilical cord blood for admission laboratory testing in 91 of those enrolled. Cord blood was successfully obtained following DCC from twins and triplets and in 8 of 9 infants born at 23 to 24 completed weeks of gestation. The intervention group in this report required vasopressors less often, experienced an increase in hemoglobin level in the first 12 to 24 hours of life, received fewer RBC transfusions per patient, and had fewer patients requiring any RBC transfusion. The rate of severe IVH was lower but was not statistically significant ($P = .115$). To date, no randomized controlled trials assessing short- and long-term outcomes following the use of umbilical cord blood for admission laboratory studies have been reported.

SUMMARY

Umbilical cord blood is an important but underutilized resource that can be used in the care of premature neonates. Utilization of this resource by adopting DCC or MUC has been endorsed as the standard of care for preterm infants. Use of umbilical cord blood for DCC/MUC results in many improved outcomes, with a decrease in IVH being one of the most notable. Utilization of umbilical cord blood for admission laboratory testing of neonates is an increasingly common practice that has demonstrated benefits. Further studies including randomized controlled trials are needed to better understand the impact of this strategy.

ACKNOWLEDGMENTS

We appreciate J.A. Widness, MD, for his editorial and technical contributions to this article.

Best Practices

What is the current practice?

Laboratory testing of premature babies admitted to the NICU is done on phlebotomized blood obtained from heel-stick, venipuncture, radial arterial puncture, umbilical venous catheter, or umbilical arterial catheter. This procedure is most often completed when the baby is in the NICU. Laboratory testing frequently includes complete blood count with manual leukocyte differential, blood type and antibody screen, and blood culture. In some circumstances, additional laboratory tests may include state newborn metabolic screen, chromosome analysis, and arterial blood gas.

Until recently, current practice was ICC following delivery of a premature infant. Recently, several organizations, including the World Health Organization, Royal College of Obstetricians and Gynaecologists (RCOG), and American College of Obstetricians and Gynecologists (ACOG), have formally endorsed DCC as standard of care for premature infants.

WHO guideline: Delayed umbilical cord clamping for improved maternal and infant health and nutrition outcomes. Geneva: World Health Organization; 2014. Available at: http://www.who.int/nutrition/publications/guidelines/cord_clamping/en/.

RCOG release: Timing of clamping the umbilical cord analyzed in new opinion paper. February 27, 2015. Available at: https://www.rcog.org.uk/en/news/rcog-release-timing-of-clamping-the-umbilical-cord-analysed-in-new-opinion-paper/.

ACOG Committee Opinion Number 543, December 2012 reaffirmed 2014 Timing of umbilical cord clamping after birth. Available at: http://www.acog.org/Resources-And-Publications/Committee-Opinions/Committee-on-Obstetric-Practice/Timing-of-Umbilical-Cord-Clamping-After-Birth.

What changes in current practice are likely to improve outcomes?

Admission laboratory tests obtained from fetal blood remaining in the umbilical cord has been shown to decrease erythrocyte transfusions and decrease vasopressor use.

DCC or MUC, although now widely accepted as current practice, has not been universally implemented. This intervention among preterm infants has been shown to decrease IVH and decrease erythrocyte transfusions among improvements in outcome.

Summary statement

Umbilical cord blood is a resource that is available to all neonates. Immediately after delivery of the fetus, cord blood can be used for the direct benefit of the premature infant. Use of umbilical cord blood for necessary laboratory testing offers the benefit of obtaining necessary results to make clinical treatment decisions without subjecting the infant to significant phlebotomy loss. DCC or MUC are 2 methods of transfusing additional fetal blood into the neonate after either vaginal or cesarean delivery. Together, these interventions should be considered important steps in the resuscitation pathway.

REFERENCES

1. Stephens BE, Vohr BR. Neurodevelopmental outcome of the premature infant. Pediatr Clin North Am 2009;56(3):631–46 Table of Contents.
2. Rasanen J, Wood DC, Weiner S, et al. Role of the pulmonary circulation in the distribution of human fetal cardiac output during the second half of pregnancy. Circulation 1996;94(5):1068–73.
3. Verhagen EA, Hummel LA, Bos AF, et al. Near-infrared spectroscopy to detect absence of cerebrovascular autoregulation in preterm infants. Clin Neurophysiol 2014;125(1):47–52.

4. Yao AC, Lind J, Tiisala R, et al. Placental transfusion in the premature infant with observation on clinical course and outcome. Acta Paediatr Scand 1969;58(6): 561–6.
5. Yao AC, Lind J. Effect of gravity on placental transfusion. Lancet 1969;2(7619): 505–8.
6. Sisson TR, Knutson S, Kendall N. The blood volume of infants. IV. Infants born by cesarean section. Am J Obstet Gynecol 1973;117(3):351–7.
7. Vain NE, Satragno DS, Gorenstein AN, et al. Effect of gravity on volume of placental transfusion: a multicentre, randomised, non-inferiority trial. Lancet 2014;384(9939):235–40.
8. Yao AC, Lind J, Lu T. Closure of the human umbilical artery: a physiological demonstration of Burton's theory. Eur J Obstet Gynecol Reprod Biol 1977;7(6): 365–8.
9. Smit M, Dawson JA, Ganzeboom A, et al. Pulse oximetry in newborns with delayed cord clamping and immediate skin-to-skin contact. Arch Dis Child Fetal Neonatal Ed 2014;99(4):F309–14.
10. Weissman A, Jakobi P, Bronshtein M, et al. Sonographic measurements of the umbilical cord and vessels during normal pregnancies. J Ultrasound Med 1994;13(1):11–4.
11. Barbieri C, Cecatti JG, Surita FG, et al. Sonographic measurement of the umbilical cord area and the diameters of its vessels during pregnancy. J Obstet Gynaecol 2012;32(3):230–6.
12. Togni FA, Araujo Junior E, Moron AF, et al. Reference intervals for the cross-sectional area of the umbilical cord during gestation. J Perinat Med 2007;35(2):130–4.
13. Hosono S, Hine K, Nagano N, et al. Residual blood volume in the umbilical cord of extremely premature infants. Pediatr Int 2015;57(1):68–71.
14. Rong Z, Liu H, Xia S, et al. Risk and protective factors of intraventricular hemorrhage in preterm babies in Wuhan, China. Childs Nerv Syst 2012;28(12): 2077–84.
15. Katheria AC, Leone TA, Woelkers D, et al. The effects of umbilical cord milking on hemodynamics and neonatal outcomes in premature neonates. J Pediatr 2014; 164(5):1045–50.e1.
16. Hosono S, Mugishima H, Fujita H, et al. Umbilical cord milking reduces the need for red cell transfusions and improves neonatal adaptation in infants born at less than 29 weeks gestation: a randomised controlled trial. Arch Dis Child 2008; 93(1):F14–9.
17. Hosono S, Mugishima H, Fujita H, et al. Blood pressure and urine output during the first 120 h of life in infants born at less than 29 weeks gestation related to umbilical cord milking. Arch Dis Child Fetal Neonatal Ed 2009;94:F328–31.
18. Rabe H, Diaz-Rossello JL, Duley L, et al. Effect of timing of umbilical cord clamping and other strategies to influence placental transfusion at preterm birth on maternal and infant outcomes. Cochrane Database Syst Rev 2012;(8): CD003248.
19. Boere I, Roest AA, Wallace E, et al. Umbilical blood flow patterns directly after birth before delayed cord clamping. Arch Dis Child Fetal Neonatal Ed 2015; 100(2):F121–5.
20. Jelin AC, Kuppermann M, Erickson K, et al. Obstetricians' attitudes and beliefs regarding umbilical cord clamping. J Matern Fetal Neonatal Med 2014;27(14): 1457–61.
21. Boere I, Smit M, Roest AA, et al. Current practice of cord clamping in the Netherlands: a questionnaire study. Neonatology 2015;107(1):50–5.

22. Katheria A, Blank D, Rich W, et al. Umbilical cord milking improves transition in premature infants at birth. PLoS One 2014;9(4):e94085.
23. Rabe H, Reynolds G, Diaz-Rossello J. Early versus delayed umbilical cord clamping in preterm infants. Cochrane Database Syst Rev 2004;(4):CD003248.
24. Backes CH, Rivera BK, Haque U, et al. Placental transfusion strategies in very preterm neonates: a systematic review and meta-analysis. Obstet Gynecol 2014;124(1):47–56.
25. Hamilton BE, Martin JA, Osterman MJ, et al. Births: preliminary data for 2013. Natl Vital Stat Rep 2014;63:1–19.
26. March of Dimes. Less than 39 weeks toolkit. Available at: http://www.marchofdimes.org/professionals/less-than-39-weeks-toolkit.aspx. Accessed April 23, 2013.
27. Patel S, Clark EA, Rodriguez CE, et al. Effect of umbilical cord milking on morbidity and survival in extremely low gestational age neonates. Am J Obstet Gynecol 2014;211(5):519.e1–7.
28. Rabe H, Jewison A, Alvarez RF, et al. Milking compared with delayed cord clamping to increase placental transfusion in preterm neonates: a randomized controlled trial. Obstet Gynecol 2011;117(2 Pt 1):205–11.
29. Committee on Obstetric Practice, American College of Obstetricians and Gynecologists. Committee Opinion No.543: Timing of umbilical cord clamping after birth. Obstet Gynecol 2012;120(6):1522–6.
30. Freise KJ, Widness JA, Veng-Pedersen P. Erythropoietic response to endogenous erythropoietin in premature very low birth weight infants. J Pharmacol Exp Ther 2010;332(1):229–37.
31. Carroll PD, Widness JA. Nonpharmacological, blood conservation techniques for preventing neonatal anemia – effective and promising strategies for reducing transfusion. Semin Perinatol 2012;36(4):232–43.
32. Carroll PD, Nankervis CA, Iams J, et al. Umbilical cord blood as a replacement source for admission complete blood count in premature infants. J Perinatol 2012;32(2):97–102.
33. Hansen A, Forbes P, Buck R. Potential substitution of cord blood for infant blood in the neonatal sepsis evaluation. Biol Neonate 2005;88:12–8.
34. Beeram MR, Loughran C, Cipriani C, et al. Utilization of umbilical cord blood for the evaluation of group B streptococcal sepsis screening. Clin Pediatr (Phila) 2012;51(5):447–53.
35. Christensen RD, Lambert DK, Baer VL, et al. Postponing or eliminating red blood cell transfusions of very low birth weight neonates by obtaining all baseline laboratory blood tests from otherwise discarded fetal blood in the placenta. Transfusion 2011;51(2):253–8.
36. Rotshenker-Olshinka K, Shinwell ES, Juster-Reicher A, et al. Comparison of hematologic indices and markers of infection in umbilical cord and neonatal blood. J Matern Fetal Neonatal Med 2014;27(6):625–8.
37. Herson VC, Block C, McLaughlin JC, et al. Placental blood sampling: an aid to the diagnosis of neonatal sepsis. J Perinatol 1998;18(2):135–7.
38. Polin JI, Knox I, Baumgart S, et al. Use of umbilical cord blood culture for detection of neonatal bacteremia. Obstet Gynecol 1981;57(2):233–7.
39. Gonsalves WI, Cornish N, Moore M, et al. Effects of volume and site of blood draw on blood culture results. J Clin Microbiol 2009;47(11):3482–5.
40. Connell TG, Rele M, Cowley D, et al. How reliable is a negative blood culture result? Volume of blood submitted for culture in routine practice in a children's hospital. Pediatrics 2007;119(5):891–6.

41. American Academy of Pediatrics Subcommittee on Hyperbilirubinemia. Management of hyperbilirubinemia in the newborn infant 35 or more weeks of gestation. Pediatrics 2004;114(1):297–316.
42. Judd WJ. Practice guidelines for prenatal and perinatal immunohematology, revisited. Transfusion 2001;41(11):1445–52.
43. Baer VL, Lambert DK, Carroll PD, et al. Using umbilical cord blood for the initial blood tests of VLBW neonates results in higher hemoglobin and fewer RBC transfusions. J Perinatol 2013;33(5):363–5.
44. Josephson C, Meyer E. Neonatal and Pediatric transfusion practice. In: Fung M, editor. American Association of Blood Banking Technical Manual. 18th edition. Bethesda, MD: AABB; 2011. p. 645–70.
45. Miller J, Tuerck J. Newborn screening guidelines for premature and/or sick newborns; proposed guidelines. Wayne (PA): Clinical and Laboratory Standards Institute; 2008.
46. Ononeze AB, Hutchon DJ. Attitude of obstetricians towards delayed cord clamping: a questionnaire-based study. J Obstet Gynaecol 2009;29(3):223–4.
47. Farrar D, Tuffnell D, Airey R, et al. Care during the third stage of labour: a postal survey of UK midwives and obstetricians. BMC Pregnancy Childbirth 2010;10:23.

Darbepoetin Administration in Term and Preterm Neonates

Shrena Patel, MD[a], Robin K. Ohls, MD[b],*

KEYWORDS

- Anemia • Transfusions • Neuroprotection • Neurodevelopment • Darbepoetin
- Erythropoiesis-stimulating agents

KEY POINTS

- Darbepoetin (Darbe), a long-acting erythropoiesis-stimulating agent (ESA), is being studied as an anemia prevention treatment for preterm infants.
- Darbe is also promising as an agent for neuroprotection in both term and preterm infants.
- Further research is needed to evaluate long-term and neurodevelopmental outcomes in term and preterm infants treated with Darbe.

INTRODUCTION

Premature infants receive a greater number of transfusions with exposure to a greater number of donors than term neonates. Transfusion guidelines are now used in many neonatal units; however, the search for the most appropriate transfusion guidelines continues,[1] and long-term outcomes of neonates previously enrolled in transfusion studies are still being analyzed.[2,3] In addition, prematurity is a significant risk factor for neurodevelopmental delay. Mental retardation, cerebral palsy, and learning disabilities are neurodevelopmental deficits identified in former premature infants.[4] Although significant progress has been made in improving survival of extremely low-birthweight (ELBW) infants, improved neurodevelopmental outcomes remain elusive.

The use of ESAs, such as erythropoietin (Epo), to improve neuroprotection has been validated in both animal and human studies.[5] Both retrospective studies and

Disclosure statement: Dr R.K. Ohls' research cited in this work was funded by the Thrasher Research Fund and the NIH (R01HD059856).
a Division of Neonatology, Department of Pediatrics, University of Utah, 296 Chipeta Way, Salt Lake City, UT 84105, USA; b Division of Neonatology, Department of Pediatrics, University of New Mexico, MSC10 5590, 1 University of New Mexico, Albuquerque, NM 87131-0001, USA
* Corresponding author.
E-mail address: rohls@salud.unm.edu

prospective randomized trials have been performed in neonatal populations at greatest risk for long-term developmental abnormalities, namely, ELBW infants and term infants with hypoxic ischemic encephalopathy (HIE). This article outlines data that support darbepoetin (Darbe) as both an ESA and a neuroprotective agent and reviews promising clinical studies that demonstrate benefit in premature infants and safety in term infants undergoing cooling for HIE.

CLINICAL STUDIES

Infants born prematurely do not increase production of endogenous Epo to make new red cells and thus are at risk for repeated transfusions.[6] Numerous studies evaluating the use of recombinant human erythropoietin (rHuEpo) to prevent and treat the anemia of prematurity show that it is successful in preterm infants in stimulating erythropoiesis, and transfusion requirements are decreased.[7]

Studies in newborn monkeys and sheep demonstrated that neonates have a larger volume of distribution and a more rapid elimination of Epo, necessitating the use of higher doses than required for adults.[8,9] In preterm infants, the volume of distribution is 3- to 4-fold greater than that seen in adults, and the clearance is also 3 to 4 times greater[8,9]; this was confirmed in very-low-birth-weight (VLBW) infants.[10] Although it was anticipated that similar pharmacokinetics would exist with Darbe, it remained to be determined clinically.

Preliminary in vitro studies of the effects of Darbe compared with rHuEpo on fetal and neonatal erythroid progenitors showed similar responsiveness.[11] Erythroid progenitor cells were isolated from 12- to 22-week fetal liver and marrow and from term (37–41 weeks) and preterm (<32 weeks) cord blood. The number of burst forming units-erythroid (BFU-E) colonies derived from fetal marrow progenitor cells increased significantly with both Darbe (P<.01, 10 vs 50, 100, and 500 ng/mL; **Fig. 1**) and rHuEpo

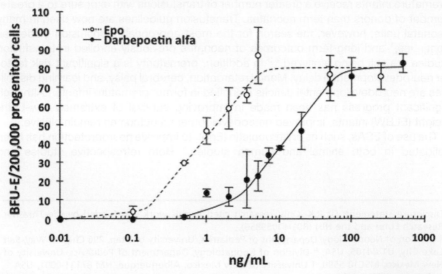

Fig. 1. Dose response curves for Epo (*open circles*) and Darbe (*solid circles*). Progenitor cells isolated from 12- to 24-week gestation fetal marrow were cultured for 10 to 14 days in increasing concentrations of Darbe (0–500 ng/mL) or protein equivalent concentrations of Epo. The number of BFU-E increased significantly (P<.01, 10 vs 50, 100, and 500 ng/mL Darbe, and P<.01, 0.05 vs 0.5, 1.0, and 2 U/mL Epo).

($P<.01$, 0.05 vs 0.5, 1.0, and 2 U/mL). BFU-E cell counts revealed similar numbers of normoblasts per colony between Darbe and rHuEpo, and BFU-E size increased with increasing concentrations of both growth factors. Progenitors isolated from fetal liver and from term and preterm cord blood were similarly responsive. When compared with term cord blood progenitors, preterm cord blood progenitors were more sensitive to Darbe at every concentration tested ($P<.01$).

DARBE DOSING AND PHARMACOKINETICS

Adult studies of Darbe pharmacokinetics demonstrated a half-life ($t_{1/2}$) of 49 hours after a single subcutaneous (SC) dose and 25 hours after intravenous (IV) dose.[12] **Table 1**[13–17] presents the area under the curve (AUC) following administration of ESAs (Darbe or Epo) in animal models and neonates. It is clear that there have been limited studies evaluating Darbe dosing and pharmacokinetics in neonates. In the following, the authors review results from trials involving preterm infants.

In a study by Warwood and colleagues,[12] neonates received a single SC dose of Darbe, 1 or 4 µg/kg. Twelve infants less than 32 weeks' gestation were enrolled, with birth weights 1129 ± 245 g and 29.2 ± 1.2 weeks' gestation at birth. Darbe concentrations peaked at 6 to 12 hours after administration. A single SC dose resulted in serum concentrations of 54 to 308 mU/mL with a 1-µg/kg dose and 268 to 980 mU/kg with a 4-µg/kg dose. The $t_{1/2}$ was 26 hours (range, 10–50 hours; mean, 29.6 for 1-µg/kg group and 21.5 for 4-µg/kg group). Clearance was 17.1 mL/h/kg for the 1-µg/kg group and 20.7 µg/h/kg for the 4-µg/kg group. Clinically, both immature (IRC) and absolute (ARC) reticulocyte counts significantly increased.

The same group analyzed pharmacokinetics after administration of a single 4-µg/kg IV dose of Darbe. Ten neonates were enrolled, with gestational ages between 26 and 40 weeks (7 neonates <32 weeks, 3 neonates >32 weeks). Doses were administered between 3 and 28 days. The $t_{1/2}$ was 10.1 hours, the volume of distribution was 0.77 L/kg (range, 0.180–3.05 L/kg), and clearance was 52.8 mL/h/kg (range, 22.4–158.0 mL/h/kg). Both volume of distribution and clearance were increased in comparison to older children and adults. In comparison to SC dosing, there was a less consistent increase in both IRC and ARC.[18] These studies suggested that dosing

Table 1
Area under the curve in ESA studies

Study	Epo 1000 U/kg	Epo 2500 U/kg	Epo 3500 U/kg	Epo 5000 U/kg	Darbe 2 µg/kg	Darbe 10 µg/kg
Rats (Statler et al[13])	—	—	—	140,331	—	—
Primates (Traudt et al[14])	94,377 (5801)	—	413,948 (39,605)	—	—	—
ELBW infants (Juul et al[15])	81,498 (7067)	317,881 (22,941)	—	—	—	—
Term HIE (Wu et al[16])	131,054 (17,083)	328,000 (61,945)	—	—	—	—
Term HIE (Baserga et al[17])	—	—	—	—	26,555 (20,049– 35,029)	180,886 (146,568– 199,680)

AUC values are in units hour per liter and are reported as mean (standard deviation) (Traudt and Wu studies), mean (standard error) (Juul), or median (IQR) (Baserga).

needed to be higher (micrograms per kilogram) and more frequent than that used in children and adults.

The authors previously evaluated reticulocyte responses to SC Darbe administration in preterm infants randomized in a blinded Darbe dose-response study.[19] Preterm infants 1500 g or less and aged 10 days or more were randomized to placebo or 2.5, 5, or 10 μg/kg/dose Darbe, given once a week SC for 4 weeks. Complete blood counts, reticulocyte counts, transfusions, and adverse events (AEs) were recorded. Eighteen preterm infants (896 ± 59 g, 28.7 ± 0.7 weeks' gestation, 13 ± 1 days of age) were enrolled (**Table 2**). Infants randomized to 10 μg/kg/dose achieved the highest reticulocyte counts by day 14 of the study (**Fig. 2**A; $P = .04$). Infants receiving any dose of Darbe maintained hematocrits at a higher level at 14 days than infants receiving placebo (see **Fig. 2**B; $P = .002$). Infants receiving 5 or 10 μg/kg/dose required fewer transfusions during the study period (see **Table 2**; $P = .006$). No AEs were noted. It was concluded that preterm infants respond to Darbe by increasing erythropoiesis in a dose-dependent fashion, with the greatest reticulocyte response occurring with 10 μg/kg/dose. Both 5 and 10 μg/kg/dose were sufficient to decrease transfusions in preterm infants.

PRETERM ERYTHROPOIESIS-STIMULATING AGENT STUDIES

Preterm infants have received fewer transfusions during the last several years compared with previous decades.[20] This decrease has been in part due to an increased awareness of morbidities, including transfusion-related lung injury, donor exposure, and transfusion-related intestinal injury.[21] The development and adherence to transfusion guidelines, cord milking/delayed cord clamping, and reduction in phlebotomy losses have all contributed to an overall decrease in transfusions.[20] Some studies have demonstrated that the more liberal use of blood transfusions may not improve outcomes.[2] In a recent quality improvement project done across 4 newborn intensive care units (NICUs), Henry and colleagues[20] demonstrated that transfusion rates are further decreased with the use of anemia prevention guidelines. Such guidelines included initiating iron and Darbe treatment, instituting delayed cord clamping/cord milking, and introducing policies for limiting phlebotomy losses. The study found that the NICUs that adhered to such anemia preventing guidelines also had lower rates of neonatal morbidities, such as necrotizing enterocolitis (Bell stage ≥2), retinopathy of prematurity (ROP) (stage ≥3), or severe intraventricular hemorrhage (grade ≥3).

Table 2
Characteristics of study infants, Darbe dose-response study

	0 μg/kg/Dose	2.5 μg/kg/Dose	5 μg/kg/Dose	10 μg/kg/Dose
Birth weight (g)	961 ± 83	872 ± 123	970 ± 138	774 ± 43
Gestation (wk)	29.0 ± 2.0	30.1 ± 1.4	27.4 ± 0.9	28.5 ± 1.3
Age (d)	14 ± 4	17 ± 2	12 ± 1	11 ± 1
Baseline hematocrit (%)	34.0 ± 3.0	32.3 ± 4.2	33.5 ± 2.7	34.7 ± 3.3
Baseline reticulocyte count ($\times 10^3$/mL)	50 ± 10	97 ± 23	95 ± 23	127 ± 61
Number of transfusions during study	1.7 ± 0.3	2.3 ± 0.3	0.5 ± 0.3[a]	1.3 ± 0.3[a]
Transfusion volume during study (mL)	27 ± 7	34 ± 6	13 ± 3	23 ± 7

[a] $P = .006$, 5 and 10 μg/kg doses versus 0 and 2.5 μg/kg.

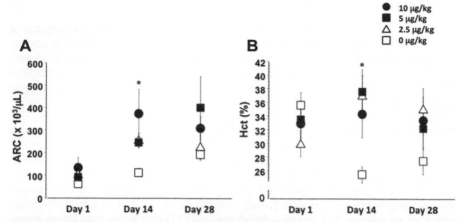

Fig. 2. Changes in reticulocyte count (*panel A*) and hematocrit (*panel B*) in preterm infants treated with 4 weekly Darbe doses (0 [placebo], 2.5, 5, and 10 μg/kg). Reticulocyte counts increased by day 14 in infants receiving either 5 or 10 μg/kg dosing. Infants receiving 10 μg/kg had the greatest reticulocyte response (*P = .04 vs placebo). Hematocrits were greater by day 14 in infants receiving any Darbe (*P = .006 vs placebo).

The results of trials in which preterm infants received Darbe as an anemia-preventing technique are reviewed later.

In a recent single-center trial by Warwood and colleagues,[21] 20 VLBW infants were randomized to receive a single, 10-μg/kg dose of Darbe or placebo within 30 minutes of initiating a transfusion. Infants were enrolled at an average age of 34.5 to 35.1 days (corresponding with physiologic hematocrit nadir). Infants in the Darbe group had a significant increase in their absolute reticulocyte count throughout the study period. The Darbe group also seemed to maintain higher hematocrit values following the transfusion. This study was a small pilot study, but the findings suggested that Darbe treatment may abrogate the transfusion-induced suppression of erythropoiesis.

Based on the authors' preliminary Darbe dose response study and previous work comparing Epo concentrations to cognitive outcome,[22] they designed a multicenter, randomized, placebo-controlled study of Darbe and Epo administration to preterm infants. Infants with birth weights between 500 and 1250 g and less than or equal to 48 hours of age were randomized to Darbe (10 μg/kg, once a week SC), Epo (400 U/kg, thrice a week SC), or placebo (sham dosing) through 35 weeks' gestation. All were transfused according to protocol and received supplemental iron, folate, and vitamin E. Transfusions (primary outcome), complete blood counts, ARC, phlebotomy losses, and AEs were recorded. Infants in the ESA groups received significantly fewer transfusions (P = .015) and were exposed to fewer donors (P = .044) than those in the placebo group (Darbe, 1.2 ± 2.4 transfusions and 0.7 ± 1.2 donors per infant; Epo, 1.2 ± 1.6 transfusions and 0.8 ± 1.0 donors per infant; placebo, 2.4 ± 2.9 transfusions and 1.2 ± 1.3 donors per infant). ESA-treated infants had a 50% reduction in transfusions and donor exposure than placebo-treated infants. Hematocrit and ARC were higher in the Darbe and Epo groups compared with placebo (P = .001, Darbe and Epo vs placebo for both hematocrit and ARC). Morbidities were similar among groups, including the incidence of ROP. The authors concluded that infants receiving ESAs received fewer transfusions and fewer donor exposures, and fewer injections were given to Darbe recipients.[23] Greater than 50% of VLBW infants in the ESA group remained transfusion-free during their NICU stay.

PRETERM NEUROPROTECTION

The authors were able to complete follow-up on 80 (29 Epo, 27 Darbe, 24 placebo) of the 99 infants enrolled and evaluated during the hospital course in the above-mentioned study (**Table 3**).[23,24] After adjusting for gender, analysis demonstrated that infants who had received Darbe or Epo had significantly higher cognitive scores (96.2 ± 7.3 and 97.9 ± 14; mean ± standard deviation) in comparison with placebo recipients (88.7 ± 13.5; P = .01 vs ESA recipients). The ESA group also scored significantly higher on object permanence, an early test of executive function (P = .05). There was no cerebral palsy among recipients of Darbe or Epo, whereas 5 cases of cerebral palsy were identified in the placebo group (P<.001). The incidence of neurodevelopmental impairment in the ESA group was significantly lower compared with placebo (odds ratio, 0.18; 95% confidence interval, 0.05–0.63).[24] There were no differences in visual or hearing impairment among groups. The significance of improved neurodevelopmental outcomes in preterm infants demonstrated by this study (when confirmed by a larger trial) would support the use of Darbe in this population, especially given Darbe's weekly dosing schedule.

There were no differences in the incidence of any stage of ROP during the hospital phase and no differences in visual impairment at 18 to 22 months corrected age. Hesitancy in the use of ESAs is linked to a 2006 meta-analysis, which suggested an

Table 3
Infant characteristics and neurodevelopmental outcomes from ESA randomized controlled trial

	Darbe (n = 27)	Epo (n = 29)	Placebo (n = 24)	P	Adjusted Odds Ratio	P
Birth weight (g)	938.3 ± 176.5	947.2 ± 212.7	953.0 ± 210.0	NS	—	—
Gestation (wk)	28.1 ± 1.8	27.8 ± 1.9	27.8 ± 1.6	NS	—	—
Corrected age at follow-up (mo)	20.5 ± 1.1	21.2 ± 2.0	20.6 ± 1.9	NS	—	—
Composite cognitive	96.2 ± 7.5	97.9 ± 14.0	88.7 ± 13.3	.01	—	—
Composite language	92.4 ± 12.8	89.9 ± 17.4	83.6 ± 13.9	.05	—	—
Object permanence	2.8 ± 0.4	2.4 ± 0.8	2.2 ± 1.0	.05	—	—
Neurodevelopmental impairment	3 (11%)	2 (7%)	9 (38%)	—	0.18 (0.05–0.63)	.01
Cerebral palsy (%)	0 (0)	0 (0)	5 (21)	.002	0 (0–0)	<.001
Visual deficit (%)	1 (4)	0 (0)	1 (4)	.09	0.23 (0.04–1.54)	NS
Hearing deficit (%)	0	1 (3)	1 (4)	.33	0.54 (0.11–2.65)	NS
Composite cognitive score <85	0	3 (10.3%)	6 (25%)	.02	0.18 (0.04–0.78)	.01
Composite cognitive score <70	0	1 (3.4%)	2 (8.3%)	.29	—	—

Odds ratios adjusted for gender. Values represent mean ± standard deviation or number (percentage). *P* values represent 3-way comparisons among groups.
Data from Ohls RK, Christensen RD, Kamath-Rayne BD, et al. A randomized, masked, placebo-controlled study of darbepoetin alfa in preterm infants. Pediatrics 2013;132:e119–27; and Ohls RK, Kamath-Rayne BD, Christensen RD, et al. Cognitive outcomes of preterm infants randomized to darbepoetin, erythropoietin, or placebo. Pediatrics 2014;133:1023–30.

association between early (first week of life) Epo administration and ROP greater than stage 2[6] compared with late Epo administration.[25] However, this meta-analysis reflected a misclassification of a single-center Epo study by Romagnoli and colleagues[26] into the early Epo administration group. When this study was correctly grouped with other studies of late Epo use, the revised meta-analysis showed no significant difference in ROP with the use of early or late Epo. Evaluation for ROP continues to be a priority in most clinical trials of ESA use for preterm infants.

TERM NEUROPROTECTION STUDIES

Based on the previous studies, several multicenter clinical trials evaluating ESAs in conjunction with hypothermia in term infants with HIE are being planned. Only 1 study to date has evaluated Darbe as a potential neuroprotective agent in term infants undergoing hypothermia as treatment of HIE. The Darbepoetin Administered to Neonates Undergoing Cooling for Encephalopathy (DANCE) study lead by Baserga[17] enrolled 30 infants ($\geq$36 weeks gestation) with moderate to severe HIE. Infants were randomized to placebo (n = 10), 2 μg/kg Darbe (n = 10), or 10 μg/kg Darbe (n = 10) IV. The first dose was administered before 12 hours of life and the second on day 7. AEs and serious AEs were documented for 1 month. Serum samples were obtained at specific time points to determine pharmacokinetics. At 2 and 10 μg/kg Darbe, $t_{1/2}$ was 24 and 32 hours, and the AUC extrapolated to infinity was 26,555 (interquartile range [IQR], 20,049–35,029) and 180,886 mU/mL (IQR, 146,568–199,680), respectively.[17] The investigators concluded that the 10 μg/kg dose achieved an AUC in the neuroprotective range and a terminal $t_{1/2}$ of 53.4 hours[5] when compared with the 2-μg/kg dose. No side effects attributable to Darbe were reported. These infants are still being followed for long-term developmental outcomes. If these outcomes are similar to those in infants treated with Epo, Darbe's longer $t_{1/2}$ and fewer number of doses needed may convey a clinical benefit.

The $t_{1/2}$ of the 10-μg/kg Darbe dose reported in the DANCE study was approximately 3 times the $t_{1/2}$ of Epo reported in the Neonatal Erythropoietin in Asphyxiated Term Newborns (NEAT) trial.[16] In the NEAT trial, Wu and colleagues[16] randomized 24 infants with moderate to severe HIE to an open label dose escalation trial of Epo (NCT00719407). Infants received 250, 500, 1000, or 2500 U/kg of Epo administered IV every other day for up to 6 doses. Pharmacokinetics were performed with the first, second, and last doses, and infants were monitored closely for any adverse effects. Epo followed nonlinear pharmacokinetics but did not accumulate with multiple dosing. The AUC was 50,306, 131,054, and 328,002 Uh/L for 500, 1000, and 2500 U/kg, respectively. No serious adverse effects or deaths were reported. They concluded that 1000 U/kg Epo administered intravenously in conjunction with hypothermia was well tolerated and produced plasma concentrations that in previous studies were neuroprotective in animals.

Several adult studies have evaluated neuroprotective properties of ESAs. The pathology of neuronal disease and patient characteristics are different; however, information on mechanism of neuroprotection may be useful in the study of neonatal neuronal injury. A study by Messé and colleagues[27] evaluating the effects of Darbe on adults undergoing aortic surgery was terminated early when the US Food and Drug Association placed a hold on all ESA studies of neuroprotection after Epo recipients in a European multicenter study of patients with stroke were found to have increased mortality.[28] Only 9 adults in Messé's study received 1 mg/kg Darbe immediately before surgery. An additional 9 untreated adult patients were added as a comparison cohort. Although this small number of enrolled patients prevented appropriate analysis, results demonstrated that the primary outcome of death or neurologic impairment between groups was nonsignificant (1 of 9, 11% in the Darbe group and 3 of 9, 33% in control group, $P = .58$). Significantly higher concentrations of cerebral spinal fluid biomarkers (S100-beta and glial fibrillary acidic protein [GFAP]) were found in patients with perioperative neurologic ischemia; however, there were no differences in these biomarkers between the Darbe and control groups (S100-beta, 214 vs 260 ng/mL, $P = .69$; GFAP, 22 vs 580 pg/mL, $P = .45$).[27]

SUMMARY

Clinical studies in preterm and term infants have shown Darbe to be safe, and evidence of neuroprotection is growing. Preterm infants administered Darbe during their NICU stay show fewer need for transfusions, higher cognitive scores, and a lower incidence of neurodevelopmental impairment. Darbe is consequently being used as an ESA across several NICUs in the country. Studies of Darbe administration in term infants with HIE being cooled for encephalopathy are ongoing. Developmental follow-up of those term infants is progressing. ESAs hold great promise in providing neuroprotection and improving neurodevelopmental outcomes of preterm neonates.

Best Practices

What is the current practice to prevent and treat the anemia of prematurity?

Best practice/guideline/care path objectives

Epo administration

  Recommendations for infants receiving total parenteral nutrition (TPN):

    200 U/kg/d, added to TPN

    Begin dosing when TPN is ordered

    IV administration (if not added to TPN) to run for at least 4 hours, use protein-containing solution to dilute

  Recommendations for SC administration

    400 U/kg given thrice a week

    Begin dosing at 7 to 10 days of life or when IV access is gone

    For preterm infants being discharged, or for infants with late anemia due to Rh or ABO isoimmunization, use a dose of 1000 U/kg SC once a week to stimulate erythropoiesis

  Recommendations for length of treatment

    Continue dosing until 34 to 36 weeks corrected gestational age

    Epo is contraindicated in infants with thromboembolic disease, hypertension, or seizures

Iron and vitamin supplementation for infants receiving Epo

  Iron: Iron dextran, 3 to 5 mg/kg once a week added to TPN solution if available (1 mg/kg/d is acceptable; check ferritin after 2 weeks of dosing)

  Iron dextran can be added to 5% Dextrose Water (D5W), 10% Dextrose Water (D10W), and normal saline (NS) and run via peripheral IV for 4 hours

  Ferrous sulfate 4 to 6 mg/kg/d: preterm formula (4 mg/kg/d); expressed breast milk (6 mg/kg/d)

  Vitamin E: 25 IU/d by mouth

  Folate: 50 μg/d by mouth

  Vitamin B_{12} (if available): 21 μg/wk SC

What changes in current practice are likely to improve outcomes?

The use of Epo in preterm infants decreases the number of transfusions in most infants and eliminates transfusions in some infants.

Major recommendations (see above-mentioned guidelines)

Rating for the strength of the evidence: category 1A, moderate

Bibliographic sources

Christensen RD, Carroll PD, Josephson CD. Evidence-based advances in transfusion practice in neonatal intensive care units. Neonatology 2014;106:245–53.

Summary statement

The use of ESAs in preterm infants continues to grow, and new indications (neuroprotection and improved neurodevelopmental outcomes) are currently being evaluated. ESA administration maintains/increases hematocrit and decreases transfusion need, thereby avoiding potential risks of red cell transfusions in preterm infants.

REFERENCES

1. Kirpalani H, Whyte RK, Andersen C, et al. The Premature Infants in Need of Transfusion (PINT) study: a randomized, controlled trial of a restrictive (low) versus liberal (high) transfusion threshold for extremely low birth weight infants. J Pediatr 2006;149:301–7.
2. McCoy TE, Conrad AL, Richman LC, et al. Neurocognitive profiles of preterm infants randomly assigned to lower or higher hematocrit thresholds for transfusion. Child Neuropsychol 2011;17:347–67.
3. Whyte RK, Kirplani H, Aszatalos EV, et al. Neurodevelopmental outcome of extremely low birth weight infants randomly assigned to restrictive or liberal hemoglobin thresholds for blood transfusion. Pediatrics 2009;123:207–13.
4. Stephens BE, Vohr BR. Protein intake and neurodevelopmental outcomes. Clin Perinatol 2014;41:323–9.
5. Juul S. Neuroprotective role of erythropoietin in neonates. J Matern Fetal Neonatal Med 2012;25(Suppl 4):105–7.
6. Ohlsson A, Aher SM. Early erythropoietin for preventing red blood cell transfusion in preterm and/or low birth weight infants. Cochrane Database Syst Rev 2006;(3):CD004863.
7. Bishara N, Ohls RK. Current controversies in the management of the anemia of prematurity. Semin Perinatol 2009;33:29–34.
8. Widness JA, Veng-Pedersen P, Peters C, et al. Erythropoietin pharmacokinetics in premature infants: developmental, nonlinearity, and treatment effects. J Appl Physiol (1985) 1996;80:140–8.
9. George JW, Bracco CA, Shannon KM, et al. Age-related differences in erythropoietic response to recombinant human erythropoietin: comparison in adult and infant rhesus monkeys. Pediatr Res 1990;28:567–71.
10. Ohls RK, Veerman MW, Christensen RD. Pharmacokinetics and effectiveness of recombinant erythropoietin administered to preterm infants by continuous infusion in parenteral nutrition solution. J Pediatr 1996;128:518–23.
11. Ohls RK, Dai A. Long-acting erythropoietin: clinical studies and potential uses in neonates. Clin Perinatol 2004;31:77–89.
12. Warwood TL, Ohls RK, Wiedmeier SE, et al. Single-dose darbepoetin administration to anemic preterm neonates. J Perinatol 2005;25:725–30.

13. Statler PA, McPherson RJ, Bauer LA, et al. Pharmacokinetics of high-dose recombinant erythropoietin in plasma and brain of neonatal rats. Pediatr Res 2007;61: 671–5.

14. Traudt CM, McPherson RJ, Bauer LA, et al. Concurrent erythropoietin and hypothermia treatment improve outcomes in a term nonhuman primate model of perinatal asphyxia. Dev Neurosci 2013;35:491–503.

15. Juul SE, McPherson RJ, Bauer LA, et al. A phase I/II trial of high-dose erythropoietin in extremely low birth weight infants: pharmacokinetics and safety. Pediatrics 2008;122:383–91.

16. Wu YW, Bauer LA, Ballard RA, et al. Erythropoietin for neuroprotection in neonatal encephalopathy: safety and pharmacokinetics. Pediatrics 2012;130:683–91.

17. Baserga MC, Beachy JC, Roberts JK, et al. DANCE (Darbe Administration in Newborns Undergoing Cooling for Encephalopathy): a safety and pharmacokinetics trial. Pediatr Res 2015, in press.

18. Warwood TL, Ohls RK, Lambert DK, et al. Intravenous administration of darbepoetin to NICU patients. J Perinatol 2006;26:296–300.

19. Roohi M, Peceny MC, Ohls RK. A randomized, masked, dose response study of darbepoetin administered to preterm infants. In: Programs and abstracts of the Pediatric Academic Society Annual Meeting. Toronto (Ontario), May 5-8, 2007. [abstract: 5899.3].

20. Henry E, Christensen RD, Sheffield MJ, et al. Why do four NICUs using identical RBC transfusion guidelines have different gestational age-adjusted RBC transfusion rates? J Perinatol 2015;35:132–6.

21. Warwood TL, Lambert DK, Henry E, et al. Very low birth weight infants qualifying for a 'late' erythrocyte transfusion: does giving darbepoetin along with the transfusion counteract the transfusion's erythropoietic suppression? J Perinatol 2011; 31:S17–21.

22. Bierer R, Peceny MC, Harenberger CH, et al. Erythropoietin concentrations and neurodevelopmental outcome in preterm infants. Pediatrics 2006;118:e635–40.

23. Ohls RK, CHristensen RD, Kamath-Rayne BD, et al. A randomized, masked, placebo-controlled study of darbepoetin alfa in preterm infants. Pediatrics 2013;132:e119–27.

24. Ohls RK, Kamath-Rayne BD, Christensen RD, et al. Cognitive outcomes of preterm infants randomized to darbepoetin, erythropoietin, or placebo. Pediatrics 2014;133:1023–30.

25. Aher S, Ohlsson A. Late erythropoietin for preventing red blood cell transfusion in preterm and/or low birth weight infants. Cochrane Database Syst Rev 2006;(3):CD004868.

26. Romagnoli C, Zecca E, Gallini F, et al. Do recombinant human erythropoietin and iron supplementation increase the risk of retinopathy of prematurity? Eur J Pediatr 2000;159:627–8.

27. Messé SR, McGarvey ML, Bavaria JE, et al. A pilot study of darbepoetin alfa for prophylactic neuroprotection in aortic surgery. Neurocrit Care 2013;18:75–80.

28. Ehrenreich H, Wessenborn K, Prange H, et al. Recombinant human erythropoietin in the treatment of acute ischemic stroke. Stroke 2009;40:e647–56.

Immunologic and Hematological Abnormalities in Necrotizing Enterocolitis

Akhil Maheshwari, MD[a,b,c,*]

KEYWORDS

- NEC • Blood counts • Inflammation • Macrophages • Signaling • Neutrophils
- Platelets • Monocytes

KEY POINTS

- Necrotizing enterocolitis (NEC) is a leading cause of morbidity and mortality in preterm infants born before 32 weeks' gestation or with a birth weight less than 1500 g.
- Bacterial flora plays a central pathophysiological role in NEC.
- Premature intestine is at risk of NEC because of mucosal sensitivity to bacterial products and paucity of mechanisms that normally limit the interaction of luminal bacteria with mucosal cells.
- The onset of NEC is associated with elevated plasma concentrations of several inflammatory cytokines. Increased circulating interleukin-8 concentrations may provide prognostic information.
- Low circulating TGF-β concentrations on the first postnatal day may predict later occurrence of NEC.
- Hematological abnormalities such as thrombocytopenia, disseminated intravascular coagulation, increased or decreased neutrophil counts, eosinophilia, and anemia occur frequently in infants with NEC.
- In a premature infant with feeding intolerance, an acute drop in peripheral blood monocyte concentrations compared with the last presymptomatic blood counts may be an early indicator of NEC.

Conflicts of Interest: The authors disclose no conflicts.

Funding: National Institutes of Health award HL124078A.

[a] Department of Pediatrics, Morsani College of Medicine, Tampa, FL 33606, USA; [b] Department of Molecular Medicine, Morsani College of Medicine, Tampa, FL 33612, USA; [c] Department of Community and Family Health, College of Public Health, University of South Florida, Tampa, FL 33612, USA

* 1 Tampa General Circle, TGH Suite F170, Tampa, FL 33606.

E-mail address: akhilm@health.usf.edu

Clin Perinatol 42 (2015) 567–585

http://dx.doi.org/10.1016/j.clp.2015.04.014

0095-5108/15/$ – see front matter © 2015 Elsevier Inc. All rights reserved.

perinatology.theclinics.com

INTRODUCTION

Necrotizing enterocolitis (NEC) is a devastating inflammatory condition of the gastro-intestinal disease that afflicts 4% to 11% of very low birth weight infants and is a lead-ing cause of morbidity and mortality in this population.[1-3] The pathogenesis of NEC is complex and is not well understood. Clinical studies associate NEC with diverse pre-natal and postnatal factors, such as placental insufficiency, prolonged/premature rupture of membranes, chorioamnionitis, gut ischemia, altered bacterial colonization, viral infections of the gastrointestinal tract, bacterial overgrowth, and red blood cell (RBC) transfusions.[1,2] Although a unifying mechanism may not be readily evident in all the risk factors of NEC, some of these conditions presumably alter/disrupt the intestinal epithelial barrier to allow bacterial translocation from the lumen into the subepithelial lamina propria, where these bacteria or their products trigger an exag-gerated, damaging mucosal inflammatory reaction.[1,4] In severe intestinal injury, bac-terial products and/or the inflammatory mediators may spill into the bloodstream, causing a systemic inflammatory response and multiorgan dysfunction.[5] In this article, we review the immunologic aspects of the pathogenesis of NEC and its hematological manifestations. A literature search was performed using the databases PubMed, EMBASE, and Scopus. To minimize bias, keywords from PubMed's Medical Subject Heading (MeSH) thesaurus were shortlisted before the actual search and combined with text words likely to be used in titles and abstracts.

IMMUNOLOGIC ASPECTS OF NECROTIZING ENTEROCOLITIS
Mucosal Sensitivity to Bacterial Products in the Premature Intestine

Several lines of evidence indicate that luminal bacteria play a central pathophysiolog-ical role in NEC: (1) bacterial overgrowth, and *pneumatosis intestinalis*, the accumula-tion of gaseous products of bacterial fermentation in the bowel wall, are prominent histopathological findings in NEC; (2) ischemic intestinal injury in the sterile in utero microenvironment may cause strictures or atresia, whereas similar insults after post-natal bacterial colonization may increase the risk of NEC[6]; (3) enteral antibiotics can reduce the incidence of NEC and NEC-related mortality.[7] Although specific bacterial species have not been causally associated with NEC, infants who go on to develop NEC often display a microbial imbalance ("dysbiosis") with abnormal abundance of gammaproteobacteria (Enterobacteriaceae and Pseudomonadaceae) and *Clostridia*, but with fewer Firmicutes, the dominant Gram-positive bacterial phylum in infants who do not develop NEC.[8,9] Gammaproteobacteria express lipopolysaccharides and other products that have unique microbial-associated molecular patterns, which engage with the Toll-like receptors (TLRs) on mucosal cells to activate downstream inflammatory signaling. As discussed in the following section, the developing intestine is at risk of inflammatory injury because of 2 major factors: (1) the epithelium and mucosal immune cells in the developing intestine are uniquely sensitive to bacterial products, and (2) a paucity of adaptive mechanisms that normally limit the interaction of luminal bacteria with the mucosa.

Intestinal Epithelium

Fetal intestinal epithelial cells (IECs) express a variety of innate response receptors and display a "hyperactive" TLR-activated transcriptional program, which manifests with exaggerated expression of cytokines and inflammatory mediators.[10-15] This epithelial sensitivity to bacterial products correlates with high levels of expression of TLR2, TLR4, downstream adaptors such as the myeloid differentiation primary response gene 88, and tumor necrosis factor receptor-associated factor 6, and the transcriptional regulator nuclear factor kappa B 1 (NF-κB1). In addition, fetal IECs are developmentally deficient in many negative regulators of TLR signaling, such as the single immunoglobulin interleukin-1-related receptor, interleukin-1 (IL-1) receptor-associated kinase (IRAK)-M, tumor necrosis factor-alpha–induced protein 3, and the Toll-interacting protein.[16] Other reports implicate low levels of inhibitor of κB.[17] NF-κB signaling may also be dampened after full-term birth due to posttranscriptional downregulation of IRAK-1, another key intermediate in TLR signaling.[18]

Goblet cells start producing mucus by week 12, but this mucus layer contains low amounts of the protective mucin 2 (muc2).[19] Expression of muc2 is further compromised during NEC, possibly through bile acid–mediated mucosal injury.[20] Paneth cells appear at about the same time as goblet cells and produce antibacterial proteins such as lysozyme and α-defensins. The number of Paneth cells is low in the premature intestine and increases with maturation until adulthood.[21] In rodents, Paneth cell ablation may trigger NEC-like injury in the developing intestine.[22] Developmental differences in secretory immunoglobulin A (sIgA) are described later in this article.

Intestinal Macrophages and Dendritic Cells

Macrophages first appear in the fetal intestine at 11 to 12 weeks. The resident macrophage population increases rapidly during the 12-week to 22-week period, and then a slower pace through early childhood.[23–25] These cells play a critical role in host defense as the first phagocytic cells of the innate immune system to encounter luminal bacteria that breach the epithelium and gain access to the lamina propria. In the adult intestine, macrophages display avid phagocytic and bacteriocidal activity but are attenuated in their inflammatory responses,[26] a unique adaptation that minimizes inflammation in the gut mucosa despite the close proximity to luminal bacteria. We have shown that macrophage precursors undergo inflammatory downregulation on recruitment to the intestinal mucosa under the influence of transforming growth factor-beta (TGF-β), particularly the TGF-β$_2$ isoform, present in the local extracellular matrix.[4] In the midgestation intestine, which is developmentally deficient in TGF-β bioactivity, macrophages are yet to acquire this inflammatory anergy and produce inflammatory cytokines on exposure to bacterial products.[4,27] These inflammatory responses of the mucosal macrophages likely add to the risk of mucosal injury during NEC. Transgenic mice with defects in tissue-specific differentiation of gut macrophages due to loss of TGF-β signaling or mutations in the signal transducer and activator of transcription pathway are at increased risk of inflammatory mucosal injury.[4,28]

There are very limited data on fetal/neonatal intestinal dendritic cells (DCs).[23] HLA-DR$^+$ DC-like cells are detected in both lamina propria and the Peyer patches after 14 weeks, but these cells may have some overlap with lamina propria macrophages.[29] In rats and nonhuman primates, DCs have been noted in the fetal lamina propria as well as in Peyer patches.[30,31] The functional importance of these DCs in NEC remains unclear, although DCs were proposed as a cause of epithelial damage in mice with *Cronobacter sakazakii*–induced NEC-like injury.[32]

Mucosa-Associated Lymphoid Tissue

Peyer patches first appear at 11 weeks and develop during mid-late gestation (**Table 1**).[33,34] At birth, these lymphoid aggregates are structurally complete but "naïve," as germinal centers take a few weeks to develop.[35] The number of Peyer patches in the ileum increases as a function of gestational maturation, and premature infants born before 32 weeks' gestation may have only half as many Peyer patches as their full-term counterparts.[36] Other mucosa-associated lymphoid tissue (MALT)

Table 1	
Development of Peyer patches in the human fetus	
11 wk gestation	PP anlagen with HLA-DR$^+$ CD4$^+$ lymphoid cells
16 wk gestation	Appearance of T and B cells
	First appearance of CD8$^+$ cells[a]
	B-cell maturation with appearance of surface IgM and IgD
16–18 wk gestation	Appearance of CD5$^+$ B-1 cells
	Surface IgA on B cells
18–20 wk gestation	Appearance of PP zonation into B-cell and T-cell areas
24 wk gestation	PP are macroscopically identifiable
0–4 wk postnatal	Germinal center formation

Abbreviations: Ig, immunoglobulin; PP, Peyer patch.
[a] Fetal PP T cells are predominantly of the CD4$^+$ phenotype.

structures, such as the lymphoid aggregates in the vermiform appendix, develop after birth following postnatal bacterial colonization.[37,38]

T Lymphocytes in the Lamina Propria and Intraepithelial Compartments

T cells are first seen in the fetal intestine at 12 to 14 weeks' gestation.[39] Outside the MALT, intestinal T cells are distributed in the lamina propria and the intraepithelial compartments. Lamina propria lymphocytes develop in the fetal intestine in utero and reach densities similar to the full-term intestine by 19 to 27 weeks' gestation.[39] In contrast, intraepithelial lymphocytes (IELs) expand mainly after birth.[40,41] Approximately 10% to 30% of IELs express the γδ T-cell receptor[34] and may serve specialized roles in epithelial homeostasis, cytotoxic activity, and antimicrobial immunity.[42–44] The fetal intestine also shows some early-lineage T-cell populations, indicating that T cells may also develop locally in a mucosal, extrathymic pathway.[34,39,40,45–49] In premature infants, the T-cell receptor shows a polyclonal repertoire that undergoes gradual restriction to a mature, oligoclonal pattern, possibly due to the emergence of a few dominant clones specific for commensal bacteria.[50,51] Although the role of T-cell subsets in NEC remains unclear, there is an overall paucity of T cells in surgically resected bowel affected by NEC and in murine models of NEC-like injury.[52–54] Consistent with this deficiency in T-cell development, infants who go on to develop NEC had lower circulating levels of T-lymphokines, such as IL-2, IL-18, CC-motif ligand (CCL) 4, and CCL5 in the preceding weeks than other premature infants who did not develop NEC.[55]

FOXP3$^+$ T regulatory cells (Treg) can be seen in both the small intestine and colonic mucosa as early as 23 weeks' gestation.[56] The role of Tregs in mucosal homeostasis is evident from the early development of enteropathy in patients lacking this subset of regulatory immune cells due to FOXP3 mutations (IPEX syndrome).[57] Interestingly, excessive innate immune activation can suppress Treg function in the preterm intestine.[58] Tregs can act via several distinct mechanisms, such as expression of anti-inflammatory cytokines (IL-10, IL-35, TGF-β); granzyme-mediated and perforin-mediated cytolysis or induction of apoptosis in T-effector cells; and inhibition of dendritic cell maturation.[59] Compared with gestational-age–matched non-NEC controls, infants with surgical NEC show decreased ratios of Tregs to effector T cells in the ileal mucosa.[60]

B Cells and Secretory Immunoglobulins

The first B cells are seen in the lamina propria at 14 weeks' gestation and display a mature B-cell phenotype similar to the thymic B cells (CD20$^+$ IgM$^+$ IgD$^+$ light chain+).[34] Some pre–B cells (IgM+ light chain− CD20−) also may be seen, indicating that the mucosa may serve as an alternative site for B-cell development.[61] During the second postnatal week, some B cells in both the lamina propria and the MALT[62] undergo IgA class-switch.[63,64] The number of IgA+ plasma cells reaches adult levels at 2 years, although serum IgA concentrations may not reach adult levels until the second decade.[40]

The sIgA is first detected in mucosal secretions at 1 to 8 weeks after birth.[65–68] In premature infants, sIgA may first appear in secretions at a similar chronologic age as in full-term infants, although the concentrations are usually lower, as sIgA concentrations rise as a function of postmenstrual age.[30,31,69,70] The IgA responses also may be functionally less robust with a predominance of monomeric (instead of polymeric) sIgA[71,72] and IgA1 (instead of the sIgA2) subclass.[73] Premature infants also show global abnormalities in their immunoglobulin responses, such as reduced antigen affinity, polyreactivity, and autoreactivity.[74,75] In addition, immunoglobulin heavy chains have short complementarity-determining regions in premature neonates,[76] which markedly lowers the potential antibody diversity available to these infants.[76]

During the neonatal period, colostrum provides an important alternative source of sIgA.[77] Milk antibodies may contribute approximately 0.5 to 1.0 g per day throughout lactation (comparable to the 2.5 g per day being produced by a 65-kg adult), and are directed against antigens present in the environment shared by the mother-infant dyad.[78] Immune cells stimulated by antigens in the maternal intestine and bronchial mucosa have been shown to migrate specifically to the mammary gland.[77,79–81] Interestingly, sIgA levels in colostrum and milk of mothers of preterm neonates may be higher than in mothers who delivered at full-term.[82]

Platelet-Activating Factor

Platelet-activating factor (PAF), an endogenous phospholipid mediator produced by platelets, leukocytes, and endothelial cells, is believed to represent a final, common effector in diverse forms of intestinal injury.[83] In rodent models, exogenous administration of PAF induces systemic hypotension, microvascular permeability, and gut mucosal necrosis, which is often most prominent in the ileum.[84] In NEC, the role of PAF is supported by several lines of evidence: (1) compared with age-matched controls, infants with NEC have elevated plasma PAF levels and decreased plasma activity of PAF-acetylhydrolase (PAF-AH), the enzyme that normally degrades PAF[85,86]; (2) human milk contains PAF-AH[87]; (3) NEC-like injury was prevented in rat pups and piglets by PAF-receptor antagonists[88,89]; (4) enteral administration and intravenous infusion of recombinant PAF-AH prevented NEC in rats[90]; (5) PAF-AH knockout mice are more susceptible to NEC-like injury[91]; and (6) ileum, the site of predilection of NEC, shows highest regional expression of PAF receptors in the gastrointestinal tract.[92]

Nitric Oxide

Nitric oxide (NO) is a key regulator of vascular tone, inflammation, neurotransmission, and tissue restitution and repair.[93] There are 3 isoforms of NO synthases (NOS): endothelial NOS (eNOS) and neuronal NOS (nNOS), which generate low (picomolar) concentrations of NO, and inducible NOS (iNOS), which produces high (micromolar) concentrations of NO. Low levels of NO play physiologic roles in epithelial homeostasis and water absorption. However, at high concentrations, NO reacts with superoxide to form peroxynitrite, a highly toxic intermediate that disrupts protein conformation, alters cellular metabolism, and can block epithelial restitution and induce apoptosis in diverse cell types.[94,95] Increased iNOS expression was noted in IECs in surgically resected intestinal tissue samples of NEC.[96] Formula-fed rat pups show increased iNOS expression in the gut mucosa, which is further increased during NEC-like injury.[97,98]

Reactive Oxygen Species

Reactive oxygen species (ROS) are believed to play a key proinflammatory role in NEC. The xanthine oxidase/dehydrogenase system is one of the main producers of ROS in the intestine. Xanthine dehydrogenase is constitutively expressed in IECs and normally catalyzes the transformation of xanthine into uric acid (Xanthine + H_2O + NAD $\rightarrow$ Uric acid + NADH + H^+). However, during ischemia, xanthine dehydrogenase is converted into xanthine oxidase, which leads to xanthine oxidation into uric acid and superoxide (Xanthine + H_2O + O_2 $\rightarrow$ Uric acid + $2O_2^-$ + $2H^+$). ROS activates the intestinal mitochondrial apoptotic signaling pathway during oxidative stress and leads to IEC apoptosis via the p38 mitogen-activated protein kinase.[99,100] Xanthine oxidase and superoxide are implicated in intestinal reperfusion injury and PAF-induced bowel necrosis, as allopurinol, a xanthine oxidase inhibitor, has been shown to be protective in these models.[101,102]

Transforming Growth Factor-β

We have shown recently that premature infants who developed NEC had lower circulating TGF-β_1 levels than their non-NEC controls since birth.[55] In this study, blood TGF-β_1 concentrations less than 1380 pg/mL on the first postnatal day predicted future onset of NEC with 64% accuracy. Although several biomarkers (such as the inter-alpha inhibitor protein, intestinal fatty acid–binding protein, hexosaminidase, proapolipoprotein CII, and des-arginine serum amyloid A) have been identified for their ability to discriminate between confirmed NEC and other causes of feeding intolerance,[103–106] blood TGF-β_1 is the first biomarker to estimate the risk of NEC in a newly born premature infant. Even though genetic factors do not seem to be a major contributor to the risk of NEC,[107] the ability of blood TGF-β_1 to identify infants at risk of NEC on day 1 is interesting because it indicates that the risk-stratification for NEC may start early, possibly in utero, before most hypoxic-ischemic events of the early neonatal period would have occurred or the microbial flora would have been established in the intestinal lumen. These findings are consistent with our previous reports indicating that preterm neonates may be at risk of inflammatory mucosal injury and NEC because of a developmental deficiency of TGF-β bioactivity in the intestine.[4,27] The reasons for low blood TGF-β levels in infants who developed NEC were unclear, although a few interesting possibilities merit consideration. The first is increased peripheral uptake of TGF-β to compensate for low tissue expression. We have previously shown that TGF-β expression is decreased in healthy margins of tissues resected for NEC.[4] A second explanation could be based on an assumption that the developing intestine is a major contributor to circulating TGF-β levels. Because TGF-β expression increases in the intestine as a function of gestational maturation,[4] lower tissue expression of TGF-β in infants who developed NEC could conceivably reflect an underlying state of arrested mucosal development, where low TGF-β expression may indicate persistence of a cytokine profile corresponding to an earlier, less mature developmental epoch. In support of this possibility, we detected lower TGF-β levels in the NEC group than in controls at the same postmenstrual age. Finally, infants who developed NEC may constitutively produce less TGF-β than controls due to genetic/epigenetic factors. Premature baboons with spontaneously occurring NEC-like injury showed histone methylation in the TGF-β nucleosome, a repressive modification associated with facultative heterochromatin assembly and transcriptional silencing.[27]

Cytokine Responses Associated with Necrotizing Enterocolitis

Several studies have investigated the cytokine response during NEC. Cytokines are attractive not only as potential biomarkers of the primary disease and the severity of inflammation in NEC, but also for possible pathophysiological roles in intestinal injury. At the tissue level, increased IL-1β and tumor necrosis factor expression have been detected in surgically resected tissue specimens of human NEC.[108–110] In preclinical models, NEC-like intestinal injury induces chemokines such as the CXC-motif ligand 5 (CXCL5), CXCL1, and CXCL2, CCL2, CCL3, CCL5, CCL20, IL-1β, IL-6, IL-12, and IL-18.[54,109–113] In plasma, the diagnosis of NEC in premature infants was associated with elevated IL-1β, IL-1 receptor antagonist, IL-6, IL-10, CXCL5, IL-8/CXCL8, CCL2, CCL3, neurotrophin-4, and C-reactive protein.[55,114–116] In one study, plasma IL-8/CXCL8, epithelial-derived neutrophil chemoattractant-78/CXCL5, and IL-10 levels were higher in infants with NEC than in those with sepsis syndrome.[117] IL-6 has a shorter half-life and may be detectable only for short periods after onset of NEC,[118] whereas IL-8/CXCL8 levels show sustained elevation[116] and correlate with the extent of NEC (NEC-totalis), the need for surgical resection of bowel, and higher 60-day mortality in infants with NEC.[114,115,117]

HEMATOLOGICAL MANIFESTATIONS OF NECROTIZING ENTEROCOLITIS

Hematological abnormalities occur frequently in infants with NEC, and in many, carry important diagnostic and prognostic information. These abnormalities remain mild and require no intervention in most infants with NEC, although some with severe disease may require blood product transfusions and monitoring for complications such as hemorrhage, infections, anemia, and even death.[5,119]

Platelet Counts

Thrombocytopenia, defined as a platelet count less than $150 \times 10^9/L$, is seen at clinical presentation in 50% to 95% of infants with NEC, and many have platelet counts in the range of $30 \times 10^9/L$ to $60 \times 10^9/L$.[120–122] Most neonates with advanced NEC develop thrombocytopenia within 24 to 72 hours of onset of disease.[121–123] The severity of thrombocytopenia correlates with the Bell clinical stage of NEC, and a rapid drop in platelet counts to less than $100 \times 10^9/L$ is a sensitive (although not specific) predictor of bowel gangrene or the need for surgical intervention.[120,124] Ververidis and colleagues[124] reviewed the clinical course of 58 neonates with advanced NEC (Bell's stages II or III, gestational age 23–41 weeks) and noted platelet counts less than $150 \times 10^9/L$ in 54 (93%) infants and counts less than $100 \times 10^9/L$ in 51 (88%). Most infants who showed a rapid drop in platelet counts to less than $100 \times 10^9/L$ were bacteremic. In patients without intestinal necrosis, platelet counts recovered to normal levels within 24 hours.[124] These data are similar to previous reports by Hutter and colleagues,[121] Patel,[122] O'Neill,[120] and Kenton and colleagues.[123]

Platelet counts provide important predictive information for the outcome in patients with NEC. In survivors, the median time to recovery to a platelet count greater than $150 \times 10^9/L$ is approximately 7 to 10 days.[121,122] Infants who die of NEC tend to have lower nadir platelet counts than survivors. In the cohort described by Ververidis and colleagues,[124] patients who died of NEC had a lower nadir in platelet counts than the survivors. All patients with a platelet count greater than $100 \times 10^9/L$ during the course of the disease survived. Ragazzi and colleagues[125] recorded platelet counts less than $150 \times 10^9/L$ in 86% of nonsurvivors versus 43.3% of the survivors ($P<.0001$). Severe thrombocytopenia ($<100 \times 10^9/L$) was noted more frequently in nonsurvivors (70%) than in survivors (33%; P<.0001). In another study, Kenton and colleagues[123] reported higher median platelet counts in survivors than in nonsurvivors (203 × 10^9/L vs 33 × 10^9/L; P<.001). Severe thrombocytopenia was a predictor of mortality (adjusted odds ratio [OR] 6.39; P = .002) and NEC-related gastrointestinal complications, such as cholestatic liver disease and short bowel syndrome (adjusted OR 5.47; P = .006).

The primary mechanism for thrombocytopenia in NEC is widely believed to be increased platelet destruction. Indirect evidence for platelet consumption is seen in the rapid drop in platelet counts in many patients, and also in the short-lived rise in platelet concentrations after transfusions lasting less than 24 to 48 hours.[126] The mechanism(s) of thrombocytopenia in NEC has not been investigated in clinical studies, but existing information from animal models indicates a likely role of PAF and circulating bacterial products, such as lipopolysaccharide.[127] These mediators stimulate endothelial cells and macrophages to release inflammatory cytokines and NO, which, along with thromboplastin released from gangrenous bowel, can increase platelet activation and aggregation in the microvasculature.[120]

Patients with NEC have higher plasma thrombopoietin (Tpo) concentrations than their healthy counterparts.[128,129] Brown and colleagues[130] measured plasma Tpo concentrations, circulating megakaryocyte progenitors, reticulated platelet counts, and the percentage of reticulated platelets in the circulating platelet pool (RP%) in 20 neonates with sepsis and/or NEC. They showed elevated concentrations of Tpo and a modest increase in circulating megakaryocyte progenitors and RP% in thrombocytopenic neonates. The investigators hypothesized that this dampening of thrombopoietic response may be due to increased levels of platelet factor 4, which is released from activated platelets and is a potent inhibitor of megakaryocytopoiesis.

Coagulopathy

Hutter and colleagues[121] noted signs of disseminated intravascular coagulation (DIC) in 14 of their 40 infants. Many infants showed decreased plasma fibrinogen, tested positive for fibrin split products, and had elevated partial thromboplastin times. These data are similar to Patel[122] and Sonntag and colleagues,[131] who described a similar frequency of DIC in their respective cohorts.

Anemia

Patients with NEC may develop anemia due to multiple pathogenetic mechanisms. In the presence of mucosal injury, thrombocytopenia, and coagulation disturbances, occult and obvious blood loss is common. Sites of bleeding may include bloody stools, peritoneal hemorrhage, pulmonary hemorrhage, hemopericardium, myocardial hemorrhage, and intracranial hemorrhage.[119] Iatrogenic anemia due to phlebotomy losses is an added problem. In some patients, hemolysis can cause further worsening of anemia. Thrombotic microangiopathy can cause red cell damage, which can often be seen on blood smears as tear drop cells, schistocytes, spherocytes, and acanthocytes. Hutter and colleagues[121] reported red cell fragmentation in 25 of their 40 patients. Another possible cause is activation of the Thomsen-Friedenreich (T) cryptantigen on the RBC surface, a naturally occurring antigen that is normally concealed by a layer of N-acetylneuraminic acid but can be exposed in NEC by bacterial or other neuraminidases. T-activation can cause hemolysis and anemia in multitransfused patients who have previously received adult blood containing anti-T antibodies.[132,133] Studies show considerable variation in the frequency of T-activation in NEC, ranging from rare occurrences to up to a third of all patients.[119,134] T-activation is associated with increased morbidity and mortality in NEC. Finally, infants with NEC may be at enhanced risk of inflammatory suppression of erythropoiesis. NEC tends to occur most frequently in extremely premature infants who show an impaired erythropoietin response for a given level of anemia and are prone to develop severe anemia of prematurity.[119] The presence of inflammation after onset of NEC in these infants can further suppress erythropoietin and red cell production.

In some situations, anemia may be a risk factor for the development of NEC rather than its effect. Infants with severe anemia related to glucose-6-phosphate dehydrogenase deficiency, hemolytic disease of newborn, and in donor twins in twin-to-twin transfusion syndrome are at increased risk of NEC.[135,136] Anemia also has been identified as a predisposing factor in patients who develop NEC after RBC transfusions. Singh and colleagues[137] investigated the association between anemia and transfusion-associated NEC in a cohort of 111 preterm infants with confirmed NEC and 222 matched controls. In a multivariate model, lower hematocrit was associated with increased odds of NEC (OR 1.10, $P = .01$) after controlling for other factors. They showed that RBC transfusions had a temporal relationship with onset of NEC, where a transfusion within the preceding 24 hours (OR 7.60, $P = .001$) and 48 hours (OR 5.55, $P = .001$) was associated with increased odds of developing NEC. Although the mechanisms by which anemia may increase the risk of NEC remain unclear, anemia has been shown to impair splanchnic perfusion and increase oxygen extraction as a compensatory mechanism.[138] Anemia also can impair the normal postnatal changes in splanchnic vascular resistance,[139] predisposing the developing intestine to hypoxemic-ischemic gut mucosal injury, and possibly, to NEC.[140]

Neutrophils

Increased neutrophil counts comprise an appropriate inflammatory response in patients with mild-moderately severe disease. In contrast, neutropenia, defined as an absolute neutrophil count (ANC) less than 1500/μL, can be seen in severe NEC and is associated with adverse outcome.[121,122,124,125] Patel[122] noted neutropenia in 14 of their 23 patients who died of NEC, compared with 6 of 24 survivors. In another study, Ragazzi and colleagues[125] noted that neutropenia in the initial blood counts at onset of NEC was associated with adverse outcome; there was a trend for a higher frequency of neutropenia in nonsurvivors (37%) than in survivors (25%; $P = .136$), and thrombocytopenia and neutropenia occurred together more frequently in nonsurvivors (39%) than in survivors (14%; $P = .0007$). In infants at greater than 34 weeks' gestation and with lower ANC, higher immature neutrophil number, and greater immature:total neutrophil ratio at onset of NEC were associated with the need for surgical intervention.[141] Although the pathophysiology of neutropenia in NEC is not well understood, depletion of the circulating neutrophil pool due to emigration into the intestines and peritoneum, and increased margination in the microvasculature are some of the possible causes.[121,124,125]

Macrophages and Monocytes

The cellular inflammatory response in NEC is characterized by the presence of a macrophage-rich infiltrate.[54] We have previously shown that gut macrophage populations are normally maintained through continuous recruitment of circulating monocytes and in situ differentiation of these cells in the lamina propria.[142,143] Because preterm infants have a limited circulating monocyte pool[144] and lack significant reservoirs of mature monocytes in the bone marrow or elsewhere,[145] we asked whether the migration of circulating monocytes into NEC lesions could result in an acute drop in peripheral blood monocyte counts that may distinguish early NEC from other causes of feeding intolerance.[146] We compared the absolute monocyte counts (AMC) at the onset of feeding intolerance with the last available presymptomatic AMC. In patients who developed stage II NEC, the AMC fell from median 1.7×10^9/L (interquartile range [IQR] 0.98–2.4) to median 0.8 (IQR 0.62–2.1, $P<.05$), whereas those who developed stage III NEC dropped their AMCs from median 2.1×10^9/L (IQR 0.15–3.2) to median 0.8 (IQR 0.6–1.9, $P<.05$). Total white cell counts, ANC, and lymphocyte counts did not change significantly. In the control group (developed feeding intolerance for a reason other than NEC), there was no change in AMC or the white cell, ANC, or lymphocyte counts.

Eosinophils

Eosinophilia, defined as a blood eosinophil count exceeding the 95th percentile upper reference limit, ranges from 1180/μL during the first postnatal week to 1560/μL after 3 weeks.[144] Christensen and colleagues[147] noted eosinophilia in 54 (19.6%) of 275 infants who were evaluated for bloody stools. They hypothesized that premature infants with bloody stools and eosinophilia were likely to have atopic enteropathy and not develop the classic signs of NEC, and were therefore, more likely to have a benign course of disease. However, the rate of pneumatosis, bowel resection, and death in infants with bloody stools and eosinophilia was similar to those with normal blood eosinophil counts. Interestingly, infants with eosinophilia were more likely to have received an RBC transfusion in a 48-hour period before passing a bloody stool. These infants with a preceding history of a blood transfusion showed a progressive rise in eosinophil counts. In contrast, infants who developed bloody stools and eosinophilia but did not have a history of a previous transfusion showed reduction in eosinophil counts once the feedings were discontinued and had a relatively benign course of disease. Although the mechanism for transfusion-associated eosinophilia is unclear, exposure to foreign antigens on donor RBCs or to medications administered during the transfusion may play a role.

Basophils

Kim and colleagues[148] showed that low basophil counts (16.5 ± 43.0/μL in the NEC group vs 60.6 ± 131.4/μL in controls, $P<.001$) at birth may predict the development of NEC. The investigators speculated that these differences in basophil hematopoiesis may reflect host interaction with commensal bacteria.[149] However, additional study is needed to understand the mechanistic basis of these findings because these differences were identifiable early, possibly before the intestinal microbial flora would have been established in these infants.

Lymphocytes

Lambert and colleagues[150] reported that infants who died of fulminant NEC within 48 hours of onset had low lymphocyte counts. They reviewed the medical records of 523 infants with a diagnosis of NEC, of whom 35 (6.7%) had a fulminant course. These infants were more likely to have a blood lymphocyte count less than 4000/μL ($P = .018$), besides having portal venous air, severe anemia, recent increase in feeding volume or introduction of human milk fortifier, and increased immature to total neutrophil ratio.

Nucleated Red Blood Cells

Infants who develop NEC may have a higher number of nucleated RBCs at birth than their gestation-matched controls. Mandel and colleagues[151] compared 23 preterm infants diagnosed with NEC with pair-matched controls who were admitted immediately after a case, had the same gestational age (±1 week), 1-minute and 5-minute Apgar scores (±1), and who did not develop NEC. Exclusion criteria included factors that may influence the absolute nucleated RBC counts at birth, such as maternal diabetes, pregnancy-induced hypertension, major congenital malformations, chromosomal abnormalities, hemolysis, and perinatal blood loss. Infants who developed NEC had higher absolute nucleated RBC counts than controls, suggesting that these neonates may have experienced intrauterine hypoxemia, which may increase the risk of NEC. These data are consistent with observations by Baschat and colleagues,[152] who showed that nucleated RBC counts greater than 30/100 white blood cells beyond 3 days were associated with increased risk of NEC.

SUMMARY

In the premature intestine, developmental limitations in both the innate and adaptive arms of the mucosal immune system increase the risk of inflammatory injury and NEC. The systemic inflammatory response during NEC is characterized by elevated circulating cytokine levels and a consistent pattern of hematological abnormalities, which may also play a direct or indirect role in augmenting the mucosal injury. Some of these immunologic and hematological abnormalities carry important prognostic information.

Best Practices

What is the current practice?

Infants who develop necrotizing enterocolitis (NEC) frequently show immunologic and hematological abnormalities, such as elevated circulating cytokine levels, thrombocytopenia, increased or decreased neutrophil counts, low monocyte counts, and anemia. These findings show high sensitivity and in some infants, might convey important diagnostic and prognostic information. In others, the clinical utility of these tests may be limited due to low specificity and the overlap with comorbidities, such as bacterial or fungal sepsis, or cholestasis.

What changes in current practice are likely to improve outcomes?

Many hematological abnormalities associated with NEC have been identified in recent years and still need confirmation in larger studies. Cytokine measurements, although straightforward and relatively inexpensive, are not routinely available yet in clinical laboratories. Further study is needed to refine these measurements and determine whether the diagnostic accuracy of these tests could be improved if used in combination.

Is there a clinical algorithm?

No. Because of low specificity, immunologic and hematological abnormalities are likely to be less useful as diagnostic tests in infants with NEC. Instead, these findings are more likely to find utility as "early-warning" systems that indicate a need for clinical monitoring and/or imaging. Elevated plasma concentrations of interleukin (IL)-8 and IL-6, low levels of TGF-β, and the detection of worsening thrombocytopenia or an acute drop in monocyte counts are some of the more promising findings. In infants at risk of transfusion-associated NEC, a rise in blood eosinophil counts may be important.

Summary statement

NEC is characterized by elevated circulating cytokine levels and a consistent pattern of hematological abnormalities. Some of these findings may provide important diagnostic and prognostic information.

REFERENCES

1. Neu J, Walker WA. Necrotizing enterocolitis. N Engl J Med 2011;364:255–64.
2. Maheshwari A, Corbin LL, Schelonka RL. Neonatal necrotizing enterocolitis. Res Rep Neonatol 2011;1:39–53.
3. Patel RM, Kandefer S, Walsh MC, et al. Causes and timing of death in extremely premature infants from 2000 through 2011. N Engl J Med 2015; 372:331–40.
4. Maheshwari A, Kelly DR, Nicola T, et al. TGF-beta(2) suppresses macrophage cytokine production and mucosal inflammatory responses in the developing intestine. Gastroenterology 2011;140:242–53.
5. Walsh MC, Kliegman RM. Necrotizing enterocolitis: treatment based on staging criteria. Pediatr Clin North Am 1986;33:179–201.
6. Hsueh W, Caplan MS, Tan X, et al. Necrotizing enterocolitis of the newborn: pathogenetic concepts in perspective. Pediatr Dev Pathol 1998;1:2–16.
7. Bury RG, Tudehope D. Enteral antibiotics for preventing necrotizing enterocolitis in low birthweight or preterm infants. Cochrane Database Syst Rev 2001;(1): CD000405.
8. de la Cochetiere MF, Piloquet H, des Robert C, et al. Early intestinal bacterial colonization and necrotizing enterocolitis in premature infants: the putative role of *Clostridium*. Pediatr Res 2004;56:366–70.
9. Wang Y, Hoenig JD, Malin KJ, et al. 16S rRNA gene-based analysis of fecal microbiota from preterm infants with and without necrotizing enterocolitis. ISME J 2009;3:944–54.
10. Maheshwari A, Lacson A, Lu W, et al. Interleukin-8/CXCL8 forms an autocrine loop in fetal intestinal mucosa. Pediatr Res 2004;56:240–9.
11. Nanthakumar NN, Young C, Ko JS, et al. Glucocorticoid responsiveness in developing human intestine: possible role in prevention of necrotizing enterocolitis. Am J Physiol Gastrointest Liver Physiol 2005;288:G85–92.
12. Fusunyan RD, Nanthakumar NN, Baldeon ME, et al. Evidence for an innate immune response in the immature human intestine: toll-like receptors on fetal enterocytes. Pediatr Res 2001;49:589–93.
13. Nanthakumar NN, Fusunyan RD, Sanderson I, et al. Inflammation in the developing human intestine: a possible pathophysiologic contribution to necrotizing enterocolitis. Proc Natl Acad Sci U S A 2000;97:6043–8.
14. Daig R, Rogler G, Aschenbrenner E, et al. Human intestinal epithelial cells secrete interleukin-1 receptor antagonist and interleukin-8 but not interleukin-1 or interleukin-6. Gut 2000;46:350–8.
15. Martin CR, Walker WA. Intestinal immune defences and the inflammatory response in necrotising enterocolitis. Semin Fetal Neonatal Med 2006;11(5): 369–77.
16. Nanthakumar N, Meng D, Goldstein AM, et al. The mechanism of excessive intestinal inflammation in necrotizing enterocolitis: an immature innate immune response. PLoS One 2011;6:e17776.
17. Claud EC, Lu L, Anton PM, et al. Developmentally regulated IkappaB expression in intestinal epithelium and susceptibility to flagellin-induced inflammation. Proc Natl Acad Sci U S A 2004;101:7404–8.
18. Lotz M, Gütle D, Walther S, et al. Postnatal acquisition of endotoxin tolerance in intestinal epithelial cells. J Exp Med 2006;203:973–84.
19. Montgomery RK, Mulberg AE, Grand RJ. Development of the human gastrointestinal tract: twenty years of progress. Gastroenterology 1999;116:702–31.

20. Martin NA, Mount Patrick SK, Estrada TE, et al. Active transport of bile acids decreases mucin 2 in neonatal ileum: implications for development of necrotizing enterocolitis. PLoS One 2011;6:e27191.
21. Mallow EB, Harris A, Salzman N, et al. Human enteric defensins. Gene structure and developmental expression. J Biol Chem 1996;271:4038–45.
22. Zhang C, Sherman MP, Prince LS, et al. Paneth cell ablation in the presence of *Klebsiella pneumoniae* induces necrotizing enterocolitis (NEC)-like injury in the small intestine of immature mice. Dis Model Mech 2012;5:522–32.
23. MacDonald TT. Accessory cells in the human gastrointestinal tract. Histopathology 1996;29:89–92.
24. Rognum TO, Thrane S, Stoltenberg L, et al. Development of intestinal mucosal immunity in fetal life and the first postnatal months. Pediatr Res 1992;32:145–9.
25. Braegger CP, Spencer J, MacDonald TT. Ontogenetic aspects of the intestinal immune system in man. Int J Clin Lab Res 1992;22:1–4.
26. Smythies LE, Sellers M, Clements RH, et al. Human intestinal macrophages display profound inflammatory anergy despite avid phagocytic and bactericidal activity. J Clin Invest 2005;115:66–75.
27. Namachivayam K, Blanco CL, MohanKumar K, et al. Smad7 inhibits autocrine expression of TGF-beta2 in intestinal epithelial cells in baboon necrotizing enterocolitis. Am J Physiol Gastrointest Liver Physiol 2013;304:G167–80.
28. Takeda K, Clausen BE, Kaisho T, et al. Enhanced Th1 activity and development of chronic enterocolitis in mice devoid of Stat3 in macrophages and neutrophils. Immunity 1999;10:39–49.
29. Spencer J, MacDonald TT, Isaacson PG. Heterogeneity of non-lymphoid cells expressing HLA-D region antigens in human fetal gut. Clin Exp Immunol 1987;67:415–24.
30. Wilders MM, Sminia T, Janse EM. Ontogeny of non-lymphoid and lymphoid cells in the rat gut with special reference to large mononuclear Ia-positive dendritic cells. Immunology 1983;50:303–14.
31. Makori N, Tarantal AF, Lü FX, et al. Functional and morphological development of lymphoid tissues and immune regulatory and effector function in rhesus monkeys: cytokine-secreting cells, immunoglobulin-secreting cells, and CD5(+) B-1 cells appear early in fetal development. Clin Diagn Lab Immunol 2003;10: 140–53.
32. Emami CN, Mittal R, Wang L, et al. Recruitment of dendritic cells is responsible for intestinal epithelial damage in the pathogenesis of necrotizing enterocolitis by *Cronobacter sakazakii*. J Immunol 2011;186:7067–79.
33. Finke D, Acha-Orbea H, Mattis A, et al. CD4+CD3- cells induce Peyer's patch development: role of alpha4beta1 integrin activation by CXCR5. Immunity 2002;17:363–73.
34. Spencer J, Finn T, Isaacson PG. Gut associated lymphoid tissue: a morphological and immunocytochemical study of the human appendix. Gut 1985;26: 672–9.
35. Husband AJ, Gleeson M. Ontogeny of mucosal immunity—environmental and behavioral influences. Brain Behav Immun 1996;10:188–204.
36. Cornes JS. Peyer's patches in the human gut. Proc R Soc Med 1965;58:716.
37. Bhide SA, Wadekar KV, Koushik SA. Peyer's patches are precocious to the appendix in human development. Dev Immunol 2001;8:159–66.
38. Gebbers JO, Laissue JA. Bacterial translocation in the normal human appendix parallels the development of the local immune system. Ann N Y Acad Sci 2004; 1029:337–43.

39. Spencer J, MacDonald TT, Finn T, et al. The development of gut associated lymphoid tissue in the terminal ileum of fetal human intestine. Clin Exp Immunol 1986;64:536–43.
40. Latthe M, Terry L, MacDonald TT. High frequency of CD8 alpha alpha homodimer-bearing T cells in human fetal intestine. Eur J Immunol 1994;24:1703–5.
41. Cerf-Bensussan N, Guy-Grand D. Intestinal intraepithelial lymphocytes. Gastroenterol Clin North Am 1991;20:549–76.
42. Komano H, Fujiura Y, Kawaguchi M, et al. Homeostatic regulation of intestinal epithelia by intraepithelial gamma delta T cells. Proc Natl Acad Sci U S A 1995;92:6147–51.
43. Boismenu R, Havran WL. Modulation of epithelial cell growth by intraepithelial gamma delta T cells. Science 1994;266:1253–5.
44. Kagnoff MF. Current concepts in mucosal immunity. III. Ontogeny and function of gamma delta T cells in the intestine. Am J Physiol 1998;274:G455–8.
45. Howie D, Spencer J, DeLord D, et al. Extrathymic T cell differentiation in the human intestine early in life. J Immunol 1998;161:5862–72.
46. Gunther U, Holloway JA, Gordon JN, et al. Phenotypic characterization of CD3-7+ cells in developing human intestine and an analysis of their ability to differentiate into T cells. J Immunol 2005;174:5414–22.
47. Spencer J, Isaacson PG, Walker-Smith JA, et al. Heterogeneity in intraepithelial lymphocyte subpopulations in fetal and postnatal human small intestine. J Pediatr Gastroenterol Nutr 1989;9:173–7.
48. Fichtelius KE. The gut epithelium–a first level lymphoid organ? Exp Cell Res 1968;49:87–104.
49. Koningsberger JC, Chott A, Logtenberg T, et al. TCR expression in human fetal intestine and identification of an early T cell receptor beta-chain transcript. J Immunol 1997;159:1775–82.
50. Williams AM, Bland PW, Phillips AC, et al. Intestinal alpha beta T cells differentiate and rearrange antigen receptor genes in situ in the human infant. J Immunol 2004;173:7190–9.
51. Holtmeier W, Witthoft T, Hennemann A, et al. The TCR-delta repertoire in human intestine undergoes characteristic changes during fetal to adult development. J Immunol 1997;158:5632–41.
52. Anttila A, Kauppinen H, Koivusalo A, et al. T-cell-mediated mucosal immunity is attenuated in experimental necrotizing enterocolitis. Pediatr Surg Int 2003;19:326–30.
53. Pender SL, Braegger C, Gunther U, et al. Matrix metalloproteinases in necrotising enterocolitis. Pediatr Res 2003;54:160–4.
54. Mohankumar K, Kaza N, Jagadeeswaran R, et al. Gut mucosal injury in neonates is marked by macrophage infiltration in contrast to pleomorphic infiltrates in adult: evidence from an animal model. Am J Physiol Gastrointest Liver Physiol 2012;303:G93–102.
55. Maheshwari A, Schelonka RL, Dimmitt RA, et al. Cytokines associated with necrotizing enterocolitis in extremely-low-birth-weight infants. Pediatr Res 2014;76:100–8.
56. Weitkamp JH, Rudzinski E, Koyama T, et al. Ontogeny of FOXP3(+) regulatory T cells in the postnatal human small intestinal and large intestinal lamina propria. Pediatr Dev Pathol 2009;12:443–9.
57. Wildin RS, Ramsdell F, Peake J, et al. X-linked neonatal diabetes mellitus, enteropathy and endocrinopathy syndrome is the human equivalent of mouse scurfy. Nat Genet 2001;27:18–20.

58. Silverstein AM, Lukes RJ. Fetal response to antigenic stimulus. I. Plasmacellular and lymphoid reactions in the human fetus to intrauterine infection. Lab Invest 1962;11:918–32.
59. Vignali DA, Collison LW, Workman CJ. How regulatory T cells work. Nature reviews. Immunology 2008;8:523–32.
60. Weitkamp JH, Koyama T, Rock MT, et al. Necrotising enterocolitis is characterised by disrupted immune regulation and diminished mucosal regulatory (FOXP3)/effector (CD4, CD8) T cell ratios. Gut 2013;62:73–82.
61. Golby S, Hackett M, Boursier L, et al. B cell development and proliferation of mature B cells in human fetal intestine. J Leukoc Biol 2002;72:279–84.
62. Fagarasan S, Kinoshita K, Muramatsu M, et al. In situ class switching and differentiation to IgA-producing cells in the gut lamina propria. Nature 2001;413:639–43.
63. Crabbe PA, Nash DR, Bazin H, et al. Immunohistochemical observations on lymphoid tissues from conventional and germ-free mice. Lab Invest 1970;22: 448–57.
64. Shroff KE, Meslin K, Cebra JJ. Commensal enteric bacteria engender a self-limiting humoral mucosal immune response while permanently colonizing the gut. Infect Immun 1995;63:3904–13.
65. Haworth JC, Dilling L. Concentration of gamma-A-globulin in serum, saliva, and nasopharyngeal secretions of infants and children. J Lab Clin Med 1966;67: 922–33.
66. Brandtzaeg P, Nilssen DE, Rognum TO, et al. Ontogeny of the mucosal immune system and IgA deficiency. Gastroenterol Clin North Am 1991;20:397–439.
67. Gleeson M, Cripps AW, Clancy RL, et al. Ontogeny of the secretory immune system in man. Aust N Z J Med 1982;12:255–8.
68. Mellander L, Carlsson B, Hanson LA. Appearance of secretory IgM and IgA antibodies to Escherichia coli in saliva during early infancy and childhood. J Pediatr 1984;104:564–8.
69. Hayes JA, Adamson-Macedo EN, Perera S, et al. Detection of secretory immunoglobulin A (SIgA) in saliva of ventilated and non-ventilated preterm neonates. Neuroendocrinol Lett 1999;20:109–13.
70. Shields CJ, O'Sullivan AW, Wang JH, et al. Hypertonic saline enhances host response to bacterial challenge by augmenting receptor-independent neutrophil intracellular superoxide formation. Ann Surg 2003;238:249–57.
71. Cripps AW, Gleeson M, Clancy RL. Ontogeny of the mucosal immune response in children. Adv Exp Med Biol 1991;310:87–92.
72. Weemaes C, Klasen I, Göertz J, et al. Development of immunoglobulin A in infancy and childhood. Scand J Immunol 2003;58:642–8.
73. Fitzsimmons SP, Evans MK, Pearce CL, et al. Immunoglobulin A subclasses in infants' saliva and in saliva and milk from their mothers. J Pediatr 1994;124: 566–73.
74. Bhat NM, Kantor AB, Bieber MM, et al. The ontogeny and functional characteristics of human B-1 (CD5+ B) cells. Int Immunol 1992;4:243–52.
75. Chen ZJ, Wheeler CJ, Shi W, et al. Polyreactive antigen-binding B cells are the predominant cell type in the newborn B cell repertoire. Eur J Immunol 1998;28: 989–94.
76. Bauer K, Zemlin M, Hummel M, et al. Diversification of Ig heavy chain genes in human preterm neonates prematurely exposed to environmental antigens. J Immunol 2002;169:1349–56.
77. Ogra PL, Losonsky GA, Fishaut M. Colostrum-derived immunity and maternal-neonatal interaction. Ann N Y Acad Sci 1983;409:82–95.

78. Hanson LA, Korotkova M. The role of breastfeeding in prevention of neonatal infection. Semin Neonatol 2002;7:275–81.
79. Hanson LA, Ahlstedt S, Andersson B, et al. The immune response of the mammary gland and its significance for the neonate. Ann Allergy 1984;53:576–82.
80. Takahashi T, Yoshida Y, Hatano S, et al. Reactivity of secretory IgA antibodies in breast milk from 107 Japanese mothers to 20 environmental antigens. Biol Neonate 2002;82:238–42.
81. Flamand V, Donckier V, Demoor FX, et al. CD40 ligation prevents neonatal induction of transplantation tolerance. J Immunol 1998;160:4666–9.
82. Araujo ED, Gonçalves AK, Cornetta Mda C, et al. Evaluation of the secretory immunoglobulin A levels in the colostrum and milk of mothers of term and pre-term newborns. Braz J Infect Dis 2005;9:357–62.
83. Caplan MS, Simon D, Jilling T. The role of PAF, TLR, and the inflammatory response in neonatal necrotizing enterocolitis. Semin Pediatr Surg 2005;14: 145–51.
84. Hsueh W, Gonzalez-Crussi F, Arroyave JL. Platelet-activating factor-induced ischemic bowel necrosis. An investigation of secondary mediators in its pathogenesis. Am J Pathol 1986;122:231–9.
85. Caplan M, Hsueh W, Kelly A, et al. Serum PAF acetylhydrolase increases during neonatal maturation. Prostaglandins 1990;39:705–14.
86. MacKendrick W, Hill N, Hsueh W, et al. Increase in plasma platelet-activating factor levels in enterally fed preterm infants. Biol Neonate 1993;64:89–95.
87. Furukawa M, Narahara H, Yasuda K, et al. Presence of platelet-activating factor-acetylhydrolase in milk. J Lipid Res 1993;34:1603–9.
88. Caplan MS, Hedlund E, Adler L, et al. The platelet-activating factor receptor antagonist WEB 2170 prevents neonatal necrotizing enterocolitis in rats. J Pediatr Gastroenterol Nutr 1997;24:296–301.
89. Ewer AK, Al-Salti W, Coney AM, et al. The role of platelet activating factor in a neonatal piglet model of necrotising enterocolitis. Gut 2004;53:207–13.
90. Caplan MS, Lickerman M, Adler L, et al. The role of recombinant platelet-activating factor acetylhydrolase in a neonatal rat model of necrotizing enterocolitis. Pediatr Res 1997;42:779–83.
91. Lu J, Pierce M, Franklin A, et al. Dual roles of endogenous platelet-activating factor acetylhydrolase in a murine model of necrotizing enterocolitis. Pediatr Res 2010;68:225–30.
92. Wang H, Tan X, Chang H, et al. Regulation of platelet-activating factor receptor gene expression in vivo by endotoxin, platelet-activating factor and endogenous tumour necrosis factor. Biochem J 1997;322(Pt 2):603–8.
93. Chokshi NK, Guner YS, Hunter CJ, et al. The role of nitric oxide in intestinal epithelial injury and restitution in neonatal necrotizing enterocolitis. Semin Perinatol 2008;32:92–9.
94. Potoka DA, Upperman JS, Nadler EP, et al. NF-kappaB inhibition enhances peroxynitrite-induced enterocyte apoptosis. J Surg Res 2002;106:7–14.
95. Stanford A, Chen Y, Zhang XR, et al. Nitric oxide mediates dendritic cell apoptosis by downregulating inhibitors of apoptosis proteins and upregulating effector caspase activity. Surgery 2001;130:326–32.
96. Ford H, Watkins S, Reblock K, et al. The role of inflammatory cytokines and nitric oxide in the pathogenesis of necrotizing enterocolitis. J Pediatr Surg 1997;32: 275–82.
97. D'Souza A, Fordjour L, Ahmad A, et al. Effects of probiotics, prebiotics, and synbiotics on messenger RNA expression of caveolin-1, NOS, and genes regulating

oxidative stress in the terminal ileum of formula-fed neonatal rats. Pediatr Res 2010;67:526–31.

98. Nadler EP, Dickinson E, Knisely A, et al. Expression of inducible nitric oxide synthase and interleukin-12 in experimental necrotizing enterocolitis. J Surg Res 2000;92:71–7.

99. Zhou Y, Wang Q, Mark Evers B, et al. Oxidative stress-induced intestinal epithelial cell apoptosis is mediated by p38 MAPK. Biochem Biophys Res Commun 2006;350:860–5.

100. Baregamian N, Song J, Papaconstantinou J, et al. Intestinal mitochondrial apoptotic signaling is activated during oxidative stress. Pediatr Surg Int 2011; 27:871–7.

101. Clark DA, Fornabaio DM, McNeill H, et al. Contribution of oxygen-derived free radicals to experimental necrotizing enterocolitis. Am J Pathol 1988;130:537–42.

102. Qu XW, Rozenfeld RA, Huang W, et al. The role of xanthine oxidase in platelet activating factor induced intestinal injury in the rat. Gut 1999;44:203–11.

103. Chaaban H, Shin M, Sirya E, et al. Inter-alpha inhibitor protein level in neonates predicts necrotizing enterocolitis. J Pediatr 2010;157:757–61.

104. Ng PC, Ang IL, Chiu RW, et al. Host-response biomarkers for diagnosis of late-onset septicemia and necrotizing enterocolitis in preterm infants. J Clin Invest 2010;120:2989–3000.

105. Edelson MB, Sonnino RE, Bagwell CE, et al. Plasma intestinal fatty acid binding protein in neonates with necrotizing enterocolitis: a pilot study. J Pediatr Surg 1999;34:1453–7.

106. Lobe TE, Richardson CJ, Rassin DK, et al. Hexosaminidase: a biochemical marker for necrotizing enterocolitis in the preterm infant. Am J Surg 1984;147: 49–52.

107. Bhandari V, Bizzarro MJ, Shetty A, et al. Familial and genetic susceptibility to major neonatal morbidities in preterm twins. Pediatrics 2006;117:1901–6.

108. Viscardi RM, Lyon NH, Sun CC, et al. Inflammatory cytokine mRNAs in surgical specimens of necrotizing enterocolitis and normal newborn intestine. Pediatr Pathol Lab Med 1997;17:547–59.

109. Caplan MS, Sun XM, Hseuh W, et al. Role of platelet activating factor and tumor necrosis factor-alpha in neonatal necrotizing enterocolitis. J Pediatr 1990;116: 960–4.

110. Tan X, Hsueh W, Gonzalez-Crussi F. Cellular localization of tumor necrosis factor (TNF)-alpha transcripts in normal bowel and in necrotizing enterocolitis. TNF gene expression by Paneth cells, intestinal eosinophils, and macrophages. Am J Pathol 1993;142:1858–65.

111. Halpern MD, Holubec H, Dominguez JA, et al. Up-regulation of IL-18 and IL-12 in the ileum of neonatal rats with necrotizing enterocolitis. Pediatr Res 2002;51: 733–9.

112. Halpern MD, Khailova L, Molla-Hosseini D, et al. Decreased development of necrotizing enterocolitis in IL-18-deficient mice. Am J Physiol Gastrointest Liver Physiol 2008;294:G20–6.

113. Maheshwari A, Christensen RD, Calhoun DA, et al. Circulating CXC-chemokine concentrations in a murine intestinal ischemia-reperfusion model. Fetal Pediatr Pathol 2004;23:145–57.

114. Benkoe T, Reck C, Pones M, et al. Interleukin-8 predicts 60-day mortality in premature infants with necrotizing enterocolitis. J Pediatr Surg 2014;49:385–9.

115. Bhatia AM, Stoll BJ, Cismowski MJ, et al. Cytokine levels in the preterm infant with neonatal intestinal injury. Am J Perinatol 2014;31:489–96.

116. Edelson MB, Bagwell CE, Rozycki HJ. Circulating pro- and counterinflammatory cytokine levels and severity in necrotizing enterocolitis. Pediatrics 1999;103: 766–71.
117. Harris MC, D'Angio CT, Gallagher PR, et al. Cytokine elaboration in critically ill infants with bacterial sepsis, necrotizing entercolitis, or sepsis syndrome: correlation with clinical parameters of inflammation and mortality. J Pediatr 2005;147: 462–8.
118. Lodha A, Asztalos E, Moore AM. Cytokine levels in neonatal necrotizing enterocolitis and long-term growth and neurodevelopment. Acta Paediatr 2010;99: 338–43.
119. Kling PJ, Hutter JJ. Hematologic abnormalities in severe neonatal necrotizing enterocolitis: 25 years later. J Perinatol 2003;23:523–30.
120. O'Neill JA Jr. Neonatal necrotizing enterocolitis. Surg Clin North Am 1981;61: 1013–22.
121. Hutter JJ Jr, Hathaway WE, Wayne ER. Hematologic abnormalities in severe neonatal necrotizing enterocolitis. J Pediatr 1976;88:1026–31.
122. Patel CC. Hematologic abnormalities in acute necrotizing enterocolitis. Pediatr Clin North Am 1977;24:579–84.
123. Kenton AB, O'Donovan D, Cass DL, et al. Severe thrombocytopenia predicts outcome in neonates with necrotizing enterocolitis. J Perinatol 2005;25:14–20.
124. Ververidis M, Kiely EM, Spitz L, et al. The clinical significance of thrombocytopenia in neonates with necrotizing enterocolitis. J Pediatr Surg 2001;36: 799–803.
125. Ragazzi S, Pierro A, Peters M, et al. Early full blood count and severity of disease in neonates with necrotizing enterocolitis. Pediatr Surg Int 2003;19: 376–9.
126. Sola MC, Del Vecchio A, Rimsza LM. Evaluation and treatment of thrombocytopenia in the neonatal intensive care unit. Clin Perinatol 2000;27:655–79.
127. Hsueh W, Caplan MS, Qu XW, et al. Neonatal necrotizing enterocolitis: clinical considerations and pathogenetic concepts. Pediatr Dev Pathol 2003;6:6–23.
128. Colarizi P, Fiorucci P, Caradonna A, et al. Circulating thrombopoietin levels in neonates with infection. Acta Paediatr 1999;88:332–7.
129. Oygur N, Tunga M, Mumcu Y, et al. Thrombopoietin levels of thrombocytopenic term and preterm newborns with infection. Am J Perinatol 2001;18:279–86.
130. Brown RE, Rimsza LM, Pastos K, et al. Effects of sepsis on neonatal thrombopoiesis. Pediatr Res 2008;64:399–404.
131. Sonntag J, Wagner MH, Waldschmidt J, et al. Multisystem organ failure and capillary leak syndrome in severe necrotizing enterocolitis of very low birth weight infants. J Pediatr Surg 1998;33:481–4.
132. Osborn DA, Lui K, Pussell P, et al. T and Tk antigen activation in necrotising enterocolitis: manifestations, severity of illness, and effectiveness of testing. Arch Dis Child Fetal Neonatal Ed 1999;80:F192–7.
133. Hall N, Ong EG, Ade-Ajayi N, et al. T cryptantigen activation is associated with advanced necrotizing enterocolitis. J Pediatr Surg 2002;37:791–3.
134. Boralessa H, Modi N, Cockburn H, et al. RBC T activation and hemolysis in a neonatal intensive care population: implications for transfusion practice. Transfusion 2002;42:1428–34.
135. Schutzman DL, Porat R. Glucose-6-phosphate dehydrogenase deficiency: another risk factor for necrotizing enterocolitis? J Pediatr 2007;151:435–7.
136. Detlefsen B, Boemers TM, Schimke C. Necrotizing enterocolitis in premature twins with twin-to-twin transfusion syndrome. Eur J Pediatr Surg 2008;18:50–2.

137. Singh R, Visintainer PF, Frantz ID 3rd, et al. Association of necrotizing enterocolitis with anemia and packed red blood cell transfusions in preterm infants. J Perinatol 2011;31:176–82.
138. Szabo JS, Mayfield SR, Oh W, et al. Postprandial gastrointestinal blood flow and oxygen consumption: effects of hypoxemia in neonatal piglets. Pediatr Res 1987;21:93–8.
139. Caplan MS, Jilling T. New concepts in necrotizing enterocolitis. Curr Opin Pediatr 2001;13:111–5.
140. Reber KM, Nankervis CA, Nowicki PT. Newborn intestinal circulation. Physiology and pathophysiology. Clin Perinatol 2002;29.23–39.
141. Schober PH, Nassiri J. Risk factors and severity indices in necrotizing enterocolitis. Acta Paediatr Suppl 1994;396:49–52.
142. Maheshwari A, Kurundkar AR, Shaik SS, et al. Epithelial cells in fetal intestine produce chemerin to recruit macrophages. Am J Physiol Gastrointest Liver Physiol 2009;297:G1–10.
143. Smythies LE, Maheshwari A, Clements R, et al. Mucosal IL-8 and TGF-beta recruit blood monocytes: evidence for cross-talk between the lamina propria stroma and myeloid cells. J Leukoc Biol 2006;80:492–9.
144. Christensen RD, Jensen J, Maheshwari A, et al. Reference ranges for blood concentrations of eosinophils and monocytes during the neonatal period defined from over 63 000 records in a multihospital health-care system. J Perinatol 2010;30:540–5.
145. van Furth R, Sluiter W. Distribution of blood monocytes between a marginating and a circulating pool. J Exp Med 1986;163:474–9.
146. Remon J, Kampanatkosol R, Kaul RR, et al. Acute drop in blood monocyte count differentiates NEC from other causes of feeding intolerance. J Perinatol 2014;34: 549–54.
147. Christensen RD, Lambert DK, Gordon PV, et al. Neonates presenting with bloody stools and eosinophilia can progress to two different types of necrotizing enterocolitis. J Perinatol 2012;32(11):874–9.
148. Kim D-H, Bae S-P, Hahn W-H, et al. Low basophil count and red cell distribution width at birth may predict the development of neonatal necrotizing enterocolitis: a matched control study. Soonchunhyang Med Sci 2013;19:61–4.
149. Hill DA, Siracusa MC, Abt MC, et al. Commensal bacteria-derived signals regulate basophil hematopoiesis and allergic inflammation. Nat Med 2012;18: 538–46.
150. Lambert DK, Christensen RD, Baer VL, et al. Fulminant necrotizing enterocolitis in a multihospital healthcare system. J Perinatol 2012;32:194–8.
151. Mandel D, Lubetzky R, Mimouni FB, et al. Nucleated red blood cells in preterm infants who have necrotizing enterocolitis. J Pediatr 2004;144:653–5.
152. Baschat AA, Gungor S, Kush ML, et al. Nucleated red blood cell counts in the first week of life: a critical appraisal of relationships with perinatal outcome in preterm growth-restricted neonates. Am J Obstet Gynecol 2007;197:286.e1–8.

Hematologic Aspects of Early and Late-Onset Sepsis in Preterm Infants

Paolo Manzoni, MD, PhD

KEYWORDS

- Preterm neonates • Infection • Hematology • Neutropenia • Thrombocytopenia
- *Candida spp* • CMV

KEY POINTS

- Hematologic changes during neonatal sepsis may occur and may be of diagnostic and prognostic help.
- Suspicion of a specific pathogen based on hematologic changes during sepsis is an open issue.
- Neutropenia and neutrophilia are frequently associated with sepsis, but correction of neutropenia is not associated with improved outcomes in sepsis.
- Thrombocytopenia is very common in sepsis and is a marker of severity with high predictivity for poor outcomes.
- *Candida spp* and cytomegalovirus are the pathogens most frequently associated with severe thrombocytopenia in preterm neonates.

INTRODUCTION

Hematologic changes during sepsis and infection in preterm neonates are frequent and may be seen as a diagnostic sign on one hand as well as a prognostic sign on the other hand.

As a preliminary consideration, it is important to remember that the reference ranges for the various blood cell elements in the neonatal period are not stable but change considerably according to gestational and postnatal age. The normal ranges established in healthy adults cannot be used; therefore, reference ranges originating from analysis of large neonatal datasets are mandatory in order to appropriately assess and guide diagnostics and treatment.[1]

Conflict of Interest Statement: The author has no commercial or financial conflicts of interest as well as no funding sources to disclose related to this article.
Division of Neonatology and NICU, Sant'Anna Hospital, Azienda Ospedaliera Universitaria Città della Salute e della Scienza, Torino 10126, Italy
E-mail address: paolomanzoni@hotmail.com

The extent of all hematologic changes ultimately depends on the severity of sepsis, on the peripheral consumption, and on the bone marrow reserve—this last being specifically decreased in preterm infants.

During neonatal sepsis, leucocytes and platelets are more frequently affected than red blood cells. **Table 1** summarizes the main trends of all possible hematologic changes that may occur during neonatal sepsis for all the different blood cells.

The most frequently encountered features are an abnormal total leukocyte count, an abnormal total neutrophil (polymorphonuclear neutrophil [PMN]) count, an elevated immature PMN count, an elevated immature to total PMN ratio, an abnormal immature to mature PMN ratio (eg, ≥ 0.3), a low platelet count (eg, $\leq 80,000/mm^3$), and the occurrence of pronounced degenerative changes in PMNs.

A specific association of each of these features with specific causative pathogens has been occasionally suggested only for some of these features.

This article reviews and updates the state of the art on this topic, discussing all hematologic changes occurring during neonatal sepsis and their implications both as diagnostic and prognostic parameters to guide clinicians at the bedside.

Red Blood Cells

In preterm neonates, anemia is commonly observed; its onset, or worsening, is not specifically related to infections, at least not in the same way that it may occur in older patients.

Nonetheless, although clearly anemia itself is not a diagnostic clue for sepsis, an episode of infection may unchain clusters of immune or nonimmune hemolysis, hemophagocytosis, or direct infection of progenitor cells (eg, by parvovirus B19), and so forth.[1]

Measurements of the red cell distribution width (RDW) ranges at birth have been evaluated for potential association with several neonatal diseases, including late-onset sepsis (LOS) in full-term, preterm, and intrauterine growth–restricted infants. Preterm newborns with such conditions feature higher RDW than others; specifically, those affected by sepsis have statistically significant higher RDW before 3 days of life; hence, some investigators speculate that high RDW might be an indication of risk for critical newborns at risk of LOS.[2] It is likely that an instable erythropoiesis can occur, and often the general inflammatory state typically occurring in the critical preterm infant may add to the sepsis-driven stress condition, thus furthermore impacting on the RDW values of septic neonates that might be higher than normal under such conditions.

Leucocytes

Neutrophils

It is well known that neonatal neutrophil function and kinetics are hugely different from those of adults, specifically during infection. The neutrophil response in such patients

Table 1
Summary of hematologic changes in neonatal sepsis

Pathogen or Group of Pathogens	RBC Count	WBC Count	Neutrophils Count	Lymphocytes Count	Platelets Count
Gram positives	a	↑ or ↓	a (rarely↓)	a	↓↓
Gram negatives	a	↑or ↓	↓	a	↓
Fungi	a	↑or ↓	↓↓	a	↓↓↓

Abbreviations: RBC, red blood cells; WBC, white blood cells.
a Inconsistent and unpredictive changes.

may be less robust and thus may not be fully effective in contrasting pathogens and protect from systemic infection.

In addition, similar to other patients, changes in neutrophil count can be associated with the occurrence of systemic infections also in preterm neonates.

In the literature, early onset neutropenia has been described as related with several pathologic features in premature neonates, including maternal hypertension, intrauterine growth restriction, severe asphyxia, periventricular hemorrhage, early onset and LOS, bronchopulmonary dysplasia, and colonization by Candida spp.[3]

During neonatal bacterial infections, increased levels of activated complement products, granulocyte colony-stimulating factor (G-CSF), and proinflammatory cytokines, such as tumor necrosis factor α, interleukin 1 (IL-1), and IL-6, may cause an initial and transient neutrophilia (more frequently) but also neutropenia.

Neutropenia is a condition of reduced PMN count, and in the normal neonate it is often identified as less than $500/mm^3$ or less than $1000/mm^3$ but rapidly decreasing.

Several studies have been conducted to establish and validate neonatal neutrophil reference ranges and to determine the usefulness of serial measurements of neutrophil values in the first days of life to screen the likelihood of developing early onset or late-onset neonatal sepsis. The most used reference value charts have historically been those published by Manroe and colleagues[4] and Mouzinho and colleagues[5] in the early 1990s.

More recently, updated reference values have been published and validated through a retrospective study on more than 2000 preterm neonates. This study provided confirming evidence that neutropenia and nonspecific neutrophilia actually occur not rarely in uninfected preterm neonates but also that the distribution of neutrophil values is significantly different between infants who would later develop infections or not. Absolute total immature neutrophils and immature to total neutrophil proportions are reported as having a very good predictability for early onset sepsis greater than 6 hours' postnatal age. As a result, serial determination of neutrophil values at 0, 12, and 24 hours, together with blood culture and clinical evaluation, may be suggested as a tool to manage discontinuation of antimicrobial therapy at 36 to 48 hours of life.[6]

Similar to other categories of patients, initial neutrophilia is related to mobilization of neutrophils from the bone marrow storage pool (mainly neutrophils and band forms) into the circulation and occurs in most neonates with gram-positive bacterial infections. Patients with gram-negative bacterial infections may present with extreme neutrophilia but may also feature neutropenia. In this last case, derangements in the neutrophil count are often associated with similar events in the platelet count, with such features occurring more frequently in the case of septic shock.[7]

Although it is recommendable to carefully evaluate the neutrophil counts in premature and critically ill neonates, the true clinical significance of these changes is still debated.

In other categories of patients, neutropenia is associated with increased risk of severe infections and sepsis-related mortality, and is a well-known risk factor for severe infections in hematology and oncology. This might not be the case with preterm neonates.

In neonates, this condition may occasionally be prolonged and translate into a serious antimicrobial deficiency in selected patients whereby it actually become a long-lasting risk factor for bacterial sepsis.[8] However, neonatal neutropenia is more often considered benign and self-limiting in most neonates.[9]

A retrospective study on 338 very-low-birth-weight (VLBW) neonates found that early neutropenia (defined in this study as an absolute neutrophil count less than

1500/µl at any time during the first week of life) was not associated with the occurrence of late-onset infections.[10]

Consistent with these findings, administration of G-CSF or granulocyte-macrophage colony-stimulating factor (GM-CSF), although likely safe and without adverse side effects, might be helpful in correcting neutropenia but not beneficial in treating and/or preventing sepsis and sepsis-related poor outcomes in preterm infants.[11] A multicenter randomized controlled trial (RCT) assessed whether GM-CSF administered as a prophylaxis (10 µg/kg/d subcutaneously for 5 days) to preterm neonates at high risk of neutropenia would reduce sepsis, mortality, and morbidity compared with standard management. The investigators found that, as expected, neutrophil counts after trial entry were increasing significantly more rapidly in infants treated with GM-CSF than in controls during the first 11 days but that there was no significant difference in sepsis-free survival for all infants.

This evidence supports the idea that early postnatal prophylactic GM-CSF can correct neutropenia but cannot reduce the incidence of sepsis or improve short-term infection-associated outcomes in preterm neonates.[12] Other RCTs added recently to this one[13,14]; but still there is an ultimate need for adequately powered, randomized controlled clinical trials of neutropenic infants to further and fully assess the efficacy of these agents as adjuncts to antibiotic therapy.[15]

Even though changes in neutrophil count may be of limited clinical value, as discussed earlier, the same changes can have some prognostic value because clinical improvement and control of sepsis is always associated with a return to normality of neutrophil counts as well as of platelet counts. In addition, there is evidence suggesting that neutrophil counts and various neutrophil indices can respond differently to different causative microorganisms, providing room for a possible usefulness of these findings in the diagnostic algorithm of neonatal sepsis. In fact, total white blood cells and neutrophil count are reported significantly lower in infants with late-onset gram-negative sepsis compared with gram-positive bacterial and fungal sepsis. Therefore, occurrence of neutropenia during sepsis in VLBW infants might be more common with gram-negative bacterial infection.[16]

Maternal preeclampsia is a condition frequently associated with premature birth, and neonates born to preeclamptic mothers often have low or very-low birth weights, therefore, featuring, per se, an increased risk for infections. Of note, maternal preeclampsia is specifically associated with neonatal neutropenia[17,18]; this condition might expose the premature neonate to an increased risk of infection, although this association has been occasionally questioned.[10] Actually, neutropenic neonates have increased risk of fungal colonization[19]; additionally, the number of sites colonized by Candida spp and the condition of neutropenia are associated with Candidaemia.[20] Because maternal preeclampsia is associated with neonatal hyperglycaemia[21] and because this last is associated with Candida systemic infection in extremely premature neonates,[22] it is clear that complex relationships exist involving the neutrophil count and the risk of developing infectious events caused specifically by Candida spp in premature neonates and that this risk might be originating, even partially, already during pregnancy.

Lymphocytes

Lymphocyte values reference ranges have been recently established by Christensen and colleagues[23] on 40,487 neonates. The lymphocyte count normally drops after birth, possibly related to the corticosteroid surge during labor and delivery; but a few hours later the count reaches a plateau and remains stable up to the first 12 to 18 hours of life.[24]

It has been suggested that low lymphocyte counts in the first hours after birth is associated with early onset sepsis.[25] However, according to recent, larger datasets, both a high count and a low count at birth can be significantly associated with early onset sepsis.[1]

Prolonged lymphopenia (absolute lymphocyte count <1000 for >7 days) is reported as associated independently with nosocomial infection and occurring more frequently in infants with multiple organ failure (MOF), possibly related to prolonged hypoprolactinemia (>7 days) leading to lymphoid depletion.[26]

Platelets

The occurrence of thrombocytopenia is not rare in the preterm neonate, and can develop or worsen abruptly from 72 hours of life onwards in preterm neonates in a neonatal intensive care unit with a frequency that is inversely correlated with the gestational age.

However, the magnitude of the occurrence of thrombocytopenia is uncertain since inconsistent definitions of this condition are reported in the literature, hence, determining difficultly comparable incidence rates in different published studies.

Thrombocytopenia should be defined as a platelet count less than the fifth percentile reference range (platelet count of 104,000/μL for infants <32 weeks' gestation and 123,000/μL for late preterm and term neonates) for gestational age and postnatal age.[27] However, in the "bedside, real-life" absolute platelet counts are used more often, making the case for different thresholds of low platelet counts that have actually been identified as *thrombocytopenia*, with this last being defined, in different studies, as at least one finding of a platelet count less than 150,000, less than 80,000, or even less than 50,000/mm^3.[28]

There is a general agreement that the smallest extremely low-birth-weight neonates (ie, those weighing less than 750 g at birth) may have the highest likelihood of featuring pathologically decreased platelet counts. In such infants, the most frequently encountered possible causative factors behind thrombocytopenia are LOS and necrotizing enterocolitis (NEC).[28] In a recent study, a platelet count less than 80,000/mm^3 was detected in 35% of all septic VLBW preterm infants.[29] A secondary analysis of prospectively collected data from an RCT on prevention of sepsis and NEC in VLBW infants with the use of bovine lactoferrin[30] provides confirming evidence of a statistically significant association between thrombocytopenia (here defined as a platelet count <80,000/mm^3) and LOS (any pathogen) in such infants but reduces the burden of this condition. At least one finding of low platelet count occurred in 5.6% of all VLBW septic neonates, compared with 2.1% of the VLBW infants who did not experience any septic episodes (P<.05). Among all pathogens, gram positives (incidence rate of thrombocytopenia = 14.7%) and gram negatives (incidence rate of thrombocytopenia = 6.5%) were the groups of pathogens most frequently and significantly associated with this feature (Manzoni and colleagues, 2015, unpublished data).

The pathways leading to a decrease in the platelet count during neonatal infections basically involve and combine exaggerated consumption and impaired production. The reticule-endothelial removal of platelets activated by endothelial damage is enhanced, and neonates respond to this trigger with an upregulation of the thrombopoiesis. Thrombocytopenia develops only after platelet production cannot fully replace platelet destruction, which is related to serum thrombopoietin levels.[31,32] It is also important to underline that the median absolute immature platelet fraction (IPF) significantly decreases soon after the onset of sepsis; therefore, low absolute IPF values during the course of neonatal sepsis suggest suppression of megakaryopoietic activity.[33]

A decrease in the platelet count usually develops with the early signs of sepsis or NEC and often progresses rapidly, with a platelet nadir reached within 24 to 48 hours.[34]

Neonatal thrombocytopenia is commonly considered as an additional marker of the severity of sepsis and has been identified as a potent predictor of sepsis-associated mortality in a recent study revealing that the need for intubation, initiation of vasopressors, hypoglycemia, and thrombocytopenia as presenting laboratory signs of infection and NEC are the most predictive, independent risk factors for sepsis-related death.[35]

What is discussed for neutrophils is also similar for platelets in that the existence of a specific response to different infectious agents has been postulated and has been the object of extensive investigation.

Some studies in the literature have illustrated a specificity of thrombocytopenia for one or more microorganisms (or a group of). A possible specificity would clearly allow hypotheses of a use of this finding as an early diagnostic, specific marker for a certain causative pathogen (or group of) in neonatal sepsis. Unfortunately the evidence in this area is controversial because the studies came to different conclusions. Currently, it is, therefore, unclear whether thrombocytopenia is suggestive of one (or more) causative agents of neonatal sepsis. Different infectious agents (gram-negative, fungi, and coagulase-negative *Staphylococcus*, in turn) have all been found to have a tendency to affect the platelet count; as a matter of fact, a low platelet count has been related in turn to gram-positive, gram-negative, or fungal sepsis.

Neonates with gram-negative sepsis might feature more thrombocytopenia and more severe illness but less thrombopoietic response (downregulation of thrombo-poietic response during severe illness) to relative hypoproliferation. The most convincing data seem to show that no major differences exist in the platelet response among LOS caused by gram-positive, gram-negative, and fungal microorganisms, thus, excluding an organism-specific role for thrombocytopenia.

Nonetheless, it is worthy to briefly mention 2 septic patterns in which thrombocyto-penia has been described as particularly frequent, specifically in the most immature preterm neonates (eg, systemic candidiasis) and systemic viral infections (first of all, acquired systemic cytomegalovirus [CMV] infection).

In this last event, similar to what occurs in any other immunosuppressed patient, thrombocytopenia may be secondary to either immune-mediated platelet destruction with or without immune-mediated megakaryocyte damage or alternatively to direct toxicity to megakaryocytes resulting from viral infection of these cells.

A low platelet count is such a frequent finding in systemic CMV perinatal disease that thrombocytopenia has often been reported as the main reason to analyze the infant's urine for diagnostic purposes because it is reported that up to 50% of CMV-affected infants may present with thrombocytopenia as the only symptom.[36] CMV can directly infect megakaryocytes and cause impaired platelet production and release. Just as in other septic situations, systemic CMV infection thrombocytopenia may be seen a marker of severity of disease, especially when associated with NEC.

As for candidiasis, its association with thrombocytopenia is so frequent and sugges-tive that thrombocytopenia (defined as a platelet count <80,000/mm^3) is one of the 3 items entered into a clinical predictive model tested at multivariable analysis for neonatal candidemia with high sensitivity and moderate specificity.[37] According to this model, when a physician obtains a blood culture, the physician should consider providing antifungal therapy to neonates who are less than 25 weeks' estimated gestational age and to neonates who have thrombocytopenia at the time of blood culture or a history of third-generation cephalosporin or carbapenem exposure in the 7 days before the blood culture. In this model, thrombocytopenia stands with high predictivity, with an odds ratio of 3.56 as a specific risk factor predictive of imminent, ongoing candidemia.

SUMMARY

Neonatal infections and sepsis are, by definition, systemic diseases in premature neonates; therefore, the involvement of blood cell elements and (to a larger extent) of the hematopoietic organs (bone marrow, liver, and spleen) can be expected and needs to be ruled out. Hematologic changes may be not only suggestive of infection but also a cluster of severity and progression of this disease. Therefore, monitoring serum values of neutrophils and platelets may provide useful information on the progression of the infection and the response to treatment and sometimes can be helpful in targeting specific pathogens as possible causative agents.

REFERENCES

1. Christensen RD, Henry E, Jopling J, et al. The CBC: reference ranges for neonates. Semin Perinatol 2009;33(1):3–11.
2. Garofoli F, Ciardelli L, Mazzucchelli I, et al. The red cell distribution width (RDW): value and role in preterm, IUGR (intrauterine growth restricted), full-term infants. Hematology 2014;19(6):365–9.
3. Del Vecchio A, Christensen RD. Neonatal neutropenia: what diagnostic evaluation is needed and when is treatment recommended? Early Hum Dev 2012; 88(Suppl 2):S19–24.
4. Manroe BL, Weinberg AG, Rosenfeld CR, et al. The neonatal blood count in health and disease. Reference values for neutrophilic cells. J Pediatr 1979;95: 89–98.
5. Mouzinho A, Rosenfeld CR, Sanchez PJ, et al. Revised reference ranges for circulating neutrophils in very low birth weight neonates. Pediatrics 1994;94: 76–82.
6. Mikhael M, Brown LS, Rosenfeld CR. Serial neutrophil values facilitate predicting the absence of neonatal early-onset sepsis. J Pediatr 2014;164(3):522–8.e1–3.
7. Funke A, Berner R, Traichel B, et al. Frequency, natural course, and outcome of neonatal neutropenia. Pediatrics 2000;106:45–51.
8. Doron MW, Makhlouf RA, Katz VL, et al. Increased incidence of sepsis at birth in neutropenic infants of mothers with preeclampsia. J Pediatr 1994; 125:452–8.
9. Maheshwari A. Neutropenia in the newborn. Curr Opin Hematol 2014;21(1):43–9.
10. Teng RJ, Wu TJ, Garrison RD, et al. Early neutropenia is not associated with an increased rate of nosocomial infection in very low-birth-weight infants. J Perinatol 2009;29(3):219–24.
11. Carr R, Modi N, Dore C. G-CSF and GM-CSF for treating or preventing neonatal infections. Cochrane Database Syst Rev 2003;(3):CD003066.
12. Carr R, Brocklehurst P, Doré CJ, et al. Granulocyte-macrophage colony stimulating factor administered as prophylaxis for reduction of sepsis in extremely preterm, small for gestational age neonates (the PROGRAMS trial): a single-blind, multicentre, randomised controlled trial. Lancet 2009;373(9659):226–33.
13. Kuhn P, Messer J, Paupe A, et al. A multicenter, randomized, placebo-controlled trial of prophylactic recombinant granulocyte-colony stimulating factor in preterm neonates with neutropenia. J Pediatr 2009;155:324–30.
14. Marlow N, Morris T, Brocklehurst P, et al. A randomised trial of granulocyte-macrophage colony-stimulating factor for neonatal sepsis: outcomes at 2 years. Arch Dis Child Fetal Neonatal Ed 2013;98:F46–53.
15. Castagnola E, Dufour C. Role of G-CSF GM-CSF in the management of infections in preterm newborns: an update. Early Hum Dev 2014;90(Suppl 2):S15–7.

16. Sarkar S, Bhagat I, Hieber S, et al. Can neutrophil responses in very low birth weight infants predict the organisms responsible for late-onset bacterial or fungal sepsis? J Perinatol 2006;26(8):501–5.

17. Procianoy RS, Silveira RC, Mussi-Pinhata MM, et al. Brazilian Network on Neonatal Research. Sepsis and neutropenia in very low birth weight infants delivered of mothers with preeclampsia. J Pediatr 2010;157:434–8.

18. Manzoni P, Rizzollo S, Mostert M, et al. Preeclampsia, neutropenia, and risk of fungal sepsis in preterm very low birth weight infants. J Pediatr 2011;158(1):173–4 [author reply: 174].

19. Manzoni P, Farina D, Monetti C, et al. Early-onset neutropenia is a risk factor for Candida colonization in very low-birth-weight neonates. Diagn Microbiol Infect Dis 2007;57:77–83.

20. Mahieu LM, Van Gasse N, Wildemeersch D, et al. Number of sites of perinatal Candida colonization and neutropenia are associated with nosocomial candidemia in the neonatal intensive care unit patient. Pediatr Crit Care Med 2010;11:240–5.

21. Manzoni P, Baù MG, Farina D. Glucose regulation in preterm infants with very low birth weight. N Engl J Med 2007;357:616–7.

22. Manzoni P, Castagnola E, Mostert M, et al. Hyperglycaemia as a possible marker of invasive fungal infection in preterm neonates. Acta Paediatr 2006;95:486–93.

23. Christensen RD, Baer VL, Gordon PV, et al. Reference ranges for lymphocyte counts of neonates: associations between abnormal counts and outcomes. Pediatrics 2012;129(5):e1165–72.

24. Shah V, Beyene J, Shah P, et al. Association between hematologic findings and brain injury due to neonatal hypoxic-ischemic encephalopathy. Am J Perinatol 2009;26(4):295–302.

25. Glavina-Durdov M, Springer O, Capkun V, et al. The grade of acute thymus involution in neonates correlates with the duration of acute illness and with the percentage of lymphocytes in peripheral blood smear. Pathological study. Biol Neonate 2003;83(4):229–34.

26. Felmet KA, Hall MW, Clark RS, et al. Prolonged lymphopenia, lymphoid depletion, and hypoprolactinemia in children with nosocomial sepsis and multiple organ failure. J Immunol 2005;174(6):3765–72.

27. Wiedmeier SE, Henry E, Sola-Visner MC, et al. Platelet reference ranges for neonates, defined using data from over 47,000 patients in a multihospital healthcare system. J Perinatol 2009;29:130–6.

28. Del Vecchio A. Evaluation and management of thrombocytopenic neonates in the intensive care unit. Early Hum Dev 2014;90(Suppl 2):S51–5.

29. Roberts I, Murray NA. Neonatal thrombocytopenia: causes and management. Arch Dis Child Fetal Neonatal Ed 2003;88:F359–64.

30. Manzoni P, Meyer M, Stolfi I, et al. Bovine lactoferrin supplementation for prevention of necrotizing enterocolitis in very-low-birth-weight neonates: a randomized clinical trial. Early Hum Dev 2014;90(Suppl 1):S60–5.

31. Brown RE, Rimsza LM, Pastos K, et al. Effects of sepsis on neonatal thrombopoiesis. Pediatr Res 2008;64(4):399–404.

32. Eissa DS, El-Farrash RA. New insights into thrombopoiesis in neonatal sepsis. Platelets 2013;24(2):122–8.

33. Cremer M, Weimann A, Szekessy D, et al. Low immature platelet fraction suggests decreased megakaryopoiesis in neonates with sepsis or necrotizing enterocolitis. J Perinatol 2013;33(8):622–6.

34. Murray NA, Howarth LJ, McCloy MP, et al. Platelet transfusion in the management of severe thrombocytopenia in neonatal intensive care unit patients. Transfus Med 2002;12:35–41.
35. Levit O, Bhandari V, Li FY, et al. Clinical and laboratory factors that predict death in very low birth weight infants presenting with late-onset sepsis. Pediatr Infect Dis J 2014;33(2):143–6.
36. Mehler K, Oberthuer A, Lang-Roth R, et al. High rate of symptomatic cytomegalovirus infection in extremely low gestational age preterm infants of 22-24 weeks' gestation after transmission via breast milk. Neonatology 2014;105(1):27–32.
37. Benjamin DK Jr, DeLong ER, Steinbach WJ, et al. Empirical therapy for neonatal candidemia in very low birth weight infants. Pediatrics 2003;112(3 Pt 1):543–7.

Stem Cells

Potential Therapy for Neonatal Injury?

Momoko Yoshimoto, MD, PhD[a], Joyce M. Koenig, MD[b,c],*

KEYWORDS

- Stem cells • Hematopoiesis • Cord blood • Transplantation • Neonate • Injury

KEY POINTS

- Umbilical cord blood (CB) contains a plethora of stem cells and multipotent progenitor cells (MPPs).
- In preclinical animal models, transplantation with CB or specific stemlike cells can limit brain and lung injury and/or preserve or restore function in part through antiinflammatory mechanisms.
- The few human studies to date suggest the short-term safety of CB-derived stem cells; however, additional preclinical and human studies are needed to establish therapeutic efficacy and long-term safety.

INTRODUCTION

Stem cell transplantation (SCT) is an established first-line or adjunctive therapy for a variety of neonatal diseases, including those involving inborn errors of metabolism, types of primary immune deficiencies, certain neutrophil disorders, and hematologic malignancies, such as neonatal leukemia. The utility of SCT in these and related conditions has been extensively discussed in the literature and is beyond the scope of the present review.[1–6] This article briefly summarizes current understanding of human stem cell biology during ontogeny and presents recent evidence of the potential role of SCT for the treatment of postinsult neonatal injury.

Disclosure Statement: The authors have no conflicts of interest relevant to the present review to disclose.
[a] Pediatrics, Wells Center for Pediatric Research, Indiana University School of Medicine, 1044 West Walnut Street, R4-W116, Indianapolis, IN 46202, USA; [b] Pediatrics, E Doisy Research Center, Saint Louis University School of Medicine, 1100 South Grand Boulevard, St Louis, MO 63104, USA; [c] Molecular Microbiology & Immunology, E Doisy Research Center, Saint Louis University School of Medicine, 1100 South Grand Boulevard, St Louis, MO 63106, USA
* Corresponding author. Pediatrics, Molecular Microbiology & Immunology, E Doisy Research Center, Saint Louis University School of Medicine, 1100 South Grand Boulevard, St Louis, MO 63104.
E-mail address: koenijm@slu.edu

STEM CELL BIOLOGY: A BRIEF REVIEW
Stem Cell Theory: Pluripotent Stem Cells and Tissue-Specific Somatic Stem Cells

Two main types of stem cells have been described: pluripotent stem cells (PSCs) and somatic stem cells. The PSCs are multipotent stem cells that can differentiate into all cell types in the body and include embryonic stem cells (ESCs) and inducible PSCs (iPSCs). Tissue-specific somatic stem cells give rise to organ-specific cell types. ESCs are first established from the inner cell mass of the blastocysts in a fertilized egg.[7-9] In vitro studies have shown that cultured ESCs display self-renewal ability and have the capacity for multilineage differentiation. ESCs can differentiate into cell types that include all 3 germ layers, and in vivo studies have shown that ESCs can form teratomas when inoculated into immune-deficient mice. Murine studies have shown that when a fertilized egg is injected with ESCs and implanted into a pseudopregnant dam, ESC-derived cells contribute to all embryonic cell types, forming a chimeric animal. The multilineage differentiation ability of ESCs both in vivo and in vitro highlights their potential utility for stem cell therapies. This therapeutic potential is accompanied, however, by ethical problems because ESCs can be derived only from fertilized eggs.

More recently, ESC-like PSCs have been established from postnatal mouse testis and adult mouse/human somatic cells after the introduction of stemness genes, such as Oct4, c-Myc, Sox2, and Klf4.[10-12] These iPSCs overcome the ethical problems associated with ESCs; thus, iPSC biology and its possibilities for clinical applications have been the focus of intensive research. Although mouse ESCs/iPSCs have been shown to differentiate into somatic stem cells in vivo in chimeric animals, the induction of tissue-specific somatic stem cells from iPSCs remains a challenging problem. One primary reason for this is the difficulty in maintaining iPSC-derived stem cells in cell lineages that require rapid cell cycling of their progenitors to maintain cellular homeostasis (such as in the blood, skin, and skeletal muscles). Thus, the use of iPSCs to produce functional progenitor cells or even mature cells may be most successful when cellular targets have slow intrinsic cycling rates and thus do not require rapid somatic cellular replacement. Recent major advances in iPSC-derived cell therapy have been reported in a nonhuman primate spinal injury model and in a clinical trial of iPSC-derived retinal pigment epithelium replacement.[13,14]

According to currently accepted stem cell theory, each tissue in the body is maintained by tissue-specific stem cells with the capacity for self-renewal and specific lineage differentiation. During embryonic organogenesis, stem cells differentiate into lineage cells that form specific tissues. These stem cells are maintained in the tissues even during adulthood: for example, cell types, such as hair, skin, melanocytes, blood, muscle, intestinal epithelium, and sperm, are continuously regenerated by tissue-specific stem/progenitor cells. Although the healthy liver does not typically undergo tissue regeneration, if damaged the liver becomes a regenerative organ. Stem/progenitor cells, which have been identified in every tissue/organ, reside in a special microenvironment, called a niche, which facilitates the maintenance of self-renewal capacity. Although the brain and nervous system were not previously considered to have regenerative abilities, recent studies have identified stem/progenitor cells and their niches even in adult animals.[15-17] These cells may play a role in the maintenance of tissue homeostasis and can acquire the ability to produce lineage-specific cells for tissue regeneration after injury.

Recent technological advances have facilitated the identification, isolation, and purification of human somatic stem cells. The hematopoietic stem cell (HSC), the first stem cell to be experimentally proved in humans, resides in the bone marrow (BM) and is thus readily accessible for clinical purposes. Blood stem/progenitor cells have a homing ability that enables their migration to and engraftment in the BM of the recipient when administered intravenously, without the need for surgical implanting procedures. HSC transplantation has been successfully performed to treat a wide spectrum of hematopoietic disorders and malignancies.

The hematopoietic system is the best in vivo example of the somatic stem cell theory. Post-transplantation bioassays have defined HSCs and confirmed their self-renewal and multilineage blood cell differentiation capacities.[18-20] Long-term (LT)-HSCs exhibit prolonged engraftment in recipient BM (more than 4 months in mice and 4–8 months In humans) and are secondary transplantable. LT-HSCs sit at the apex of the hematopoietic hierarchy system (**Fig. 1**) and give rise to short-term (ST)-HSCs, or MPPs, that engraft recipient BM for less than 4 months. ST-HSCs/MPPs differentiate into lymphoid-primed progenitor cells (LMPPs) and common myeloid progenitor cells (CMPs) in mice or into multilymphoid progenitors (MLPs) and CMP in humans. Murine LMPPs and human MLPs are primarily lymphoid progenitors that produce B and T cells but retain myeloid potential. The more lineage-specific CMPs give rise to erythrocyte, megakaryocytes, granulocytes, monocytes/macrophages, and dendritic cells. Thus, HSCs produce a wide variety of blood cells and are maintained by self-renewal mechanisms within the hematopoietic BM niche.

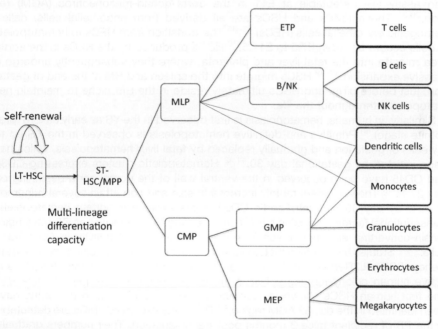

Fig. 1. Hematopoietic hierarchy system. Long-term hematopoietic stem cells (LT-HSCs) sit on the apex of the hematopoietic hierarchy system and maintain self-renewal capacity residing in the niche, and multi-lineage differentiation capacity by asymmetric cell division. B/NK, B cells and natural killer cells; CMP, common myeloid progenitor cell; ETP, earliest T lymphoid progenitor cell; GMP, granulocyte-macrophage progenitor cell; MEP, megakaryocyte and erythroid progenitor cell; MLP, multilymphoid progenitor cell; MPP, multipotent progenitor cell; NK cells, natural killer cells; ST-HSC, short-term hematopoietic stem cell.

Since the discovery of HSCs in umbilical CB and the first successful CB transplantation in a patient with Fanconi anemia in 1989, CB has been widely used for HSC transplantation in addition to BM or mobilized peripheral blood (PB) HSCs.[21–23] This article describes the development of HSCs in the human embryo/fetus and other stem/progenitor cells found in CB. Ongoing and possible clinical applications using CB and related stem cells are also discussed.

Hematopoietic Stem Cell Development in Mouse and Human Embryos

The first HSCs are produced during embryogenesis but are also found in the adult BM niche at steady state. Human CB contains proportionately greater numbers of circulating CD34+ HSCs than does the PB of adults.[24]

Developmental hematopoiesis has been well described in mice, an ideal model given a short (19-day) gestation.[25] The first site of hematopoiesis, the extraembryonic yolk sac (YS) at embryonic day (E) 7.5, consists of mainly large erythroid cells, called primitive erythrocytes.[26] Primitive erythrocytes express embryonic-type hemoglobin molecules and have a large nucleus.[27] Erythroid progenitor cells that express adult type hemoglobin molecules are called definitive erythroid progenitor cells and are detected from E8.0 YS together with myeloid progenitors.[28] The progenitors of definitive erythroid cells and myeloid cells are called erythromyeloid progenitors (EMPs) and are produced mainly in the YS during E8 to 10.[29] The first murine HSCs that can reconstitute lethally irradiated adult marrow by transplantation assay are detectable at E11 in the aorta-gonad-mesonephros (AGM) region.[30,31] These EMPs and HSCs are all derived from endothelial cells, called hemogenic endothelial cells (HECs).[32–35] The transition from HECs to hematopoietic cells occurs between E7.5 to E11.5.[36] HSCs produced by the HECs in the aortic area migrate into the fetal liver and placenta, where they subsequently undergo a massive expansion.[37–39] HSCs migrate into the spleen and BM at the end of gestation, just before birth, and HSCs ultimately reside in the BM niche to maintain hematopoiesis throughout the life.

Similarly, in humans, hematopoiesis is first observed in the YS as early as E18 (presomite stage).[40] Primitive and definitive hematopoiesis is observed in the YS up to 7 weeks of gestation and gradually replaced by fetal liver hematopoiesis, which has been initiated by gestational day 30.[41,42] Hematopoietic clusters expressing CD34 and CD45 have been observed in the ventral wall of the dorsal aorta beginning on day 27.[43–45] These clusters rapidly increase in size and can attain several hundreds of cells by day 36. The intra-aortic CD34+ cells express important hematopoietic transcriptional factors, including tal/SCL, c-myb, and GATA2 as well as CD143 (angiotensin-converting enzyme), which is known to enrich HSC activity in CB CD34+ cells.[46,47] Studies have shown that nonobese diabetic/severe combined immune deficiency (SCID)/IL2Rγcnull (NSG) mice can be reconstituted with human HSC,[48] and active human colony-forming activities are detectable in the recipient mouse BM. The first human HSCs shown to reconstitute NSG mice for up to 8 months have been identified in the day 32 AGM region.[49] These AGM-derived HSCs are detectable in the PB of recipient mice 3 months post-transplantation. Their numbers gradually increase over time, reaching up to 90% of chimerism by 8 months after transplantation.

Human AGM-derived cells also reconstitute secondary recipient mice and display self-renewal capacity (a key measure of stem cell function), generating at least 300 daughter HSCs.[49] HSCs in the AGM region express CD34, CD45, vascular endothelial (VE)-cadherin, c-kit, thy-1, and endoglin but not CD38.[50] Because VE-cadherin is an endothelial-specific marker, these observations suggest that human HSCs are derived from HECs as has been observed in murine HSCs. Fetal liver HSCs are first detected on gestational day 42 and express CD34, CD45. VE-cadherin is also initially expressed on these HSCs, although this is lost after 10 weeks of gestation.[51]

Circulating CD34+ HSCs are found in both full-term and preterm CB.[52,53] The proportions of CD34+ cells in preterm CB are generally higher than in full-term CB, although the absolute numbers of CD34+ cells reported have been variable. Although preterm CB CD34+ cells exhibit higher colony-forming ability than full-term CB CD34+ cells,[52] preterm CD34+ cells may have lower repopulating ability.[51] The ability of transplanted CD34+ cells to repopulate the BM in patients with SCID has been shown to correlate with the expression level of CXCR4, a surface receptor involved in cellular migration and homing to the BM.[42] Thus, functional differences between preterm and term CD34+ cells may be linked to a relative developmental deficiency of CXCR4 in preterm CD34+ cells.[52]

Mesenchymal Stem Cells

Original observations showed that implantation of BM cells (without bone) into nonhematopoietic tissues (such as under skin or peritoneal cavity) induced the development of reticular tissue followed by bone formation that could sustain ectopic hematopoiesis.[54-56] This ectopic bone formation is derived from a nonhematopoietic cell population that forms a clonal fibroblastic colony in vitro, the CFU-F.[57] The progeny of CFU-F contribute to bone formation after transplantation and can differentiate into multiple skeletal tissues, including bone, cartilage, adipose tissue, and fibroblastic tissue in vivo. This rare BM population was first named an osteogenic stem cell or a BM stromal stem cell.[58,59] The discovery of this cell type was important in that it identified the presence of a second stem cell population in the BM in addition to HSCs. The currently used term, mesenchymal stem cell (MSC), was first proposed in 1991 based on the capacity to differentiate into cells of the mesenchymal lineage (bone, cartridge, tendon, ligament, BM stroma, adipocytes, dermis, muscle, and connective tissue).[60] The multipotency of MSCs remains, however, controversial.[59,61] Furthermore, although MSCs are often referred to as stem cells, they do not meet strict criteria regarding self-renewal capacity and multilineage potential at the single cell level.[58] A more conservative definition of MSCs (mesenchymal stromal cells[62] or skeletal stem/progenitors[63]) includes the following: (1) they possess CFU-F (colony forming units-fibroblast) that can form fibroblastic colonies in vitro; (2) they have the capacity to differentiate into adipocytes, osteocytes, and chondrocytes in vivo and in vitro; and (3) they support hematopoietic development.

MSCs can be derived from embryonic limbs, postnatal BM, umbilical CB, and other tissues in mice and humans,[54,60,64-66] including the perivascular area or BM sinusoids.[67] Their developmental origins are primarily from mesoderm but they also originate in part from neuroepithelium.[68] MSCs express unique surface antigens, including Sto-1, CD271, and CD146, but lack hematopoietic and endothelial markers (CD45, CD14, CD11b, CD79, CD19, HLA-DR, CD34, and CD31).

MSCs exhibit poor engraftment capacity after intravenous injection, and the small number that do engraft survive for only a short time in the recipient animals.[69] Despite this shortcoming, MSCs may be useful for (1) direct cell replacement for tissue regeneration and (2) indirect effects on damaged tissue related to MSC secretion of immunosuppressive factors. The therapeutic benefit of MSCs seems greatest for the treatment of inflammatory diseases through the release of antiinflammatory cytokines.

Endothelial Progenitors: Endothelial Colony-Forming Cells

The first putative endothelial progenitors were isolated from human adult PB in 1997 by Asahara and colleagues.[70] The major discovery that endothelial progenitor cells

(EPCs) circulate in the PB led to the concept that these EPCs contribute to the repair of vascular injuries. This nomenclature was unfortunate, however, because it has created long-standing confusion regarding the true definition of EPCs: the cells originally defined as EPCs have since been designated as hematopoietic cells, not endothelial cells.[71] The term that now most reliably defines circulating endothelial progenitors obtained from human PB or CB is *endothelial colony-forming cell (ECFC)*.[72] ECFCs are strictly defined as endothelial progenitors based on specific criteria. These include (1) the in vitro ability of cloned cells to form large colonies with high proliferative potential (HPP) that can be recultured to form secondary colonies; (2) the in vivo capacity to form capillaries that anastomose with host vessels; (3) the in vitro capacity to form tubes with lumens when plated in collagen; (4) absence of hematopoietic surface markers but surface expression of other unique markers, including CD31, CD146, CD144, CD105, CD34 (partially), KDR, vWF, and lectins; and (5) lack of phagocytic function. ECFCs or endothelial cells do not have phagocytic function whereas hematopoietic cell-derived EPCs or macrophages easily phagocytize *Escherichia coli* fragments.

ECFCs are rare in CB (2 of 10^8 CB mononuclear cells [MNCs]); however, their numbers are enriched in CB compared with adult PB. CB ECFCs have long telomeres and their proliferative potential is also much higher than for adult PB ECFC.[72] Although the cells currently designated as EPCs are not true endothelial cells, they share similarities to the recently reported proangiogenic $AC133^+CD34^+CD45^{dim}lin^-$ hematopoietic stem/progenitor cells and may contribute to neovascularization in cardiovascular disease or tumor progression.[73–75]

Inducible Pluripotent Stem Cells and Inducible Pluripotent Stem Cell–Derived Endothelial Colony-Forming Cells

Human iPSCs have been established in various human cells. Although CB does not contain true PSCs, CB can be induced into iPSCs when cultured in the presence of defined factors.[76,77] CB iPSCs are hardy: a recent report showed that CB MNCs cryopreserved for more than 20 years could still be used for HSC transplantation, ECFC isolation, and the induction of iPSCs.[78] In addition, a novel culture system to produce ECFCs from human iPSCs has been established.[79] Human iPSC-derived ECFCs display high clonal proliferative ability and have the capacity to form human vessels in mice. These pluripotent cells can repair ischemic regions in mouse retina and limb injury models without inducing secondary teratoma formation. Thus, CB is useful not only for its stem cell populations but also for the induction of iPSCs that can be stored for future clinical use.

STEM CELLS FOR THE TREATMENT OF POSTINSULT INJURY IN NEONATES

Neonates are highly susceptible to inflammatory and/or ischemic insults, particularly to critical organs, such as the brain and lungs; this risk is considerably higher in the most immature, preterm infants.[80–82] The damaging and often permanent effects related to these newborn insults are associated with high economic and societal costs, whereas the personal suffering of the afflicted and their families is incalculable.[83,84] Thus, the successful prevention or treatment of insult-related injury is of utmost and immediate importance.

Neonatal injury and its inherent complications have been intensively studied for many years. Investigations in relevant animal models and human studies have advanced understanding of the underlying mechanisms; however, treatments to prevent or to arrest injury as a result of these insults in many cases have been disappointing, until recently. A growing body of evidence and exciting new discoveries indicate the potential (and in some cases, actual) regenerative role of SCT in the treatment of neonatal injury (discussed briefly).

Brain Injury and Stem Cell Transplantation

Hypoxic-ischemic encephalopathy

Studies in animal models have been critical to defining the mechanisms underlying postinsult brain injury. These models have been based on approaches that focus on either cellular/molecular mechanisms or that recapitulate the physiologic events that produce injury; these have been recently elegantly reviewed.[85] Existing evidence has been distilled, however, from studies using a spectrum of animal models and SCT approaches, primarily involving human amnion epithelial-derived cells (hAECs), MSCs, whole CB, and neural stem cells. Thus, the reparative benefits of SCT for postinsult brain injury and the specific cells involved remain unclearly defined (reviewed by Castillo-Melendez and colleagues[86]).

Umbilical CB is a repository of a plethora of stem cell types, including those of hematopoietic, endothelial, and mesenchymal origin (discussed previously). Rodent models of neonatal hypoxic-ischemic brain injury have exhibited structural and behavioral improvements after transplantation with human CB cells, including measurable improvements in cognition.[87–89] The specific stem cell type(s) or cell combinations in CB that confer therapeutic properties have not been well defined. The underlying mechanisms are also unclear; evidence of poor engraftment in animals that respond positively to SCT suggest that the ameliorative effects are not due to the regenerative capabilities of the administered stem cells.[90] A relationship has been established between neuroprotection and indirect (paracrine and trophic) modulatory effects of administered stem cells, including MSCs and hAECs, on inflammatory and excitotoxic neural responses.[91,92] Administration of hAECs to sheep fetuses was also shown to confer protection from inflammation-induced brain injury.[93]

Studies of CB SCT in humans, although sparse, are increasing. In a recently reported prospective trial, 23 infants with hypoxic-ischemic encephalopathy received both head cooling and autologous CB transfusion within the first 72 hours of life.[94] The investigators concluded that this form of SCT was both safe and feasible even in outborn infants transferred to a tertiary care hospital. No firm conclusions could be made, however, regarding hospital and developmental outcomes or 1-year survival. In a feasibility pilot study, the transfusion of autologous CB from private CB banks to young children with neurologic disorders was found safe.[95] In a Korean study of 96 infants and children with cerebral palsy, subjects who received matched allogeneic CB cells with erythropoietin fared better developmentally 6 months later than did their counterparts given erythropoietin only or placebo.[96] This study highlights the potential therapeutic utility of banked allogeneic donor CB cells in SCT of brain injury.

Neonatal stroke

Stroke is a primarily ischemic event that occurs in the fetal or neonatal periods and involves ischemia of cerebral arteries or periventricular venous infarction.[97] Strokes in the perinatal period commonly (60% of cases) result in neurologic deficits, with hemiplegic cerebral palsy a frequent complication. A variety of preclinical studies have shown potential therapeutic value of stem cell populations derived from human umbilical CB in limiting injury and in promoting functional recovery. In rodent stroke models, the administration of neural stem cells led to glial and neuronal differentiation at sites of injury, whereas transplanted MSCs were indirectly beneficial by inducing the release of neuroprotective trophic factors that dampened inflammation.[98,99] Human

CB-derived AC133[+] EPCs limited infarct size and shortened the resolution period in a rat stroke model.[100] Stem cells from other sources in addition to those derived from CB may also be of value. The administration of amniotic fluid—derived stem cells to adult rats with ischemic stroke also resulted in significant functional recovery.[101] The most beneficial stem cell type for the treatment of stroke remains, however, unclear. Transplantation with the broader array of stem cells contained in human CD34[+] cells bestowed a limited benefit in one rodent stroke model, whereas another study showed greater therapeutic effect and less inflammation in animals receiving CB mononuclear cells compared with CB MSCs.[102,103] Although the potential therapeutic usefulness of SCT in neonates with stroke is supported by preclinical studies, its actual utility in human neonates remains to be defined.[104]

Lung Injury and Stem Cell Transplantation

Extremely preterm infants are at high risk for numerous long-term complications, of which bronchopulmonary dysplasia (BPD) is the most common.[105] The new BPD is associated with lung growth arrest as well as abnormal vascularization and fibrosis, and it can result in disabling lung abnormalities that persist into adulthood.[82] Studies in neonatal animal models of BPD have shown that transplantation with MSC or soluble MSC-derived proteins (the MSC secretome) can modulate BPD by dampening inflammatory processes.[99,106–108] In a recently reported phase I dose-escalation trial, a small group of extremely preterm infants who received intratracheal autologous MSC had diminished BPD severity and lowered inflammatory cytokine levels in tracheal aspirates compared with historical controls.[109] MSC treatment was clinically well tolerated in these tiny babies and was not associated with discernable short-term safety issues. The potential benefits of CB MSCs have stimulated numerous ongoing clinical trials addressing their use for the treatment of diverse disorders in adults and several in preterm infants.

Intestinal Injury and Stem Cell Transplantation

Necrotizing enterocolitis (NEC), an intestinal inflammatory disorder with infectious components, is a common and potentially devastating complication of prematurity.[110] The etiology of NEC is multifactorial and includes ischemia-reperfusion injury, disturbances of the intestinal microbiome, and prior inflammatory exposure. The potential role of SCT in the treatment of neonatal NEC has only recently been addressed. In an in vivo neonatal rat model of NEC, intraperitoneal administration of BM-derived MSCs was associated with attenuated histologic intestinal injury, improved weight gain, and decreased clinical illness scores.[111] MSC homing to intestinal tissue was enhanced in the pups with NEC compared with normal controls, suggesting a potentiating role for inflammation in the engraftment of MSC. In another study, neonatal rats with NEC that were treated with amniotic fluid stem cells showed improved gut structure and survival and reduced inflammatory mechanisms mediated via cyclooxygenase-2.[112] Despite these encouraging preclinical data, a role for SCT in the treatment of NEC in human neonates has not been reported to date.

UTILITY OF NEONATAL STEM CELL TRANSPLANTATION: GENERAL CONSIDERATIONS

Several critical questions remain to be answered through well-designed preclinical large animal models and human clinical trials before the use of umbilical CB or specific stem cells affords reasonable therapeutic options. One issue is that of the optimal timing of SCT administration in the context of the injury. Studies in infants with brain injury have shown a secondary postinjury period during which inflammatory and excitatory mechanisms become pronounced; thus, the time between the initial insult and this later phase may be the ideal window to institute SCT as a therapeutic measure.[113] Conversely, a Korean study showed benefit of SCT in children with cerebral palsy, even in those who were 10 years of age,[114] which suggests a possible benefit despite long-standing neurologic injury.

Another key issue to be addressed is the identification of the ideal stem cell source for a specific type of tissue injury. As discussed previously, umbilical CB contains numerous stem cell types, including those of hematopoietic, endothelial, and mesenchymal origins. It remains unclear, however, if and how the perinatal factors contributing to neonatal hypoxic-ischemic encephalopathy or other injury could potentially influence the functionality and intrinsic properties of the CB stem cells themselves.[115]

The role of specific stem cell types in various target organs also remains incompletely defined. MSCs derived from developing humans exhibit a high degree of mesodermal pluripotency (the capacity to differentiate into multiple cell types); in addition, these MSCs are associated with a low induction of immune responses in the recipient and exhibit antiinflammatory properties.[99,116] Another type of cell with pluripotent properties is the hAEC.[117] Like MSCs, hAECs are antiinflammatory and seem immunologically well tolerated.[118,119] Studies in fetal sheep showed that hAEC administration was protective against brain inflammation, including periventricular white matter injury.[93] As also observed with MSCs, the beneficial effect of hAECs may be related primarily to the release of soluble protective factors.[90]

In addition to the optimal stem cell type and timing of administration necessary for therapeutic efficacy, other issues that remain to be addressed involve the most ideal stem cell sources (autologous vs allogeneic, CB vs isolated stem cells, primary cells vs derived, or genetically modified cells), host tolerance, and safety, among others.[113,120] Although short-term safety may be acceptable, as suggested by the few recent human studies, long-term effects remain unknown. This latter point may be of particular importance to very preterm infants who are still undergoing developmental maturation, including of the immune and hematopoietic systems. Another critical safety feature to be defined involves the potential tumorigenicity or cancerous conversion of the transplanted stem cells, a question that remains enigmatic.

SUMMARY

True stem cells or cells with pluripotent properties are found in a variety of tissues and organs. Umbilical CB can provide a spectrum of stem or pluripotent progenitor cells, many of which have a greater potential for proliferation (although not necessarily engraftment) compared with similar cells mobilized from the BM into the PB of adults. Preclinical studies have shown a therapeutic benefit of SCT in perinatal and neonatal injuries, including those involving the brain, lungs, and intestines. The few human studies to date suggest short-term safety of MSCs or CB (both autologous and allogeneic) SCT and have variably shown measurable improvements in functional or inflammatory parameters. The therapeutic mechanisms remain incompletely defined, however, and the optimal usage of SCT for a particular type of injury is also unclear. Thus, despite its exciting potential for currently untreatable neonatal disorders, extensive studies in both preclinical models and in humans are necessary before SCT becomes an accepted form of therapy. Although still limited relative to studies in adults, an increasing number of human trials now address these issues in neonates (https://ClinicalTrials.gov).

Best Practices

What is the current practice?

Devastating postnatal brain or lung injury occurs commonly, particularly in preterm infants, although no successful preventive or therapeutic strategies currently exist.

Summary Statement

SCT for postnatal brain or lung injury has undergone exploration in animal models, and the few clinical trials to date seem promising. Extensive testing in large animal models and in humans, however, is required before the utility and safety of SCT for the treatment of postnatal injury can be established.

REFERENCES

1. Boelens JJ, Orchard PJ, Wynn RF. Transplantation in inborn errors of metabolism: current considerations and future perspectives. Br J Haematol 2014; 167:293–303.
2. Westgren M, Ringden O, Bartmann P, et al. Prenatal T-cell reconstitution after in utero transplantation with fetal liver cells in a patient with X-linked severe combined immunodeficiency. Am J Obstet Gynecol 2002;187:475–82.
3. Van de Vijver E, van den Berg TK, Kuijpers TW. Leukocyte adhesion deficiencies. Hematol Oncol Clin North Am 2013;27:101–16.
4. Moyer MW. Cell banks: life blood. Nature 2013;498:S16.
5. Sison EA, Brown P. Does hematopoietic stem cell transplantation benefit infants with acute leukemia? Hematology Am Soc Hematol Educ Program 2013;2013: 601–4.
6. Peffault de LR, Porcher R, Dalle JH, et al. Allogeneic hematopoietic stem cell transplantation in Fanconi anemia: the European Group for Blood and Marrow Transplantation experience. Blood 2013;122:4279–86.
7. Evans MJ, Kaufman MH. Establishment in culture of pluripotential cells from mouse embryos. Nature 1981;292:154–6.
8. Martin GR. Isolation of a pluripotent cell line from early mouse embryos cultured in medium conditioned by teratocarcinoma stem cells. Proc Natl Acad Sci U S A 1981;78:7634–8.
9. Thomson JA, Itskovitz-Eldor J, Shapiro SS, et al. Embryonic stem cell lines derived from human blastocysts. Science 1998;282:1145–7.
10. Kanatsu-Shinohara M, Inoue K, Lee J, et al. Generation of pluripotent stem cells from neonatal mouse testis. Cell 2004;119:1001–12.
11. Takahashi K, Yamanaka S. Induction of pluripotent stem cells from mouse embryonic and adult fibroblast cultures by defined factors. Cell 2006;126:663–76.
12. Takahashi K, Tanabe K, Ohnuki M, et al. Induction of pluripotent stem cells from adult human fibroblasts by defined factors. Cell 2007;131:861–72.
13. Kobayashi Y, Okada Y, Itakura G, et al. Pre-evaluated safe human iPSC-derived neural stem cells promote functional recovery after spinal cord injury in common marmoset without tumorigenicity. PLoS One 2012;7(12):e52787.
14. Kamao H, Mandai M, Okamoto S, et al. Characterization of human induced pluripotent stem cell-derived retinal pigment epithelium cell sheets aiming for clinical application. Stem Cell Reports 2014;2:205–18.
15. Song HJ, Stevens CF, Gage FH. Neural stem cells from adult hippocampus develop essential properties of functional CNS neurons. Nat Neurosci 2002;5: 438–45.

16. Doetsch F, Caille I, Lim DA, et al. Subventricular zone astrocytes are neural stem cells in the adult mammalian brain. Cell 1999;97:703–16.
17. Tavazoie M, Van der Veken L, Silva-Vargas V, et al. A specialized vascular niche for adult neural stem cells. Cell Stem Cell 2008;3:279–88.
18. Doulatov S, Notta F, Eppert K, et al. Revised map of the human progenitor hierarchy shows the origin of macrophages and dendritic cells in early lymphoid development. Nat Immunol 2010;11:585–93.
19. Doulatov S, Notta F, Laurenti E, et al. Hematopoiesis: a human perspective. Cell Stem Cell 2012;10:120–36.
20. Notta F, Doulatov S, Laurenti E, et al. Isolation of single human hematopoietic stem cells capable of long-term multilineage engraftment. Science 2011;333:218–21.
21. Nakahata T, Ogawa M. Hemopoietic colony-forming cells in umbilical cord blood with extensive capability to generate mono- and multipotential hemopoietic progenitors. J Clin Invest 1982;70:1324–8.
22. Broxmeyer HE, Douglas GW, Hangoc G, et al. Human umbilical cord blood as a potential source of transplantable hematopoietic stem/progenitor cells. Proc Natl Acad Sci U S A 1989;86:3828–32.
23. Gluckman E, Broxmeyer HA, Auerbach AD, et al. Hematopoietic reconstitution in a patient with Fanconi's anemia by means of umbilical-cord blood from an HLA-identical sibling. N Engl J Med 1989;321:1174–8.
24. Bender JG, Unverzagt K, Walker DE, et al. Phenotypic analysis and characterization of CD34+ cells from normal human bone marrow, cord blood, peripheral blood, and mobilized peripheral blood from patients undergoing autologous stem cell transplantation. Clin Immunol Immunopathol 1994;70:10–8.
25. Lin Y, Yoder MC, Yoshimoto M. Lymphoid progenitor emergence in the murine embryo and yolk sac precedes stem cell detection. Stem Cells Dev 2014;23:1168–77.
26. Moore MA, Metcalf D. Ontogeny of the haemopoietic system: yolk sac origin of in vivo and in vitro colony forming cells in the developing mouse embryo. Br J Haematol 1970;18:279–96.
27. Barker JE. Development of the mouse hematopoietic system. I. Types of hemoglobin produced in embryonic yolk sac and liver. Dev Biol 1968;18:14–29.
28. Palis J, Robertson S, Kennedy M, et al. Development of erythroid and myeloid progenitors in the yolk sac and embryo proper of the mouse. Development 1999;126:5073–84.
29. Lux CT, Yoshimoto M, McGrath K, et al. All primitive and definitive hematopoietic progenitor cells emerging before E10 in the mouse embryo are products of the yolk sac. Blood 2008;111:3435–8.
30. Muller AM, Medvinsky A, Strouboulis J, et al. Development of hematopoietic stem cell activity in the mouse embryo. Immunity 1994;1:291–301.
31. Medvinsky A, Dzierzak E. Definitive hematopoiesis is autonomously initiated by the AGM region. Cell 1996;86:897–906.
32. Nishikawa SI, Nishikawa S, Kawamoto H, et al. In vitro generation of lymphohematopoietic cells from endothelial cells purified from murine embryos. Immunity 1998;8:761–9.
33. de Bruijn MF, Ma X, Robin C, et al. Hematopoietic stem cells localize to the endothelial cell layer in the midgestation mouse aorta. Immunity 2002;16:673–83.
34. Chen MJ, Yokomizo T, Zeigler BM, et al. Runx1 is required for the endothelial to haematopoietic cell transition but not thereafter. Nature 2009;457:887–91.

35. Chen MJ, Li Y, De Obaldia ME, et al. Erythroid/myeloid progenitors and hemato-poietic stem cells originate from distinct populations of endothelial cells. Cell Stem Cell 2011;9:541–52.
36. Tober J, Yzaguirre AD, Piwarzyk E, et al. Distinct temporal requirements for Runx1 in hematopoietic progenitors and stem cells. Development 2013;140: 3765–76.
37. Ema H, Nakauchi H. Expansion of hematopoietic stem cells in the developing liver of a mouse embryo. Blood 2000;95:2284–8.
38. Gekas C, Dieterlen-Lievre F, Orkin SH, et al. The placenta is a niche for hemato-poietic stem cells. Dev Cell 2005;8:365–75.
39. Ottersbach K, Dzierzak E. The murine placenta contains hematopoietic stem cells within the vascular labyrinth region. Dev Cell 2005;8:377–87.
40. Bloom W, Bartelmez GW. Hematopoiesis in young human embryos. Am J Anat 1940;67:21–53.
41. Huyhn A, Dommergues M, Izac B, et al. Characterization of hematopoietic pro-genitors from human yolk sacs and embryos. Blood 1995;86:4474–85.
42. Migliaccio G, Migliaccio AR, Petti S, et al. Human embryonic hemopoiesis. Ki-netics of progenitors and precursors underlying the yolk sac—liver transition. J Clin Invest 1986;78:51–60.
43. Tavian M, Hallais MF, Peault B. Emergence of intraembryonic hematopoietic pre-cursors in the pre-liver human embryo. Development 1999;126:793–803.
44. Tavian M, Coulombel L, Luton D, et al. Aorta- associated CD34+ hematopoietic cells in the early human embryo. Blood 1996;87:67–72.
45. Tavian M, Robin C, Coulombel L, et al. The human embryo, but not its yolk sac, generates lympho-myeloid stem cells: mapping multipotent hematopoietic cell fate in intraembryonic mesoderm. Immunity 2001;15:487–95.
46. Jokubaitis VJ, Sinka L, Driessen R, et al. Angiotensin-converting enzyme (CD143) marks hematopoietic stem cells in human embryonic, fetal, and adult hematopoietic tissues. Blood 2008;111:4055–63.
47. Labastie MC, Cortes F, Romeo PH, et al. Molecular identity of hematopoietic pre-cursor cells emerging in the human embryo. Blood 1998;92:3624–35.
48. Ito M, Hiramatsu H, Kobayashi K, et al. NOD/SCID/gamma(c)(null) mouse: an excellent recipient mouse model for engraftment of human cells. Blood 2002; 100:3175–82.
49. Ivanovs A, Rybtsov S, Welch L, et al. Highly potent human hematopoietic stem cells first emerge in the intraembryonic aorta-gonad-mesonephros region. J Exp Med 2011;208:2417–27.
50. Ivanovs A, Rybtsov S, Anderson RA, et al. Identification of the niche and pheno-type of the first human hematopoietic stem cells. Stem Cell Reports 2014;2: 449–56.
51. Oberlin E, Fleury M, Clay D, et al. VE-cadherin expression allows identification of a new class of hematopoietic stem cells within human embryonic liver. Blood 2010;116:4444–55.
52. Nakajima M, Ueda T, Migita M, et al. Hematopoietic capacity of preterm cord blood hematopoietic stem/progenitor cells. Biochem Biophys Res Commun 2009;389:290–4.
53. Wisgrill L, Schuller S, Bammer M, et al. Hematopoietic stem cells in neonates: any differences between very preterm and term neonates? PLoS One 2014; 9(9):e106717.
54. Friedenstein AJ, Piatetzky S II, Petrakova KV. Osteogenesis in transplants of bone marrow cells. J Embryol Exp Morphol 1966;16:381–90.

55. Friedenstein AJ, Chailakhyan RK, Latsinik NV, et al. Stromal cells responsible for transferring the microenvironment of the hemopoietic tissues. Cloning in vitro and retransplantation in vivo. Transplantation 1974;17:331–40.
56. Tavassoli M, Crosby WH. Transplantation of marrow to extramedullary sites. Science 1968;161:54–6.
57. Friedenstein AJ, Chailakhjan RK, Lalykina KS. The development of fibroblast colonies in monolayer cultures of guinea-pig bone marrow and spleen cells. Cell Tissue Kinet 1970;3:393–403.
58. Friedenstein AJ. Precursor cells of mechanocytes. Int Rev Cytol 1976;47: 327–59.
59. Bianco P, Robey PG, Simmons PJ. Mesenchymal stem cells: revisiting history, concepts, and assays. Cell Stem Cell 2008;2:313–9.
60. Caplan AI. Mesenchymal stem cells. J Orthop Res 1991;9:641–50.
61. Kluth SM, Radke TF, Kogler G. Potential application of cord blood-derived stromal cells in cellular therapy and regenerative medicine. J Blood Transfus 2012; 2012:365182.
62. Dominici M, Le Blanc K, Mueller I, et al. Minimal criteria for defining multipotent mesenchymal stromal cells. The International Society for Cellular Therapy position statement. Cytotherapy 2006;8:315–7.
63. Bianco P, Robey PG, Saggio I, et al. "Mesenchymal" stem cells in human bone marrow (skeletal stem cells): a critical discussion of their nature, identity, and significance in incurable skeletal disease. Hum Gene Ther 2010;21: 1057–66.
64. Erices A, Conget P, Minguell JJ. Mesenchymal progenitor cells in human umbilical cord blood. Br J Haematol 2000;109:235–42.
65. Crisan M, Yap S, Casteilla L, et al. A perivascular origin for mesenchymal stem cells in multiple human organs. Cell Stem Cell 2008;3:301–13.
66. Yamamoto N, Akamatsu H, Hasegawa S, et al. Isolation of multipotent stem cells from mouse adipose tissue. J Dermatol Sci 2007;48:43–52.
67. Sacchetti B, Funari A, Michienzi S, et al. Self-renewing osteoprogenitors in bone marrow sinusoids can organize a hematopoietic microenvironment. Cell 2007; 131:324–36.
68. Takashima Y, Era T, Nakao K, et al. Neuroepithelial cells supply an initial transient wave of MSC differentiation. Cell 2007;129:1377–88.
69. Wang Y, Chen X, Cao W, et al. Plasticity of mesenchymal stem cells in immunomodulation: pathological and therapeutic implications. Nat Immunol 2014;15: 1009–16.
70. Asahara T, Murohara T, Sullivan A, et al. Isolation of putative progenitor endothelial cells for angiogenesis. Science 1997;275:964–7.
71. Yoder MC, Mead LE, Prater D, et al. Redefining endothelial progenitor cells via clonal analysis and hematopoietic stem/progenitor cell principals. Blood 2007; 109:1801–9.
72. Ingram DA, Mead LE, Tanaka H, et al. Identification of a novel hierarchy of endothelial progenitor cells using human peripheral and umbilical cord blood. Blood 2004;104:2752–60.
73. Estes ML, Mund JA, Mead LE, et al. Application of polychromatic flow cytometry to identify novel subsets of circulating cells with angiogenic potential. Cytometry A 2010;77:831–9.
74. Pradhan KR, Mund JA, Johnson C, et al. Polychromatic flow cytometry identifies novel subsets of circulating cells with angiogenic potential in pediatric solid tumors. Cytometry B Clin Cytom 2011;80:335–8.

75. Hill JM, Zalos G, Halcox JP, et al. Circulating endothelial progenitor cells, vascular function, and cardiovascular risk. N Engl J Med 2003;348:593–600.
76. Ye Z, Zhan H, Mali P, et al. Human-induced pluripotent stem cells from blood cells of healthy donors and patients with acquired blood disorders. Blood 2009;114:5473–80.
77. Okita K, Yamakawa T, Matsumura Y, et al. An efficient nonviral method to generate integration-free human-induced pluripotent stem cells from cord blood and peripheral blood cells. Stem Cells 2013;31:458–66.
78. Broxmeyer HE, Lee MR, Hangoc G, et al. Hematopoietic stem/progenitor cells, generation of induced pluripotent stem cells, and isolation of endothelial progenitors from 21- to 23.5-year cryopreserved cord blood. Blood 2011;117: 4773–7.
79. Prasain N, Lee MR, Vemula S, et al. Differentiation of human pluripotent stem cells to cells similar to cord-blood endothelial colony-forming cells. Nat Biotechnol 2014;32:1151–7.
80. Kurinczuk JJ, White-Koning M, Badawi N. Epidemiology of neonatal encephalopathy and hypoxic-ischaemic encephalopathy. Early Hum Dev 2010;86: 329–38.
81. Malaeb S, Dammann O. Fetal inflammatory response and brain injury in the preterm newborn. J Child Neurol 2009;24:1119–26.
82. Jobe AH. The new bronchopulmonary dysplasia. Curr Opin Pediatr 2011;23: 167–72.
83. Johnston KM, Gooch K, Korol E, et al. The economic burden of prematurity in Canada. BMC Pediatr 2014;14:93.
84. Flood K, Malone FD. Prevention of preterm birth. Semin Fetal Neonatal Med 2012;17:58–63.
85. Fleiss B, Guillot PV, Titomanlio L, et al. Stem cell therapy for neonatal brain injury. Clin Perinatol 2014;41:133–48.
86. Castillo-Melendez M, Yawno T, Jenkin G, et al. Stem cell therapy to protect and repair the developing brain: a review of mechanisms of action of cord blood and amnion epithelial derived cells. Front Neurosci 2013;7:194.
87. de Paula S, Greggio S, Marinowic DR, et al. The dose-response effect of acute intravenous transplantation of human umbilical cord blood cells on brain damage and spatial memory deficits in neonatal hypoxia-ischemia. Neuroscience 2012;210:431–41.
88. Wasielewski B, Jensen A, Roth-Harer A, et al. Neuroglial activation and Cx43 expression are reduced upon transplantation of human umbilical cord blood cells after perinatal hypoxic-ischemic injury. Brain Res 2012;1487:39–53.
89. Geissler M, Dinse HR, Neuhoff S, et al. Human umbilical cord blood cells restore brain damage induced changes in rat somatosensory cortex. PLoS One 2011;6: e20194.
90. Tan JL, Chan ST, Wallace EM, et al. Human amnion epithelial cells mediate lung repair by directly modulating macrophage recruitment and polarization. Cell Transplant 2014;23:319–28.
91. Meier C, Middelanis J, Wasielewski B, et al. Spastic paresis after perinatal brain damage in rats is reduced by human cord blood mononuclear cells. Pediatr Res 2006;59:244–9.
92. Pimentel-Coelho PM, Magalhaes ES, Lopes LM, et al. Human cord blood transplantation in a neonatal rat model of hypoxic-ischemic brain damage: functional outcome related to neuroprotection in the striatum. Stem Cells Dev 2010;19: 351–8.

93. Yawno T, Schuilwerve J, Moss TJ, et al. Human amnion epithelial cells reduce fetal brain injury in response to intrauterine inflammation. Dev Neurosci 2013; 35:272–82.
94. Cotten CM, Murtha AP, Goldberg RN, et al. Feasibility of autologous cord blood cells for infants with hypoxic-ischemic encephalopathy. J Pediatr 2014;164: 973–9.
95. Sun J, Allison J, McLaughlin C, et al. Differences in quality between privately and publicly banked umbilical cord blood units: a pilot study of autologous cord blood infusion in children with acquired neurologic disorders. Transfusion 2010;50:1980–7.
96. Min K, Song J, Kang JY, et al. Umbilical cord blood therapy potentiated with erythropoietin for children with cerebral palsy: a double-blind, randomized, placebo-controlled trial. Stem Cells 2013;31:581–91.
97. Kirton A, Shroff M, Pontigon AM, et al. Risk factors and presentations of periventricular venous infarction vs arterial presumed perinatal ischemic stroke. Arch Neurol 2010;67:842–8.
98. Kim ES, Ahn SY, Im GH, et al. Human umbilical cord blood-derived mesenchymal stem cell transplantation attenuates severe brain injury by permanent middle cerebral artery occlusion in newborn rats. Pediatr Res 2012;72: 277–84.
99. Cheng Q, Zhang Z, Zhang S, et al. Human umbilical cord mesenchymal stem cells protect against ischemic brain injury in mouse by regulating peripheral immunoinflammation. Brain Res 2015;1594:293–304.
100. Iskander A, Knight RA, Zhang ZG, et al. Intravenous administration of human umbilical cord blood-derived AC133+ endothelial progenitor cells in rat stroke model reduces infarct volume: magnetic resonance imaging and histological findings. Stem Cells Transl Med 2013;2:703–14.
101. Tajiri N, Acosta S, Glover LE, et al. Intravenous grafts of amniotic fluid-derived stem cells induce endogenous cell proliferation and attenuate behavioral deficits in ischemic stroke rats. PLoS One 2012;7:e43779.
102. Karlupia N, Manley NC, Prasad K, et al. Intraarterial transplantation of human umbilical cord blood mononuclear cells is more efficacious and safer compared with umbilical cord mesenchymal stromal cells in a rodent stroke model. Stem Cell Res Ther 2014;5:45.
103. Tsuji M, Taguchi A, Ohshima M, et al. Effects of intravenous administration of umbilical cord blood CD34(+) cells in a mouse model of neonatal stroke. Neuroscience 2014;263:148–58.
104. Basu AP. Early intervention after perinatal stroke: opportunities and challenges. Dev Med Child Neurol 2014;56:516–21.
105. McEvoy CT, Jain L, Schmidt B, et al. Bronchopulmonary dysplasia: NHLBI Workshop on the Primary Prevention of Chronic Lung Diseases. Ann Am Thorac Soc 2014;11(Suppl 3):S146–53.
106. Aslam M, Baveja R, Liang OD, et al. Bone marrow stromal cells attenuate lung injury in a murine model of neonatal chronic lung disease. Am J Respir Crit Care Med 2009;180:1122–30.
107. van Haaften T, Byrne R, Bonnet S, et al. Airway delivery of mesenchymal stem cells prevents arrested alveolar growth in neonatal lung injury in rats. Am J Respir Crit Care Med 2009;180:1131–42.
108. Abman SH, Matthay MA. Mesenchymal stem cells for the prevention of bronchopulmonary dysplasia: delivering the secretome. Am J Respir Crit Care Med 2009;180:1039–41.

109. Chang YS, Ahn SY, Yoo HS, et al. Mesenchymal stem cells for bronchopulmonary dysplasia: phase 1 dose-escalation clinical trial. J Pediatr 2014;164:966–72.
110. Neu J. Necrotizing enterocolitis. World Rev Nutr Diet 2014;110:253–63.
111. Tayman C, Uckan D, Kilic E, et al. Mesenchymal stem cell therapy in necrotizing enterocolitis: a rat study. Pediatr Res 2011;70:489–94.
112. Zani A, Cananzi M, Fascetti-Leon F, et al. Amniotic fluid stem cells improve survival and enhance repair of damaged intestine in necrotising enterocolitis via a COX-2 dependent mechanism. Gut 2014;63:300–9.
113. Kourembanas S. Stem cell-based therapy for newborn lung and brain injury: feasible, safe, and the next therapeutic breakthrough? J Pediatr 2014;164: 954–6.
114. Lee YH, Choi KV, Moon JH, et al. Safety and feasibility of countering neurological impairment by intravenous administration of autologous cord blood in cerebral palsy. J Transl Med 2012;10:58.
115. Wu CF, Huang FD, Sui RF, et al. Preeclampsia serum upregulates CD40/CD40L expression and induces apoptosis in human umbilical cord endothelial cells. Reprod Biol Endocrinol 2012;10:28.
116. English K, Wood KJ. Mesenchymal stromal cells in transplantation rejection and tolerance. Cold Spring Harb Perspect Med 2013;3:a015560.
117. Parolini O, Alviano F, Bagnara GP, et al. Concise review: isolation and characterization of cells from human term placenta: outcome of the first international Workshop on Placenta Derived Stem Cells. Stem Cells 2008;26:300–11.
118. Solomon A, Wajngarten M, Alviano F, et al. Suppression of inflammatory and fibrotic responses in allergic inflammation by the amniotic membrane stromal matrix. Clin Exp Allergy 2005;35:941–8.
119. Solomon A, Espana EM, Tseng SC. Amniotic membrane transplantation for reconstruction of the conjunctival fornices. Ophthalmology 2003;110:93–100.
120. Munoz J, Shah N, Rezvani K, et al. Concise review: umbilical cord blood transplantation: past, present, and future. Stem Cells Transl Med 2014;3:1435–43.

Platelet Transfusions in the Neonatal Intensive Care Unit

Katherine Sparger, MD[a], Emoke Deschmann, MD[b],
Martha Sola-Visner, MD[c],*

KEYWORDS

• Platelet transfusions • Neonatal intensive care unit • Thrombocytopenia

KEY POINTS

• Although platelet transfusions are currently administered on the basis of platelet counts or platelet mass, the evidence strongly suggests that factors other than the degree of thrombocytopenia determine the bleeding risk.

• Thus, larger studies are needed to better characterize the platelet function and the hemostatic profile of preterm infants, and their changes over time and in response to illness.

• It will be important to develop and validate tests that can be used in preterm infants and that incorporate both platelet count and function to evaluate hemostasis, rather than individual platelet counts alone.

• Intrauterine growth restriction, pregnancy-induced hypertension or diabetes, perinatal infection, and transplacental passage of maternal allo- or autoantibodies are frequently associated with early onset thrombocytopenia.

INTRODUCTION

Thrombocytopenia, generally defined as a platelet count less than 150×10^9/L, is (after anemia) the second most common hematologic disorder of infants admitted to neonatal intensive care units (NICUs). It affects 18% to 35% of all patients admitted to NICUs and approximately 70% of extremely low birth weight (ELBW) infants with a birth weight less than 1000 g.[1-4] The incidence of thrombocytopenia is inversely proportional to the gestational age, and it represents a risk factor for poor neonatal outcomes.[5]

Disclosures: None.
[a] Department of Pediatrics, Massachusetts General Hospital, 55 Fruit Street, Boston, MA 02114, USA; [b] Department of Neonatology, Astrid Lindgren Children's Hospital, Karolinska University Hospital, 171 76 Stockholm, Sweden; [c] Division of Newborn Medicine, Boston Children's Hospital, Enders Research Building, Room 961, 300 Longwood Avenue, Boston, MA 02115, USA
* Corresponding author.
E-mail address: Martha.Sola-Visner@childrens.harvard.edu

Clin Perinatol 42 (2015) 613–623
http://dx.doi.org/10.1016/j.clp.2015.04.009   perinatology.theclinics.com

Recently, Wiedmeier and colleagues published the largest study on neonatal platelet counts conducted to date, which included approximately 47,000 infants delivered between 22 and 42 weeks gestation.[6] This study showed that platelet counts at birth increased with advancing gestational age (**Fig. 1**). Linear regression analysis showed that, for each week increase in gestational age, there was a corresponding increase in mean platelet count of approximately 2×10^9/L. Importantly, while the mean platelet count was $\geq 200 \times 10^9$/L even in the most preterm infants, the fifth percentile in this large epidemiologic study was 104×10^9/L for those no more than 32 weeks gestation and 123×10^9/L for late-preterm and term neonates (see **Fig. 1**).[6] These findings indicate that different definitions of thrombocytopenia should be applied to preterm infants.

The etiologies of thrombocytopenia are highly diverse, as is the natural history. Clinically, a distinction is frequently made between early onset (≤ 3 days of life) and late-onset (≥ 4 days of life) neonatal thrombocytopenia. Intrauterine growth restriction, pregnancy-induced hypertension or diabetes, perinatal infection, and transplacental passage of maternal allo- or autoantibodies are frequently associated with early onset thrombocytopenia. Late-onset neonatal thrombocytopenia is most commonly caused by bacterial infection or necrotizing enterocolitis.

PLATELET TRANSFUSION PRACTICES

Platelet transfusion remains the primary treatment modality for neonatal thrombocytopenia, but there is lack of agreement regarding the platelet count below which a newborn infant should be transfused. Nevertheless, it has been widely accepted that neonates should be transfused at higher platelet counts than older children and adults, and thus platelet transfusions are a frequent intervention in the NICU. In an earlier study of a single NICU in the United States with liberal transfusion practices, 9% of infants admitted received at least 1 platelet transfusion during their NICU stay.[7] Extrapolating data from a single institution to the number of North American

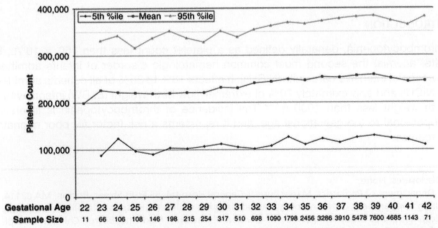

Fig. 1. First recorded platelet counts, obtained in the first 3 days after birth, in neonates born at 22 to 42 weeks gestation. Mean values are indicated by the red line, and the 5th and 95th percentiles are shown in the blue and green lines, respectively. (*From* Wiedmeier SE, Henry E, Sola-Visner MC, et al. Platelet reference ranges for neonates, defined using data from over 47,000 patients in a multihospital healthcare system. J Perinatol 2009;29:132; with permission.)

NICU admissions over a 1-year period, it was calculated that 80,000 platelet transfusions are administered annually to neonates in the United States (John Widness, personal communication, 2011). A recent survey of platelet transfusion practices among US and Canadian neonatologists revealed wide practice differences in regard to platelet transfusion thresholds in different clinical scenarios, and suggested that many platelet transfusions were given to nonbleeding neonates with platelet counts between 50 and 100 × 10⁹/L, particularly in the first week of life.[8]

In order to compare transfusion practices in North America with those in Europe, the same survey was translated to German and sent to all NICU directors in German-speaking European countries (Germany, Austria, and Switzerland). The transfusion thresholds chosen by North American and European neonatologists in each clinical scenario were then compared. In this study, European neonatologists selected substantially lower platelet transfusion thresholds than North American neonatologists in nearly all case scenarios (**Fig. 2**), with the exception of neonatal alloimmune thrombocytopenia and prior to invasive procedures. It was estimated from survey responses that practice differences alone would account for 1.8 times more platelet transfusions given in US compared with European NICUs.[9] In a subsequent prospective multicenter observational study performed in the United Kingdom, thrombocytopenic neonates were transfused at a median platelet count of 27 × 10⁹/L, confirming the use of more restrictive transfusion thresholds in European countries.[10] A single retrospective study of platelet transfusions in a Mexican NICU suggested that practices in that country resembled the European restrictive approach.[11]

The reasons underlying this practice variability are probably multifactorial, but most likely involve the lack of solid evidence from randomized controlled trials to guide neonatal transfusion decisions, the high incidence of bleeding in this population, and the known platelet hyporeactivity of neonates.

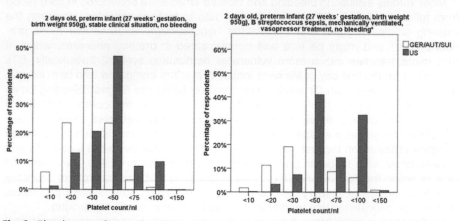

Fig. 2. Platelet transfusion thresholds selected by neonatologists in German-speaking European countries (AUT/GER/SUI, *white bars*) versus U.S. neonatologists (*black bars*) in 2 different clinical scenarios. Neonatologists were asked when they would transfuse a 2-day old stable preterm infant (*left panel*), or the same infant with bacterial sepsis (*right panel*). *$P<0.0001$ derived by Mann-Whitney U test to compare GER/AUT/SUI to US neonatologists. (*From* Cremer M, Sola-Visner M, Roll S, et al. Platelet transfusions in neonates: practices in the United States vary significantly from those in Austria, Germany, and Switzerland. Transfusion 2011;51:2636–7; with permission.)

PRIMARY HEMOSTASIS IN THE NEONATE

Multiple studies evaluating platelet activation and aggregation clearly demonstrated that neonatal platelets are hyporesponsive in vitro to most agonists (including adenosine diphosphate (ADP), epinephrine, collagen, thrombin, and thromboxane analogs), compared with adult platelets.[12,13] The underlying mechanisms responsible for the decreased platelet responses are different for each agonist. Specifically, the lack of response to epinephrine is explained by the presence of fewer α2-adrenergic receptors on neonatal platelets.[14] The diminished response to collagen is likely a consequence of impaired calcium mobilization,[15] and the reduced response to thromboxane is due to differences in signaling downstream from the receptor in neonatal platelets.[12] Recently, decreased expression of PAR-1 and PAR-4 receptors was described in neonatal platelets, thus explaining the decreased response to thrombin.[16,17] Although this platelet hyporeactivity would have been expected to result in a bleeding tendency, Andrew and colleagues[18] in 1999 reported that full-term neonates had shorter bleeding times (BTs) than healthy adults. Subsequent studies using the Platelet Function Analyzer (PFA-100), an objective in vitro test of primary hemostasis, also showed that PFA-100 closure times were shorter in full-term infants compared with healthy adults. Taken together, these studies demonstrated that full-term neonates have adequate primary hemostasis, despite their in vitro platelet hyporeactivity.[19,20] This seemingly paradoxic finding is because of the presence of compensatory factors in neonatal blood that enhance clot formation and perfectly balance the hyporeactivity of neonatal platelets, leading to normal BTs and closure times. These compensatory factors include the high hematocrits in neonatal blood, the high MCV (mean corpuscular volume) of neonatal red cells, and the predominance of ultralong polymers of von Willebrand factor, which is also present at high concentrations in neonatal plasma. Thus, the hyporeactivity of neonatal platelets should not be considered a developmental deficiency or a factor that confers a bleeding tendency, but rather part of a carefully balanced and unique hemostatic system.

Most studies evaluating bleeding and closure times were conducted in cord blood from full-term infants, and there are limited data in preterm neonates. However, the existing studies suggest that the platelet hyporeactivity is somewhat more pronounced[21,22] and might be less well compensated in preterm neonates, which in turn might translate into a more vulnerable hemostatic system. Specifically, BTs performed on the first day of life were longer in preterm compared with term infants, with neonates less than 33 weeks gestation exhibiting the longest bleeding times (approximately double those from adults).[23] Saxonhouse and colleagues[24] found that PFA-100 closure times from nonthrombocytopenic neonates were inversely correlated to gestational age in both cord blood and neonatal peripheral blood samples obtained on the first day of life. Importantly, however, while these BTs and closure times were longer in preterm compared with term neonates, they were still near or within the normal range for adults, suggesting that healthy preterm neonates also have adequate primary hemostasis. Data regarding how disease processes perturb this delicate system, particularly in the preterm neonate, are lacking.

In vitro studies using flow cytometry or the cone and platelet analyzer showed that the neonatal platelet function improves significantly and nearly normalizes by 10 to 14 days, even in preterm infants.[21,22,25] Consistent with this, Del Vecchio and colleagues[23] found that, by day of life 10, all infants had shorter BTs than at birth, and early gestational age-related differences had disappeared. Moreover, little or no further shortening occurred between days 10 and 30. Although no causal association has been demonstrated, these findings correlate well with the clinical observation that the highest risk of bleeding among NICU patients is found in preterm neonates during the first 10 days of life.[10]

RELATIONSHIP BETWEEN SEVERITY OF THROMBOCYTOPENIA AND BLEEDING RISK

The combination of thrombocytopenia and platelet dysfunction in neonates has been invoked as a potential contributor to the high incidence of intraventricular hemorrhage (IVH) in preterm infants. In that regard, several studies have shown an association between thrombocytopenia and IVH, although this does not establish causality. Importantly, most neonates who experience IVH have normal or minimally decreased platelet counts at the time of their bleeds, highlighting the fact that the pathogenesis of IVH in this patient population is complex and multifactorial, likely primarily involving cardiovascular instability and vascular fragility.

The relationship between degree of thrombocytopenia and bleeding risk has been assessed in a number of neonatal studies. The first large prospective observational study to evaluate this was published by Andrew and colleagues in 1992. This study used a hemorrhagic score to evaluate bleeding in neonates, and found that thrombocytopenic infants were 2.5 times more likely to bleed than nonthrombocytopenic infants. Among very low birthweight (VLBW) infants (<1500 g), thrombocytopenia was associated with a higher incidence of grade III or IV IVH (44% vs 16% in nonthrombocytopenic neonates).[1] Although there was a moderate inverse correlation between platelet count and hemorrhagic scores, this was confounded by the fact that the infants with the lowest platelet counts were more likely to have DIC (disseminated intravascular coagulation) than the nonthrombocytopenic neonates.[1]

A contemporary prospective multicenter observational study by Stanworth and colleagues[10] (PlaNeT-1 study) found that approximately 25% of thrombocytopenic neonates had platelet counts <60 × 10^9/L, and 9% of them experienced clinically significant bleeding (most commonly intracranial). Eighty-seven percent of these hemorrhages occurred during the first 2 weeks of life, and 87% were in neonates younger than 28 weeks gestation. However, nadir platelet counts were similar in infants who had either no bleeding, only minor bleeding, or severe bleeding (see Fig. 3 in Ref.[10]; Available at: http://pediatrics.aappublications.org/content/124/5/e826.full). Furthermore, a secondary analysis found that a lower nadir platelet count was associated with only a slightly increased number of bleeding events. The strongest predictors of hemorrhage were gestational age less than 28 weeks, postnatal age less than 10 days, and diagnosis of NEC.[26]

Two other recent retrospective studies have assessed bleeding in neonates with thrombocytopenia. One of them reported an association between severity of thrombocytopenia and cutaneous and gastrointestinal bleeding. However, neither study found a correlation between severity of thrombocytopenia and other types of major bleeding, including IVH.[27,28]

Taken together, the evidence indicates that, while thrombocytopenia is a risk factor for bleeding in neonates, there is a poor correlation between severity of thrombocytopenia and clinically significant bleeding. This suggests that thrombocytopenia might be a marker of severity of illness, and that factors other than the platelet count determine the bleeding risk. The latter is supported by the finding that gestational age less than 28 weeks, postnatal age less than 10 days, and diagnosis of NEC are far stronger predictive factors of bleeding among thrombocytopenic neonates than the platelet count itself. The lack of inverse correlation between platelet counts and bleeding risk has also been reported in recent studies of children with thrombocytopenia secondary to chemotherapy or myeloablation.[29]

DO PLATELET TRANSFUSIONS DECREASE THE INCIDENCE OF BLEEDING?

Platelet transfusions constitute the only readily available specific treatment for thrombocytopenia in neonates. Although platelet transfusions are frequently given to neonates with platelet counts below a certain arbitrary trigger, there is no good evidence to determine which neonate would benefit from a transfusion. In contrast to the multiple platelet transfusion trigger studies that have been performed in thrombocytopenic adults, the only platelet transfusion trigger trial performed in preterm infants was underpowered and was conducted more than 20 years ago.[30]

This landmark trial assessed the effects of prophylactic platelet transfusions in 152 VLBW infants with mild-to-moderate thrombocytopenia (platelet counts 50–150 $\times$ 10^9/L) in the first week of life, and found that the incidence of IVH was not different when the platelet count was maintained above 150 $\times$ 10^9/L compared with being allowed to fall to 60 $\times$ 10^9/L prior to transfusion (28% vs 26%, respectively).[30] Unfortunately, patients with severe thrombocytopenia (<50 $\times$ 10^9/L) and infants older than 7 days were excluded from the study. Thus, while this trial clearly indicated that transfusing VLBW infants with platelet counts >60 $\times$ 10^9/L in the first week of life does not reduce the incidence or severity of IVH, it remained unclear whether lower platelet counts could be safely tolerated in this population.

In the prospective observational PlaNeT-1 study, conducted in the United Kingdom, platelet transfusions were administered at a median platelet count of 27 $\times$ 10^9/L. In a secondary analysis, the temporal association between platelet transfusions and minor bleeding was assessed. This analysis showed that neonates had 21% fewer bleeding events during the 12 hours following a platelet transfusion compared with the 12 hours prior to transfusion.[26] However, these findings should be interpreted with caution, partly because of the study design (observational study being prone to confounders and lacking control group), and because these results were part of a secondary analyses. More recently, von Lindern and colleagues compared the bleeding outcomes in NICUs that used liberal transfusion thresholds with NICUs that used restrictive indications for platelet transfusions. These investigators found no significant differences between units.

Although there is limited evidence for the efficacy of platelet transfusions in neonates, several studies have reported a strong correlation between number of platelet transfusions and increased neonatal morbidity and mortality,[7,11,31,32] and at least 1 study has suggested that this increased mortality can be partially attributed to the platelet transfusions.[33] In the specific case of necrotizing enterocolitis, a common cause of thrombocytopenia, patients who developed short bowel syndrome or cholestasis received more platelet transfusions than those who did not (9 vs 1.5 platelet transfusions, $P = .01$).[32] Is remains unclear, however, whether this association simply reflects the fact that sicker infants receive more transfusions, or whether platelets contribute to the disease process in NEC. In that regard, it has become increasingly clear that platelets are active participants in immune and inflammatory processes.[34] It is also noteworthy that a multi-institutional analysis of complications from blood transfusions in children demonstrated that platelet transfusions were associated with the highest incidence of complications among all blood components.[35] Data collected over 10 years from the UK Serious Hazards of Transfusion national hemovigilance scheme also indicated that neonates experience a disproportionately high number of overall transfusion adverse events, compared with pediatric and adult patients.[36] Among all of the potential risks associated with platelet transfusions, transfusion-related acute lung injury (TRALI) deserves special consideration, because (given the frequency with which neonates experience respiratory deterioration in the NICU) it is likely to be under-recognized and under-reported in this population.

CURRENT RECOMMENDATIONS

At this point, it is clear that additional well designed randomized controlled trials are needed to help identify safe and effective platelet transfusion thresholds for neonates. The PlaNeT-2 study is a large multicenter study conducted in several European countries that is comparing liberal versus restrictive prophylactic platelet transfusion strategies in thrombocytopenic preterm Infants (50 vs 25 × 10^9/L, respectively).[37] Approximately 350 infants have been enrolled to date, of a planned total of 600 infants (Simon Stanworth, personal communication, 2015).

While awaiting for results from PlaNeT-2, several guidelines have been published, which in general adhere to somewhat restrictive practices. In the United Kingdom, current advice is based on expert opinion. The recommendation is that prophylactic platelet transfusion be given to all neonates (term or preterm) with a platelet count <20 × 10^9/L, to stable preterm infants if the platelet count falls below 30 × 10^9/L, and to all infants with a birth weight less than 1000 g if the platelets are below 50 × 10^9/L during the first week of life. Of note, a threshold of 50 × 10^9/L is commonly used in the United Kingdom for infants who are clinically unstable, have had a previous major bleed, or have other known risk factors (ie, NEC).[38] Christensen and colleagues recently published a compilation of evidence-based advances in transfusion practices in US NICUs, and graded the quality of the evidence and the strength of their recommendations. Based on the guidelines from Intermountain Healthcare in Utah, these investigators recommended that stable NICU patients receive a platelet transfusion if the platelet count falls below 20 × 10^9/L, and unstable patients should receive a transfusion for platelet counts <50 × 10^9/L. However, the strengths of these recommendations were low and moderate, respectively, due to the lack of solid data to guide them.[39]

The same group pioneered the application of platelet mass, which is the result of platelet count (per microliter) X mean platelet volume. In a study conducted in 2 Intermountain Healthcare NICUs, platelet count-based guidelines were used for 1 year, and then switched to platelet mass-guided transfusion guidelines. Fewer transfusions were administered to neonates during the period of time using platelet mass-guided transfusions, and no differences were found in bleeding outcomes.[40] This approach has never been tested in a prospective randomized trial, however, and thus the strength of the recommendation was moderate/small. A pilot randomized trial conducted in 30 infants concluded that such a study would be feasible, although it would likely require a very large sample size.[41]

Acknowledging the paucity of solid evidence to guide transfusion decisions, and while awaiting the results of the PlaNeT 2 trial,[37] the authors currently recommend transfusing neonates according to the levels shown in **Table 1**.

FUTURE DIRECTIONS

Although currently platelet transfusions are administered on the basis of platelet counts or platelet mass, the evidence strongly suggests that factors other than the degree of thrombocytopenia determine the bleeding risk. Thus, larger studies are needed to better characterize the platelet function and the hemostatic profile of preterm infants, and their changes over time and in response to illness. Along these lines, it will also be important to develop and validate tests that can be used in preterm

Table 1
Recommended transfusion levels for neonates

Platelet Count ($\times 10^9$/L)	Guidelines
<30	Transfuse all
30–49	Transfuse if: • Birth weight <1500 g and ≤7 d old • Clinically unstable • Concurrent coagulopathy • Previous significant hemorrhage (ie, grade 3 or 4 IVH) • Prior to surgical procedure • Post-operative period (72 h)
50–100	Transfuse if: • Active bleeding • NAIT with intracranial bleed • Before or after neurosurgical procedures

Abbreviation: NAIT, Neonatal Alloimmune Thrombocytopenia.

infants and that incorporate both platelet count and function to evaluate hemostasis, rather than individual platelet factors alone.

The PFA-100 is an in vitro test of primary hemostasis that provides a quantitative measurement of platelet adhesion, activation, and aggregation in whole blood.[42] As PFA-100 closure times represent global measurements of primary hemostasis, they are particularly attractive in neonates, since many factors contribute to their finely balanced hemostatic system. A recent pilot study by Deschmann and colleagues,[43] measuring PFA-100 closure times in thrombocytopenic neonates of various gestational and postnatal ages, showed that CT-ADP was a better marker for evaluating neonatal platelet function than CT-Epi, and identified a threshold effect of platelet counts on CT-ADP: all infants with platelet counts >90 $\times$ 10^9/L had normal CTs-ADP, and most infants with platelet counts <90 $\times$ 10^9/L had normal or minimally prolonged CTs-ADP; a few, however, exhibited significant prolongations. A prospective observational study to evaluate whether a prolonged CT-ADP is a better marker of bleeding risk than the platelet count alone is currently in progress (Neo-HAT).

Best Practices

What is the current practice?

1. Platelet transfusions are given to thrombocytopenic neonates at extremely variable platelet count thresholds, depending on gestational age, postnatal age, clinical condition, and individual preferences.

2. Surveys and observational studies suggest that platelet transfusion practices are significantly more liberal in North American compared with European NICUs.

3. Most platelet transfusions are given prophylactically to nonbleeding neonates with a platelet count below a certain threshold, based on minimal evidence. The only randomized controlled trial in the field demonstrated that VLBW infants in the first week of life who were transfused for any platelet count <150 $\times$ 10^9/L had the same incidence and severity of IVH than infants transfused for platelet counts <50 $\times$ 10^9/L.

4. A prospective observational study of neonates with platelet counts <60 $\times$ 10^9/L showed that severity of thrombocytopenia was not a good predictor of bleeding. Gestational age less than 28 weeks, age less than 10 days, and diagnosis of necrotizing enterocolitis were far stronger predictors of bleeding than the platelet count.

What changes in current practice are likely to improve outcomes?

1. Surveys suggest that sick neonates in North American NICUs are frequently transfused for platelet counts between 50 and 100 $\times$ 10^9/L, despite data from a randomized controlled trial indicating no benefit for transfusions at these counts.

2. Additional controlled randomized trials are needed to identify safe platelet transfusion thresholds in neonates of different gestational and postnatal ages. One such trial is currently comparing the safety and efficacy of using 50 versus 25 $\times$ 10^9/L as neonatal platelet transfusion thresholds (PlaNeT-2 trial).

3. Several studies have shown a poor correlation between platelet counts and bleeding risk, suggesting that other factors are more important determinants of bleeding. Thus, additional studies are needed to understand platelet function in preterm neonates, and to develop tests that better assess primary hemostasis and identify neonates at risk of bleeding.

Summary Statement

There is significant world-wide variability in platelet transfusion thresholds used to transfuse thrombocytopenic neonates. A large multicenter randomized controlled trial comparing 2 different platelet transfusion thresholds in neonates is currently ongoing, and should provide data to guide transfusion practice. However, several studies have found that factors other than the degree of thrombocytopenia determine the bleeding risk. Thus, it will be important to develop better tests to assess primary hemostasis and bleeding risk in neonates.

REFERENCES

1. Andrew M, Castle V, Saigal S, et al. Clinical impact of neonatal thrombocytopenia. J Pediatr 1987;110:457–64.
2. Castle V, Andrew M, Kelton J, et al. Frequency and mechanism of neonatal thrombocytopenia. J Pediatr 1986;108:749–55.
3. Mehta P, Vasa R, Neumann L, et al. Thrombocytopenia in the high-risk infant. J Pediatr 1980;97:791–4.
4. Christensen RD, Henry E, Wiedmeier SE, et al. Thrombocytopenia among extremely low birth weight neonates: data from a multihospital healthcare system. J Perinatol 2006;26:348–53.
5. Christensen RD, Henry E, Jopling J, et al. The CBC: reference ranges for neonates. Semin Perinatol 2009;33:3–11.
6. Wiedmeier SE, Henry E, Sola-Visner MC, et al. Platelet reference ranges for neonates, defined using data from over 47,000 patients in a multihospital healthcare system. J Perinatol 2009;29:130–6.
7. Del Vecchio A, Sola MC, Theriaque DW, et al. Platelet transfusions in the neonatal intensive care unit:factors predicting which patients will require multiple transfusions. Transfusion 2001;41:803–8.
8. Josephson CD, Su LL, Christensen RD, et al. Platelet transfusion practices among neonatologists in the United States and Canada: results of a survey. Pediatrics 2009;123:278–85.
9. Cremer M, Sola-Visner M, Roll S, et al. Platelet transfusions in neonates: practices in the United States vary significantly from those in Austria, Germany, and Switzerland. Transfusion 2011;51:2634–41.
10. Stanworth SJ, Clarke P, Watts T, et al. Prospective, observational study of outcomes in neonates with severe thrombocytopenia. Pediatrics 2009;124:e826–34.
11. Garcia MG, Duenas E, Sola MC, et al. Epidemiologic and outcome studies of patients who received platelet transfusions in the neonatal intensive care unit. J Perinatol 2001;21:415–20.

12. Israels SJ, Odaibo FS, Robertson C, et al. Deficient thromboxane synthesis and response in platelets from premature infants. Pediatr Res 1997;41:218–23.
13. Rajasekhar D, Barnard MR, Bednarek FJ, et al. Platelet hyporeactivity in very low birth weight neonates. Thromb Haemost 1997;77:1002–7.
14. Corby DG, O'Barr TP. Decreased alpha-adrenergic receptors in newborn platelets: cause of abnormal response to epinephrine. Dev Pharmacol Ther 1981;2: 215–25.
15. Gelman B, Setty BN, Chen D, et al. Impaired mobilization of intracellular calcium in neonatal platelets. Pediatr Res 1996;39:692–6.
16. Schlagenhauf A, Schweintzger S, Birner-Gruenberger R, et al. Newborn platelets: lower levels of protease-activated receptors cause hypoaggregability to thrombin. Platelets 2010;21:641–7.
17. Schlagenhauf A, Schweintzger S, Birner-Grunberger R, et al. Comparative evaluation of PAR1, GPIb-IX-V, and integrin alphaIIbbeta3 levels in cord and adult platelets. Hamostaseologie 2010;30(Suppl 1):S164–7.
18. Andrew M, Paes B, Bowker J, et al. Evaluation of an automated bleeding time device in the newborn. Am J Hematol 1990;35:275–7.
19. Boudewijns M, Raes M, Peeters V, et al. Evaluation of platelet function on cord blood in 80 healthy term neonates using the Platelet Function Analyser (PFA-100); shorter in vitro bleeding times in neonates than adults. Eur J Pediatr 2003;162:212–3.
20. Israels SJ, Cheang T, McMillan-Ward EM, et al. Evaluation of primary hemostasis in neonates with a new in vitro platelet function analyzer. J Pediatr 2001;138: 116–9.
21. Sitaru AG, Holzhauer S, Speer CP, et al. Neonatal platelets from cord blood and peripheral blood. Platelets 2005;16:203–10.
22. Ucar T, Gurman C, Arsan S, et al. Platelet aggregation in term and preterm newborns. Pediatr Hematol Oncol 2005;22:139–45.
23. Del Vecchio A, Latini G, Henry E, et al. Template bleeding times of 240 neonates born at 24 to 41 weeks gestation. J Perinatol 2008;28:427–31.
24. Saxonhouse MA, Garner R, Mammel L, et al. Closure times measured by the platelet function analyzer PFA-100 are longer in neonatal blood compared to cord blood samples. Neonatology 2010;97:242–9.
25. Bednarek FJ, Bean S, Barnard MR, et al. The platelet hyporeactivity of extremely low birth weight neonates is age-dependent. Thromb Res 2009;124:42–5.
26. Muthukumar P, Venkatesh V, Curley A, et al. Severe thrombocytopenia and patterns of bleeding in neonates: results from a prospective observational study and implications for use of platelet transfusions. Transfus Med 2012; 22:338–43.
27. Baer VL, Lambert DK, Henry E, et al. Severe thrombocytopenia in the NICU. Pediatrics 2009;124:e1095–100.
28. von Lindern JS, van den Bruele T, Lopriore E, et al. Thrombocytopenia in neonates and the risk of intraventricular hemorrhage: a retrospective cohort study. BMC Pediatr 2011;11:16.
29. Josephson CD, Granger S, Assmann SF, et al. Bleeding risks are higher in children versus adults given prophylactic platelet transfusions for treatment-induced hypoproliferative thrombocytopenia. Blood 2012;120:748–60.
30. Andrew M, Vegh P, Caco C, et al. A randomized, controlled trial of platelet transfusions in thrombocytopenic premature infants. J Pediatr 1993;123:285–91.
31. Bonifacio L, Petrova A, Nanjundaswamy S, et al. Thrombocytopenia related neonatal outcome in preterms. Indian J Pediatr 2007;74:269–74.

32. Kenton AB, Hegemier S, Smith EO, et al. Platelet transfusions in infants with necrotizing enterocolitis do not lower mortality but may increase morbidity. J Perinatol 2005;25:173–7.
33. Baer VL, Lambert DK, Henry E, et al. Do platelet transfusions in the NICU adversely affect survival? Analysis of 1600 thrombocytopenic neonates in a multi-hospital healthcare system. J Perinatol 2007;27:790–6.
34. Semple JW, Italiano JE Jr, Freedman J. Platelets and the immune continuum. Nat Rev Immunol 2011;11:264–74.
35. Slonim AD, Joseph JG, Turenne WM, et al. Blood transfusions in children: a multi-institutional analysis of practices and complications. Transfusion 2008;48:73–80.
36. Stainsby D, Jones H, Wells AW, et al. Adverse outcomes of blood transfusion in children: analysis of UK reports to the serious hazards of transfusion scheme 1996–2005. Br J Haematol 2008;141:73–9.
37. Curley A, Venkatesh V, Stanworth S, et al. Platelets for neonatal transfusion—study 2: a randomised controlled trial to compare two different platelet count thresholds for prophylactic platelet transfusion to preterm neonates. Neonatology 2014;106:102–6.
38. Carr R, Kelly AM, Williamson LM. Neonatal thrombocytopenia and platelet trans-fusion—a UK perspective. Neonatology 2015;107:1–7.
39. Christensen RD, Carroll PD, Josephson CD. Evidence-based advances in trans-fusion practice in neonatal intensive care units. Neonatology 2014;106:245–53.
40. Gerday E, Baer VL, Lambert DK, et al. Testing platelet mass versus platelet count to guide platelet transfusions in the neonatal intensive care unit. Transfusion 2009;49:2034–9.
41. Zisk JL, Mackley A, Clearly G, et al. Transfusing neonates based on platelet count vs. platelet mass: a randomized feasibility-pilot study. Platelets 2014;25:513–6.
42. Kundu SK, Heilmann EJ, Sio R, et al. Description of an in vitro platelet function analyzer—PFA-100. Semin Thromb Hemost 1995;21(Suppl 2):106–12.
43. Deschmann E, Sola-Visner M, Saxonhouse MA. Primary hemostasis in neonates with thrombocytopenia. J Pediatr 2014;164:167–72.

Neonatal Platelet Function

Antonio Del Vecchio, MD[a],*, Mario Motta, MD[b],
Costantino Romagnoli, MD[c]

KEYWORDS

- Platelets • Megakaryocytes • Primary hemostasis • Platelet hyporeactivity
- Neonatal hemostasis • Thrombocytopoiesis

KEY POINTS

- Platelets are crucial hemostatic components and the regulation of their production and function highly affects primary hemostasis.
- In addition to the classic role in hemostasis and thrombosis, platelets have an important role in the immune response.
- The hyporesponsiveness of neonatal platelets correlates with gestational age, concomitant with maturation of the entire hemostatic system.
- Genetic disorders of platelet function are rarely identified in neonates. Temporary acquired disorders, secondary to medications or hypothermia, are typically associated with mild to moderate clinical symptoms.

INTRODUCTION

Platelets arise from the fragmentation of megakaryocytes in the bone marrow, and circulate in the blood as disk-shaped anucleate elements. They have an average diameter of about 1.5 μm, 20% of the diameter of erythrocytes, and a lifespan of 7 to 10 days. Once released from the bone marrow, young platelets enter the circulation where a proportion of them pool in the spleen. A small pool of platelets, on the order of 10% to 15% of the total, stays in the pulmonary vasculature, and these, similarly to those in the spleen, can enter the circulation after exercise or epinephrine administration.[1] Platelets are crucial hemostatic components and the regulation of their production and function is highly relevant to clinical bleeding issues.

Disclosures: The authors have no conflict of interest to declare.
[a] Neonatal Intensive Care Unit, Di Venere Hospital, Via Ospedale Di Venere n.1, Bari 70131, Italy; [b] Neonatology and Neonatal Intensive Care Unit, Children's Hospital of Brescia, Brescia, Italy; [c] Neonatal Intensive Care Unit, Division of Neonatology, Department of Pediatrics, Catholic University of the Sacred Heart, Rome, Italy
* Corresponding author.
E-mail address: a.delvecchio@asl.bari.it

Clin Perinatol 42 (2015) 625–638
http://dx.doi.org/10.1016/j.clp.2015.04.015
0095-5108/15/$ – see front matter © 2015 Elsevier Inc. All rights reserved.

Platelets adhere to sites of vascular injury, generate biologic mediators, secrete their granule contents, form multicellular aggregates, and serve as a nucleus for plasma coagulation reactions. When the vascular endothelium is damaged, platelets adhere to the exposed basement membrane collagen, initiating the process of primary hemostasis, and interacting with subendothelium-bound von Willebrand factor (vWf) via the membrane glycoprotein (GP) Ib complex. Afterward, platelets secrete and release proaggregatory substances, such as ADP, and they synthesize thromboxane A_2 from arachidonic acid. As a consequence, additional platelets are recruited and form aggregates with those platelets that have adhered to the vessel wall, and consolidate the initial hemostatic plug. The platelet GPIIb/IIIa complex mediates platelet-to-platelet interactions. As a result, the primary hemostatic plug is formed, and bleeding is arrested.[2] Platelets also provide an extensive phospholipid surface for the interaction and activation of clotting factors in the coagulation cascade. Enzymes and cofactors of the coagulation system, and a fibrin mesh, further stabilize the initial hemostatic plug. Collectively they help maintain the integrity of the vascular system.[3]

In addition to their classic role in hemostasis and thrombosis, recent studies reveal an important role in inflammation and the immune response.[4] Platelets produce and contain various cytokines and proinflammatory molecules, such as interleukin-1β, P-selectin, CD40L, transforming growth factor-β, and thrombospondin-1, supporting leukocyte-platelet interaction. Furthermore, in association with various functional Toll-like receptors (eg, Toll-like receptors 2, 4, and 9) on their surface, platelets likely act as sentinels, recognizing invading microorganisms, thus linking innate immunity with hemostasis.[5] In addition, activated platelets can directly affect B-cell differentiation and proliferation, which ultimately influence germinal center formation and antibody production.[6] Platelets can actively bind circulating gram-positive bacteria and consign them to splenic CD8α[+] dendritic cells, supporting antibacterial CD8[+] T-cell expansion.[7] Thus, the effects of platelets on adaptive immunity may play an important role in host defense. Therefore, defects of platelet function mighty not only result in hemostatic abnormalities but theoretically could adversely affect innate and adaptive immune responses.

PLATELET PRODUCTION IN NEONATES

The complex process of platelet production, from megakaryocyte progenitors to megakaryocytes and then to platelets, initiates early during fetal life. At 8 weeks postconception megakaryocytes are detected in the liver and circulatory system. Platelets increase in number during fetal life, reaching near adult concentrations in the blood around 22 weeks of gestation.[2,8]

Sola-Visner[8] schematically described the process of platelet production as consisting of four steps: (1) production of thrombopoietic factors (mainly thrombopoietin), (2) proliferation of megakaryocyte progenitors, (3) maturation of megakaryocytes, and (4) production and release of platelets into the circulation. These four steps are essentially the same in neonates as in adults, even though substantial developmental differences in megakaryocyte biology exist and may be responsible for the unique responses of fetal/neonatal megakaryocytes to thrombocytopenia.[8]

Plasma thrombopoietin concentrations are higher in healthy neonates than in healthy adults, but neonates with thrombocytopenia usually have lower thrombopoietin concentrations than do adults with thrombocytopenia.[9] Additionally, whereas neonatal megakaryocyte progenitors have a higher proliferative potential than those of adults and are more sensitive to thrombopoietin than adult progenitors, neonatal megakaryocytes are smaller and of lower ploidy than adult megakaryocytes, and produce fewer platelets per megakaryocyte. Thus, neonates with thrombocytopenia typically increase megakaryocyte number but not size.[10] The small size and lower DNA content of neonatal megakaryocytes are probably related to their microenvironment and intrinsic factors. It has been hypothesized that these developmental differences contribute to an increased susceptibility of neonates to thrombocytopenia.[10–12]

PLATELET FUNCTION IN NEONATES

Plasma coagulation has been well studied in neonates, but because of the difficulty obtaining adequate volumes of blood for various platelet function tests, scanty data are available on neonatal platelet function. Although preterm infants are at greater risk of bleeding than are term infants, most research on neonatal platelet function has been accomplished from the blood of term neonates, and most of those studies used umbilical cord blood samples. However, it is not yet clear whether platelets from cord blood are an accurate model for neonatal platelet function over the subsequent hours and days.[13,14]

Similarly to the development of the plasma coagulation system, which matures during the early weeks and months of life, it may be assumed that age-dependent mechanisms and developmental changes influence platelet production and function.[15] In the immediate newborn period, platelet adhesion is enhanced, compared with adults: GPIb appears early on fetal platelets, around 18 to 26 weeks gestation, and similar to plasma concentrations of vWf, are present in concentrations higher than those found in adults. Neonatal plasma also contains an increased proportion of functional high-molecular-weight vWf forms, which result in an enhanced platelet adhesion that might compensate for the decreased intrinsic platelet activation in healthy neonates, but may leave sick neonates at increased risk of bleeding.[8]

Regarding platelet activation and aggregation, platelets express GPIIb/IIIa early in gestation, and at early gestation fibrinogen is found in concentrations similar to those in adults and it binds normally to newborn platelets. Although platelet adhesion and aggregation are difficult to assess in neonates, it seems that responses to various physiologic agonists are reduced.[13,16] For instance, flow cytometric analysis of cord blood and peripheral blood demonstrates a generalized platelet hyporeactivity during the first days of life to thrombin, collagen, ADP, and U46619 (a stable thromboxane A_2 analogue). This reactivity reaches normal adult levels between the fifth and ninth day of life. It is not clear whether this neonatal platelet hyporeactivity causes a clinically important reduced hemostatic effectiveness, but persistence of hyporeactivity after the 10th day of life might indeed suggest a platelet disorder.[17] The degree of hyporesponsiveness of neonatal platelets depends on gestational age. Perhaps this transient developmental dysfunction protects neonates from harmful effects of birth stresses on the coagulation system.[1,17]

The transient hyporeactivity of neonatal platelets was formerly considered to be the result of platelet activation and degranulation during labor and delivery, but more recent studies have not supported that theory.[18,19] The most accepted explanations include relative deficiencies of phospholipid metabolism and thromboxane production, different regulation of GPIIb/IIIa activation, impaired mobilization of calcium and intracellular signaling, granule secretion, and aggregation.[18,20] Morphologic modifications of neonatal platelets following activation have not been reported.

Certain maternal diseases might influence neonatal platelet function. For instance, neonates born to mothers with pregnancy-induced hypertension can have thrombocytopenia and impaired platelet function. Pregnancy-induced hypertension can also activate maternal platelets. Various mechanisms have been hypothesized to explain the effects of pregnancy-induced hypertension on platelets. These include altered metabolism of calcium, alteration of platelet membrane GPs, increased release of plasma β-thromboglobulin, and altered nitric oxide (NO) bioavailability.[21] Neonates born to mothers with pregnancy-induced hypertension can have decreased platelet surface expression of P-selectin and CD63, GPIIb/IIIa, and CD9.[22,23]

Similarly, platelets of patients with diabetes are hyperactive.[24] In gestational diabetes, maternal hyperglycemia can be accompanied by fetal hyperinsulinemia, which in animal studies has been associated with impaired platelet function. Proposed mechanisms include inhibition of platelet-activating factor biosynthesis, reduction of the levels of platelet-activating factor, and impairment of thromboxane synthesis.[23,25] It is unknown whether these conditions may be responsible for or contribute to the frequency and severity of neonatal intraventricular hemorrhage.

With regard to involvement of platelets in the activity of the innate and adaptive immune system, recent studies conducted in adults demonstrated that the lethal effects of platelets on Plasmodium falciparum parasites require platelet activation[26] and that thrombocytopenia in patients with primary chronic autoimmune thrombocytopenia is associated with a significantly higher long-term risk of infection.[27]

It is unknown whether developmental changes in platelet production and function in neonates influences their immune responses. We speculate that, especially in preterm infants,[17–19] thrombocytopenia and disorders of platelet function are responsible for increased susceptibility to infections.

DISORDERS OF NEONATAL PLATELET FUNCTION

Most disorders of neonatal platelet function are rare, have mild to moderate clinical symptoms, and are classified as either hereditary or acquired (**Box 1**). Congenital defects can be diagnosed in early childhood but it is unusual to detect them at birth. Genetic causes are typically mutations resulting in deficient or defective relevant GPs. Two genetic disorders with moderate to severe symptoms that can present at birth are Glanzmann thromboasthenia and Bernard-Soulier syndrome. Glanzmann thromboasthenia can present in the neonatal period. It involves deficiency of the GPIIb/IIIa complex, inherited in an autosomal-recessive pattern, and resulting in platelets that do not aggregate in response to normal stimuli, except ristocetin. The platelet count and morphology with light microscopy are normal.[28,29]

Bernard-Soulier syndrome is an autosomal-recessive disorder resulting from a deficiency of platelet GPIb, which mediates the initial interaction of platelets to the subendothelial components via the von Willebrand protein. This syndrome can result in a severe bleeding disorder. Platelets do not aggregate in response to ristocetin. In this condition the platelet count is low, but characteristically the platelets are large, often the size of red blood cells.[30] Secretory platelet disorders have defective platelet granules and cause mild to moderate bleeding. Included in this subset of disorders are gray platelet syndrome, dense granule deficiency, Chédiak-Higashi syndrome, and Hermansky-Pudlak syndrome.[1]

Unlike hereditary defects, acquired disorders of platelet function are common. A primary hemostatic defect can occur as a result of drugs given to the mother or neonate. The inhibition of cyclooxygenase enzyme can be produced by aspirin, often given to the mother; indomethacin; and ibuprofen, commonly used for the closure of patent ductus arteriosus.

The influence of these drugs on platelet function is transitory, generally lasting about 24 hours. Ibuprofen, administered to neonates with a patent ductus arteriosus, has little adverse effect on platelet plug formation, and prolongs the bleeding time

Box 1			
Platelet function disorders in neonates			
	Functional Platelet Disorders		**Laboratory Findings**
Inherited (rare) (because of diagnostic difficulties frequency is probably underestimated)			
Adhesion defects	Bernard-Soulier syndrome	Absence or decreased expression of GPIb/IX/V on the surface of platelets	Prolonged bleeding time Moderate thrombocytopenia (↓ platelet lifespan) Platelet aggregometry: decreased in response to ristocetin; normal with ADP, collagen, arachidonic acid, epinephrine Extraordinarily large platelets
	"Platelet type" von Willebrand disease (pseudo von Willebrand disease)	Defect of platelet GPIba → increased avidity for normal vWf → binding of the largest vWf multimers to resting platelets and clearance from the circulation → thrombocytopenia and adhesion defect	Prolonged bleeding time Moderate thrombocytopenia Loss of large vWf multimers Enhanced ristocetin-induced platelet aggregation
	Collagen receptor deficiency	Abnormalities of platelet GPVI and GPIa/IIa (receptors for collagen) → adhesion and collagen-induced platelet aggregation defects	—
Aggregation defects	Glanzmann thrombasthenia	Abnormalities of platelet GPIIb/IIIa (fibrinogen receptor) → platelets less able to adhere to each other and to the underlying tissue of damaged blood vessels	Normal platelet count and morphology Platelet aggregation in response to ristocetin, but not to other agonists (ie, ADP, thrombin, collagen, or epinephrine) Clot retraction absent
	Afibrinogenemia	Combined bleeding disorder (platelets and clotting are abnormal)	Absence of fibrinogen from the blood Abnormal platelet aggregation, bleeding time, APTT, PT, TT Moderate thrombocytopenia
			(continued on next page)

	Functional Platelet Disorders		Laboratory Findings
Secretion disorders	Abnormalities of platelet granules (α,δ,α+δ)	α: Gray platelet syndrome, Quebec platelet disorder (FV Quebec), Jacobsen syndrome, Paris-Trousseau syndrome δ: Storage pool disease, Hermansky-Pudlak syndrome, Chédiak-Higashi syndrome, Wiskott-Aldrich syndrome α and δ combined deficiency	—
	Abnormalities of the signal transduction and secretion	Impaired liberation of arachidonic acid from membrane phospholipids Cyclooxygenase deficiency ("aspirin-like disease") Thromboxane synthetase deficiency Thromboxane A$_2$ receptor abnormalities	—
Defects of platelet coagulant activity	Scott syndrome	Lack of exposure of procoagulant phosphatidylserine to the external leaflet of the plasma membrane of activated platelets and other hematologic lineages → impaired thrombin formation	—
Acquired (common)			
Drug-induced platelet dysfunction	Aspirin Nonsteroidal anti-inflammatory drugs β-Lactam antibiotics	—	—
Disease-associated platelet dysfunction	Uremia Antiplatelet antibodies Others (diabetes mellitus, liver disease, DIC) Hematopoietic disorders (paraproteinemias, myeloproliferative disorders, myelodysplastic syndrome, leukemia)	—	—

Abbreviations: APTT, activated partial thromboplastin time; DIC, disseminated intravascular coagulation; PT, prothrombin time; TT, thrombin time.

less than does indomethacin.[31,32] Inhaled NO also may reduce platelet reactivity and in premature infants, inhaled NO may decrease platelet aggregation, and inhibit platelet adhesion to endothelial cells, thus increasing the risk for intraventricular hemorrhage.[33]

Impaired platelet function and thrombocytopenia have been reported in neonates with persistent pulmonary hypertension, meconium aspiration, and congenital diaphragmatic hernia treated with extracorporeal membrane oxygenation. During extracorporeal membrane oxygenation, platelet dysfunction persists despite platelet transfusions, and platelet function returns to normal 8 hours after extracorporeal membrane oxygenation is discontinued.[1,34]

Other circumstances that can cause platelet dysfunction include hyperbilirubinemia and phototherapy, and uremia and/or renal failure.[1] Excessive production of NO by endothelial cells inhibits platelet function, and may be responsible for bleeding in patients with uremia. Because the prolonged bleeding time and the hemostatic abnormalities are in part corrected by red blood cell transfusion or erythropoietin therapy, the failure of hemoglobin to deactivate excessive NO synthesis has been suggested as involved in the platelet dysfunction. A further explanation considers that platelets arrive at exposed vascular subendothelium, being pushed there by blood flow, largely by erythrocytes, and these latter release ADP to activate the platelets following vessel injury. Consequently, a low hematocrit may be responsible for a prolongation in the bleeding time.[35,36]

EVALUATION OF PLATELET FUNCTION IN NEONATES

The objective of platelet function testing is to determine the cause of abnormal bleeding. Assessment of neonatal platelet function is hampered by the difficulty obtaining adequate blood samples, and lack of rigorous gestational-age reference intervals.[13,14] This is true particularly for aggregometry and flow cytometric evaluation of platelet activation. Clinical evaluation of platelet function begins with a complete blood count and examination of the peripheral smear to evaluate platelet clumping or platelets adhering to neutrophils (platelet satellitism), or Bernard-Soulier syndrome with giant platelets (Table 1).

Platelet Aggregometry

Aggregometry has been the most frequently reported method for evaluating neonatal platelet function, but despite its diagnostic potential it is rarely used clinically for neonates because of the limitations mentioned in the volume of blood needed for analysis (generally 10 mL).[37] Platelet aggregometry measures the transmission of light through a platelet suspension. Initially, because of platelet shape changes, there is an increase in optical density, but subsequent platelet aggregation in response to agonists, such as ADP, epinephrine, and collagen, reduces the optical density. Using these methods platelets of neonates do not have the high level of aggregations characteristic of adult platelets.[38,39] These differences are more marked in platelets of preterm infants.[40] In contrast, aggregation in response to thrombin is modestly decreased in neonatal platelets, and the ristocetin-induced agglutination of neonatal platelets is actually enhanced compared with adult control subjects.[41] Agglutination of platelets by ristocetin depends on the higher levels and enhanced activity of circulating neonatal plasma vWF and its platelet receptor GPIb/IX/V.[40,42]

The lack of appropriate neonatal reference intervals and limited availability of the technology significantly reduce clinical application to neonates.[43]

Table 1
Assessment of neonatal platelet function and possible clinical implications

Test	Findings	Possible Implication
Peripheral smear	Large platelet size, platelet clumping, platelet satellitism Platelet granularity	Bernard-Soulier syndrome Platelets adhering to neutrophils Gray platelet syndrome
Platelet aggregometry	Aggregation response to various agonists: ADP, collagen, epinephrine, thrombin ristocetin	Storage pool disorders (aggregation only with ADP, collagen, epinephrine) von Willebrand disease (impaired ristocetin aggregation) Glanzmann thrombasthenia (platelets do not aggregate in response to normal stimuli, except ristocetin)
Flow cytometric evaluation of platelet activation	Detection of platelet surface glycoproteins	Bernard-Soulier syndrome (low or absent GPIb) α granule dysfunction (low or absent P-selectin) Glanzmann thrombasthenia (low or absent GPIIb/IIIa)
Whole-blood hemostasis		
Bleeding time	Measures the time required to generate a hemostatically effective platelet plug	A prolonged bleeding time with a normal platelet count indicates a qualitative platelet disorder
Surface coverage cone and platelet analyzer	Assessment of platelet adhesion and aggregation on a polystyrene surface under near physiologic shear conditions using a cone-and-plate viscometer	Percentage of total area covered by platelets (surface coverage) indicates the extent of platelet adhesion
Closure time platelet function analyzer 100	Closure time for collagen/ADP or collagen/Epi	Shorter in neonates than in adults and healthy children Prolonged in neonates undergoing therapeutic hypothermia, but returns to normal on rewarming Prolonged in neonates after several days of treatment with ampicillin, ibuprofen, or indomethacin
Thromboelastography	Dynamics of clot development, stabilization, and dissolution	Begins gathering results exactly where conventional tests end, the first fibrin network formation

Flow Cytometric Evaluation of Platelet Activation

Whole-blood flow cytometry is an accurate way to measure neonatal platelet activation, and has addressed many of the problems encountered in neonatal aggregometry studies. A total of 5 to 100 μL of blood is required, with minimal sample manipulation before analysis. Detection of platelet surface GPs by flow cytometry, using monoclonal antibodies directed at platelet activation markers, such as P-selectin and the fibrinogen binding site exposed on the GPIIb/IIIa complex, provides insights into platelet function. Flow cytometric studies from cord blood or from neonates have confirmed the early neonatal platelet hyporesponsiveness and the resolution by Day 10.[18,20] An advantage of flow cytometric studies is the evaluation of the basal status of platelet activation and the reactivity of various agonists, such as epinephrine, thrombin, ADP, and U46619.[18] Disadvantages of this method include high costs of equipment and reagents, need for qualified laboratory staff, length of time needed for testing, and lack of neonatal reference intervals appropriate for gestational and postnatal age.

Whole-Blood Hemostasis: Bleeding Time, Surface Coverage, and Closure Time

The bleeding time measures the time required to generate a hemostatically effective platelet plug, which occurs through the interaction of platelets with the subendothelial structures of a damaged vessel, arresting bleeding from a standardized superficial skin incision (**Fig. 1**). It is a useful clinical tool to detect quantitative or qualitative platelet disorders or microvascular defectiveness. Its diagnostic value in neonates is controversial, mainly because of limited experience in executing the test and high operator-dependency.[44,45]

A prolonged bleeding time with a normal platelet count indicates a qualitative platelet disorder, because cessation of bleeding involves platelet adhesion, activation, and aggregation. This test is not useful in assessing platelet function in patients with severe thrombocytopenia, because at platelet counts lower than about 75,000 to 100,000/μL, the bleeding time is typically prolonged proportionally to the severity of thrombocytopenia.[44] Bleeding times measured on the first day of life are longer in preterm compared with full-term infants, with neonates born at less than 33 weeks gestation having the longest bleeding times (approximately twice as long as those from full-term neonates).[46]

The cone and platelet analyzer is a device developed to test platelet adhesion and aggregation on a polystyrene surface under close to physiologic shear conditions using a cone-and-plate viscometer, which requires a small amount of blood

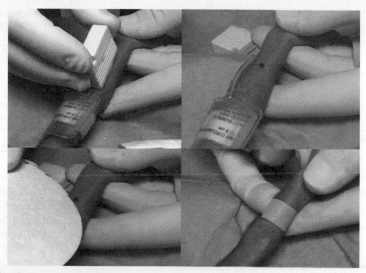

Fig. 1. Bleeding time procedure.

(about 200-μL samples of citrated whole blood).[47] The percentage of total area covered by platelets (surface coverage) indicates the extent of platelet adhesion.[48,49]

The platelet function analyzer 100 (PFA-100, Siemens Healthcare Diagnostics Inc, Deerfield, IL, USA) is an in vitro method to assess primary hemostasis under shear stress. In this system, primary hemostasis is simulated with a quantitative measurement of platelet adhesion, activation, and aggregation in whole blood.[50] The PFA-100 uses a disposable test cartridge that contains a membrane coated with collagen and either ADP (Col/ADP membrane) or epinephrine (Col/Epi membrane), thus mimicking exposed subendothelium. A blood sample of 0.8 mL of citrated blood is placed in a cup and is aspirated through the aperture. The shear stress and the agonists in the membrane activate platelets, leading to platelet aggregation. The end point, expressed as "closure time," is when blood flow stops because of occlusion of the aperture by platelet aggregates, obtaining a measure of platelet-dependent hemostasis.[51,52] The closure times, similarly to bleeding times, are significantly shorter in neonates than in adults and healthy children. The advantages of this instrument include simplicity and reproducibility. The results of the PFA-100 closure times and the cone and platelet analyzer are affected by platelet count and hematocrit.[36,47] Bleeding times and PFA-100 closure times become prolonged in neonates undergoing therapeutic hypothermia, but return to normal on rewarming.[48] Likewise, bleeding times and PFA-100 closure times become prolonged in neonates after several days of treatment with ampicillin,[53] ibuprofen,[29] and indomethicin.[32]

Surface coverage in healthy term neonates is higher than that of adults, and in preterm infants is lower compared with term infant, but higher than that of adults.

Thromboelastogram and Rotating Thromboelastogram

Thromboelastography is a point-of-care coagulation monitoring device that provides overall information on the dynamics of clot development, stabilization, and dissolution, reflecting in vivo hemostasis, using whole blood and testing small volumes. Thromboelastography analyzes the initiation of clot formation, actual clot firmness, and fibrinolysis. Interestingly, it begins gathering results exactly where conventional tests end: the first fibrin network formation. Technologic developments have now led to good standardization and improved reproducibility.[54] The use of thromboelastography and rotating thromboelastogram to evaluate clot formation in neonates has recently been reported[55–57] and reference values for rotating thromboelastogram clot formation parameters were established in cord blood of full-term and preterm infants.[58]

Best Practices

What is current practice?

- In vitro testing of platelet function indicates hypofunction of platelets of neonates, compared with platelets of adults. This finding is sometimes interpreted as suggesting a functional defect in neonatal hemostasis. This has influenced neonatologists to want relatively higher platelet counts as neonatal platelet "transfusion triggers" to avoid serious hemorrhagic problems.

- In vivo testing of platelet function indicates normal or hyperfunction of platelets of neonates, compared with platelets of adults. How this finding should influence neonatal transfusion practice remains to be determined.

What changes in current practice are likely to improve outcomes?

• Reconciliation of the in vitro and in vivo platelet function testing differences might moderate the concern that platelet hemostasis in neonates is defective, and might give confidence that platelet transfusion "trigger levels" may not have to be as high as they have been in traditional neonatal intensive care unit transfusion practice.

• Better definition of developmental aspects of all hemostatic elements will facilitate designing best practices to prevent hemostatic problems in extremely low birth weight neonates.

• The clinical value of neonatal intensive care unit platelet function testing using the thromboelastogram and the rotating thromboelastogram requires more study and better definition, because this testing might provide new and relevant information to help direct therapy and predict outcomes.

Summary statement

Tests, techniques, and approaches reviewed in this article should assist clinicians to evaluate platelet function in neonates, and should suggest means of identifying common and rare congenital and acquired abnormalities of platelet function.

REFERENCES

1. Sola MC, Christensen RD. Developmental aspects of platelets and disorders of platelets in the neonatal period. In: Christensen RD, editor. Hematologic problems of the neonate. Philadelphia: Saunders; 2000. p. 273–309.
2. Kühne T, Imbach P. Neonatal platelet physiology and pathophysiology. Eur J Pediatr 1998;157:87–94.
3. Kuhle S, Male C, Mitchell L. Developmental hemostasis: pro- and anticoagulant systems during childhood. Semin Thromb Hemost 2003;29:329–38.
4. Li C, Li J, Li Y, et al. Crosstalk between platelets and the immune system: old systems with new discoveries. Adv Hematol 2012;2012:384685.
5. Semple JW, Freedman J. Platelets and innate immunity. Cell Mol Life Sci 2010;67: 499–511.
6. Elzey BD, Grant JF, Sinn HW, et al. Cooperation between platelet-derived CD154 and CD4+ T cells for enhanced germinal center formation. J Leukoc Biol 2005; 78:80–4.
7. Verschoor A, Neuenhahn M, Navarini AA, et al. A platelet-mediated system for shuttling blood-borne bacteria to CD8α+ dendritic cells depends on glycoprotein GPIb and complement C3. Nat Immunol 2011;12:1194–201.
8. Sola-Visner M. Platelets in the neonatal period: developmental differences in platelet production, function, and hemostasis and the potential impact of therapies. Hematology Am Soc Hematol Educ Program 2012;2012:506–11.
9. Murray NA, Watts TL, Roberts IA. Endogenous thrombopoietin levels and effect of recombinant human thrombopoietin on megakaryocyte precursors in term and preterm babies. Pediatr Res 1998;43:148–51.
10. Sola MC, Calhoun DA, Hutson AD, et al. Plasma thrombopoietin concentrations in thrombocytopenic and non-thrombocytopenic neonates in a neonatal intensive care unit. Br J Haematol 1999;104:90–2.
11. Hegyi E, Nakazawa M, Debili N, et al. Developmental changes in human megakaryocyte ploidy. Exp Hematol 1991;19:87–94.
12. Murray NA, Roberts IA. Circulating megakaryocytes and their progenitors in early thrombocytopenia in preterm neonates. Pediatr Res 1996;40:112–9.

13. Israels SJ, Rand ML, Michelson AD. Neonatal platelet function. Semin Thromb Hemost 2003;29:363–72.
14. Haley KM, Recht M, McCarty OJ. Neonatal platelets: mediators of primary hemostasis in the developing hemostatic system. Pediatr Res 2014;76:230–7.
15. Andrew M, Vegh P, Johnston M, et al. Maturation of the hemostatic system during childhood. Blood 1992;80:1998–2005.
16. Strauss T, Sidlik-Muskatel R, Kenet G. Developmental hemostasis: primary hemostasis and evaluation of platelet function in neonates. Semin Fetal Neonatal Med 2011;16:301–4.
17. Bednarek FJ, Bean S, Barnard MR, et al. The platelet hyporeactivity of extremely low birth weight neonates is age-dependent. Thromb Res 2009;124:42–5.
18. Rajasekhar D, Barnard M, Bednarek FJ, et al. Platelet hyporeactivity in very low birth weight neonates. Thromb Haemost 1997;77:1002–7.
19. Saxonhouse MA, Sola MC. Platelet function in term and preterm neonates. Clin Perinatol 2004;31:15–8.
20. Hezard N, Amory C, Leroux B, et al. Platelet hyporeactivity in healthy children remains beyond the neonatal period [abstract]. Blood 2002;100:69a.
21. El Haouari M, Rosado JA. Platelet function in hypertension. Blood Cells Mol Dis 2009;42:38–43.
22. Kuhne T, Ryan G, Blanchette V, et al. Platelet-surface glycoproteins in healthy and preeclamptic mothers and their newborn infants. Pediatr Res 1996;40:876–80.
23. Strauss T, Maayan-Metzger A, Simchen MJ, et al. Impaired platelet function in neonates born to mothers with diabetes or hypertension during pregnancy. Klin Padiatr 2010;222:154–7.
24. Knobler H, Savion N, Shenkman B, et al. Shear-induced platelet adhesion and aggregation on subendothelium are increased in diabetic patients. Thromb Res 1998;90:181–90.
25. Kudolo GB, Koopmans SJ, Haywood JR, et al. Chronic hyperinsulinemia inhibits platelet-activating factor (PAF) biosynthesis in the rat kidney. J Lipid Mediat Cell Signal 1997;16:23–37.
26. McMorran BJ, Marshall VM, de Graaf C, et al. Platelets kill intraerythrocytic malarial parasites and mediate survival to infection. Science 2009;323:797–800.
27. Nørgaard M, Jensen AØ, Engebjerg MC, et al. Long-term clinical outcomes of patients with primary chronic immune thrombocytopenia: a Danish population-based cohort study. Blood 2011;117:3514–20.
28. Nair S, Ghosh K, Kulkarni B, et al. Glanzmann's thrombasthenia: updated. Platelets 2002;13:387–93.
29. Nurden AT, Pillois X, Wilcox DA. Glanzmann thrombasthenia: state of the art and future directions. Semin Thromb Hemost 2013;39:642–55.
30. Diz-Küçükkaya R. Inherited platelet disorders including Glanzmann thrombasthenia and Bernard-Soulier syndrome. Hematology Am Soc Hematol Educ Program 2013;2013:268–75.
31. Sheffield MJ, Schmutz N, Lambert DK, et al. Ibuprofen lysine administration to neonates with a patent ductus arteriosus: effect on platelet plug formation assessed by in vivo and in vitro measurements. J Perinatol 2009;29:39–43.
32. Del Vecchio A, Sullivan SE, Christensen RD, et al. Indomethacin prolongs the bleeding time in neonates significantly more than ibuprofen. Pediatr Res 2002;51:466A.
33. Cheung PY, Salas E, Schulz R. Nitric oxide and platelet function: implications for neonatology. Semin Perinatol 1997;21:409–17.
34. Konkle BA. Acquired disorders of platelet function. Hematology Am Soc Hematol Educ Program 2011;2011:391–6.

35. Sola MC, Del Vecchio A, Edwards TJ, et al. The relationship between hematocrit and bleeding time in very low birth weight infants during the first week of life. J Perinatol 2001;21:368–71.
36. Eugster M, Reinhart WH. The influence of the haematocrit on primary haemostasis in vitro. Thromb Haemost 2005;94:1213–8.
37. Gader AM, Bahakim H, Jabbar FA, et al. Dose-response aggregometry in maternal/neonatal platelets. Thromb Haemost 1988;60:314–8.
38. Israels SJ, Daniels M, McMillan EM. Deficient collagen-induced activation in the newborn platelet. Pediatr Res 1990;27:337–43.
39. Louden KA, Broughton Pipkin F, Heptinstall S, et al. Neonatal platelet reactivity and serum thromboxane B2 production in whole blood: the effect of maternal low-dose aspirin. Br J Obstet Gynaecol 1994;101:203–8.
40. Israels SJ, Odaibo FS, Robertson C, et al. Deficient thromboxane synthesis and response in platelets from premature infants. Pediatr Res 1997;41:218–23.
41. Ts'ao CH, Green D, Schultz K. Function and ultrastructure of platelets of neonates: enhanced ristocetin aggregation of neonatal platelets. Br J Haematol 1976;32:225–33.
42. Katz JA, Moake JL, McPherson PD, et al. Relationship between human development and disappearance of unusually large von Willebrand factor multimers from plasma. Blood 1989;73:1851–8.
43. Halimeh S, Angelis GD, Sander A, et al. Multiplate whole blood impedance point of care aggregometry: preliminary reference values in healthy infants, children and adolescents. Klin Padiatr 2010;222:158–63.
44. Del Vecchio A. Use of the bleeding time in the neonatal intensive care unit. Acta Paediatr Suppl 2002;91(438):82–6.
45. Del Vecchio A, Sola MC. Performing and interpreting the bleeding time in the neonatal intensive care unit. Clin Perinatol 2000;27:643–54.
46. Del Vecchio A, Latini G, Henry E, et al. Template bleeding times of 240 neonates born at 24 to 41 weeks gestation. J Perinatol 2008;28:427–31.
47. Kenet G, Lubetsky A, Shenkman B, et al. Cone and platelet analyser (CPA): a new test for the prediction of bleeding among thrombocytopenic patients. Br J Haematol 1998;101:255–9.
48. Levy-Shraga Y, Maayan-Metzger A, Lubetsky A, et al. Platelet function of newborns as tested by cone and plate(let) analyzer correlates with gestational age. Acta Haematol 2006;115:152–6.
49. Shenkman B, Einav Y, Salomon O, et al. Testing agonist-induced platelet aggregation by the Impact-R [Cone and plate(let) analyzer (CPA)]. Platelets 2008;19:440–6.
50. Kundu SK, Heilmann EJ, Sio R, et al. Description of an in vitro platelet function analyzer–PFA-100. Semin Thromb Hemost 1995;21(Suppl 2):106–12.
51. Roschitz B, Sudi K, Köstenberger M, et al. Shorter PFA-100 closure times in neonates than in adults: role of red cells, white cells, platelets and von Willebrand factor. Acta Paediatr 2001;90:664–70.
52. Saxonhouse MA, Garner R, Mammel L, et al. Closure times measured by the platelet function analyzer PFA-100 are longer in neonatal blood compared to cord blood samples. Neonatology 2010;97:242–9.
53. Christensen RD, Sheffield MJ, Lambert DK, et al. Effect of therapeutic hypothermia in neonates with hypoxic-ischemic encephalopathy on platelet function. Neonatology 2012;101:91–4.
54. Radicioni M, Bruni A, Bini V, et al. Thromboelastographic profiles of the premature infants with and without intracranial hemorrhage at birth: a pilot study. J Matern Fetal Neonatal Med 2014;17:1–5.

55. Chan KL, Summerhayes RG, Ignjatovic V, et al. Reference values for kaolin-activated thromboelastography in healthy children. Anesth Analg 2007;105: 1610–3.
56. Radicioni M, Mezzetti D, Del Vecchio A, et al. Thromboelastography: might work in neonatology too? J Matern Fetal Neonatal Med 2012;25(Suppl 4):18–21.
57. Strauss T, Levy-Shraga Y, Ravid B, et al. Clot formation of neonates tested by thromboelastography correlates with gestational age. Thromb Haemost 2010; 103:344–50.
58. Edwards RM, Naik-Mathuria BJ, Gay AN, et al. Parameters of thromboelastography in healthy newborns. Am J Clin Pathol 2008;130:99–102.

Fresh Frozen Plasma Administration in the Neonatal Intensive Care Unit
Evidence-Based Guidelines

Mario Motta, MD[a],*, Antonio Del Vecchio, MD[b],
Gaetano Chirico, MD[a]

KEYWORDS

• Fresh frozen plasma • Transfusion • Guidelines • Coagulation tests • Neonate

KEY POINTS

• Fresh frozen plasma (FFP) administration is a common intervention in neonatal intensive care units (NICUs), with a high level of inappropriate use.

• The use of FFP in neonatology should primarily be in neonates with active bleeding and associated coagulopathy.

• Interpretation of coagulation tests in the neonate is a crucial step in the decision-making process for FFP administration.

• Health care information technology provides the ability to acquire and analyze large amounts of transfusion-related data and can be used to improve neonatal transfusion management.

INTRODUCTION

The use of fresh frozen plasma (FFP) is a frequent intervention in neonatal intensive care units (NICUs), especially among critically ill neonates. Current guidelines for FFP administration in neonates are mainly based on poor-quality evidence and this contributes to the high level of inappropriate FFP use. In addition, the age-related changes of coagulation proteins during infancy make it difficult to correctly diagnose coagulopathy in neonates and subsequently determine when FFP should be used.

Declaration of Interest: The authors disclaim any competing interest. The authors have not received any honorarium, grant, or other form of payment from any funding agency in the public, commercial, or not-for-profit sectors for producing the article.
a Neonatology and Neonatal Intensive Care Unit, Children's Hospital of Brescia, Spedali Civili of Brescia, P.le Spedali Civili, Brescia 25123, Italy; b Neonatal Intensive Care Unit, Division of Neonatology, Department of Women's and Children's Health, Di Venere Hospital, ASL Bari, Bari 70012, Italy
* Corresponding author.
E-mail address: mario.motta@spedalicivili.brescia.it

Clin Perinatol 42 (2015) 639–650
http://dx.doi.org/10.1016/j.clp.2015.04.013
0095-5108/15/$ – see front matter © 2015 Elsevier Inc. All rights reserved.

In this review we

1. Examine the available studies that test the use of FFP and we synthesize the relevant information by grading the quality of evidence and strength of recommendations
2. Discuss the role of laboratory tests of hemostasis in decision-making for FFP administration, and
3. Evaluate possible strategies for reducing inappropriate FFP utilization.

EPIDEMIOLOGY OF FRESH FROZEN PLASMA USE IN THE NEONATAL INTENSIVE CARE UNIT

FFP administration continues to be a common practice in the NICU, but concern has been raised about the appropriateness of its use. In studies by Baer and colleagues[1] and Puetz and colleagues[2] the rate of FFP transfusion was 6% and 12% of patients in the NICU, respectively. Both studies reported a significant proportion of use outside of published recommendations. Altuntas and colleagues[3] reported a lower rate of 2%, with more than 20% of the FFP administrations given for reasons not compliant with recommendations. Stanworth and colleagues[4] reported that 2.3% of all patients receiving FFP were children (aged 1–15 years) and 4.4% of these were younger than 1 year. They also reported that 62% of infants who received FFP did not have clinical bleeding and 14% of infants treated with FFP did not have coagulation tests before the FFP administration. Puetz and colleagues[5] reported that FFP was administered to 2.85% of admissions to pediatric hospitals in the United States and that 29% of these transfusions were given to neonates. Recently, in a study involving 17 Italian NICUs, we found that FFP administration was a relatively frequent intervention, with 8% of admitted neonates receiving 1 or more FFP transfusion.[6] Our study showed that a remarkably high proportion (60%) of transfusions were not compliant with guidelines present in our NICUs, and 63% of transfused neonates received FFP prophylactically, without any evidence of bleeding.

RECOMMENDATIONS DERIVED FROM CLINICAL STUDIES ON THE APPROPRIATE USE OF FRESH FROZEN PLASMA IN NEONATES

Clinical studies in which the intervention was transfusion of FFP in neonates were identified by consulting the National Library of Medicine's MEDLINE, EMBASE, and the Cochrane Library. The methodology used to score the literature and transform it into level of evidence and strength of recommendation was that proposed by the Grading of recommendation, assessment, development, and evaluation (GRADE) Working Group (**Box 1**).[7] Recommendations for plasma administration to neonates, based on scientific evidence and according to the GRADE system, are summarized in **Table 1**.

Various studies have evaluated the potential usefulness of plasma transfusions in neonates across different clinical settings. The characteristics and results of randomized controlled trials identified from the literature search are summarized in **Tables 2** and **3**. One study addressed the effectiveness of FFP in disseminated intravascular coagulation and no differences in improvement of coagulation tests or in survival rate were observed.[8] A possible beneficial effect of FFP administration in neonates with disseminated intravascular coagulation was described only in case reports.[9,10] Four studies evaluated the hypothesis that FFP for early volume expansion would reduce morbidity and mortality in preterm neonates.[11–14] In one of these studies, a significant reduction in intracranial hemorrhage was found.[12] In contrast, the other

---

Box 1
Criteria for assigning grade of evidence and strength of recommendations

Quality of Evidence	Type of Clinical Study	Consistency of Results
A = High	Randomized trial without important limitations	Considerable confidence in the estimate of effect
B = Moderate	Randomized trial with important limitations or exceptionally observational studies with strong evidence	Further research likely to have impact on the confidence in estimate, may change estimate
C = Low	Observational studies or case series	Further research is very likely to have impact on confidence, likely to change the estimate

Strength of Recommendations	Balance Between Benefits and Harms
1 = Strong	Certainty of imbalance
2 = Weak	Uncertainty of imbalance

The grading scheme classifies the quality of evidence as high (grade A), moderate (grade B), or low (grade C) according to the study design and to the consistency of results. The strength of recommendations was further classified as either strong (1) or weak (2) according to the balance between desirable and undesirable outcomes.
From Atkins D, Best D, Briss PA, et al. Grading quality of evidence and strength of recommendations. BMJ 2004;328:1490–4.

---

3 reported a similar rate of intracranial hemorrhage and/or cerebral ultrasound abnormalities.[11,13,14] A meta-analysis that included these 4 studies showed no significant differences in any grade of intraventricular hemorrhage or mortality rate.[15] In the Northern Neonatal Nursing Initiative Trial, the largest of these 4 studies, in which a 2-year follow-up was performed, no significant difference in severe disability was observed between neonates receiving FFP and controls.[16]

Controlled studies did not identify a benefit of FFP administration to neonates with sepsis, respiratory distress syndrome, and hypotension.[17–20] Good-quality information for blood product usage in neonatal extracorporeal life support is limited to one study. In a randomized trial on infants undergoing cardiopulmonary bypass for heart surgery, the circuit priming with a combination of packed red cells and FFP was superior to using fresh whole blood, regarding the outcomes of reduction in hospital stay and improvement in cumulative fluid balance.[21] An intervention study on the effect of prophylactic FFP administration on extracorporeal membrane oxygenation circuit longevity is ongoing; however, results are not yet available.[22]

Partial exchange transfusion is traditionally used as the method of lowering the hematocrit and treating hyperviscosity in neonates with polycythemia. Although there is no evidence that this procedure improves long-term outcome,[23] in many NICUs the standard of care for polycythemic neonates with worsening symptoms continues to be partial exchange transfusion. Three randomized trials compared the efficacy of crystalloid solution versus FFP for partial exchange transfusion in neonates with polycythemia (see **Table 3**).[24–26] Two meta-analyses, which included all these studies, showed no significant difference in the reduction of postexchange hematocrit.[27,28] In addition, crystalloid solution and plasma were reported to be equally effective in the alleviation of symptoms.

Table 1
Clinical settings in which the use of FFP is recommended (A) or not recommended (B) in neonates

(A) The Use of FFP Is Recommended	Level of Evidence	Strength of Recommendations
Treatment of acute bleeding in combination with the following:		
1. Coagulopathy[a] due to multiple coagulation factor deficiencies (ie, DIC, liver failure)	C	1
2. Single inherited clotting factor deficiency without safer replacement product available[b]	C	1
3. Vitamin K deficiency[c]	C	1
Prophylaxis of bleeding for an invasive procedure in the presence of coagulopathy	C	2
Blood reconstitution (in conjunction with PRBC) for the following:		
1. Circuit priming for cardiopulmonary bypass	A	1
2. Circuit priming for ECMO	C	1
3. Exchange transfusion for hyperbilirubinemia	C	1

(B) The Use of FFP Is Not Recommended	Level of Evidence	Strength of Recommendations
Prevention of mortality and morbidity in preterm infants	A	1
Replacement fluid for partial exchange transfusion for polycythemia/hyperviscosity	B	1
Treatment of sepsis	C	1
Treatment of RDS	B	1
Volume replacement for hypotension	B	1
Treatment of coagulopathy without bleeding during therapeutic hypothermia for asphyxia	C	2

Abbreviations: DIC, disseminated intravascular coagulation; ECMO, extracorporeal membrane oxygenation; FFP, fresh frozen plasma; PRBC, peripheral red blood cell; RDS, respiratory distress syndrome.

[a] Coagulopathy is defined as coagulation tests outside the 95% confidence limits of the age-related hemostatic parameters (see **Table 4**).

[b] Currently, this applies only to Factor V. However, FFP may be also given if treatment is urgently required before the diagnosis of inherited clotting factor deficiency (ie, hemophilia) has been confirmed.

[c] The administration of FFP should be combined with intravenous infusion of vitamin K. Methods for grading evidence and formulating recommendation according to the GRADE system.[7]

EFFECT OF FRESH FROZEN PLASMA DOSE ON CLOTTING TIMES

Studies have examined the volume of FFP on clotting times. For instance, Hambleton and Appleyard treated asphyxiated low birth weight neonates with 2 infusions of FFP (10 mL/kg).[11] The administration did not improve either the Thrombotest or prothrombin time (PT), although there was a significant change in the activated partial thromboplastin time (APTT) among small for dates neonates so treated. Johnson and colleagues[29] reported the effects of FFP infusions (10 mL/kg) on coagulation screening tests in preterm neonates with respiratory distress syndrome and a prolonged PT (greater than 18 seconds) or APTT (greater than 70 seconds). The infusion of FFP produced a full correction of both PT and APTT in only 7 of 23 treated neonates. In our clinical audit on the use of FFP in NICUs, the mean dose of FFP administered

Table 2
Controlled studies evaluating the effectiveness of FFP administration in neonates

Study	Design	Clinical Setting	Intervention	Outcome
Gross et al,[8] 1982	Single-center RCT	DIC	FFP + PLTs vs ET vs control	No differences in survival, or resolution of DIC
Hambleton & Appleyard,[11] 1973	Single-center RCT	Prevention of IVH in LBW neonates	FFP for 2 d vs control	No evidence of beneficial effect
Beverley et al,[12] 1985[a,b]	Single-center RCT	Prevention of IVH in preterm neonates	FFP for 2 d vs control	Decreased rate of IVH
Ekblad et al,[13] 1991[b]	Single-center RCT	Prevention of IVH and improvement of renal function in preterm neonates	FFP for 3 d vs control	No evidence of beneficial effect
NNNI Trial Group,[14,15] 1996[a]	Multicenter RCT	Prevention of mortality, cerebral ultrasound abnormality, and disability in preterm neonates	FFP for 2 d vs Gelofusin vs dextrose-saline	No evidence of beneficial effect
Emery et al,[20] 1992	Single-center RCT	Hypotension in preterm neonates	FFP vs 20% albumin vs 4.5% albumin	No benefit in blood pressure levels in any group
Gottuso et al,[19] 1976[a]	Multicenter RCT	Prevention of mortality in LBW neonates with RDS	FFP vs ET vs control	No evidence of beneficial effect in FFP group, possible benefit for ET
Acunas et al,[17] 1994	Multicenter RCT	Sepsis	FFP vs IVIG vs control	No evidence of immunity function improvement in FFP group
Mou et al,[21] 2004	Single-center RCT	Priming of the cardiopulmonary bypass circuit	FFP + PRBC vs whole blood	Decreased length of stay and perioperative fluid overload in FFP + PRBC group

Abbreviations: DIC, disseminated intravascular coagulation; ET, exchange transfusion; FFP, fresh frozen plasma; IVH, intraventricular hemorrhage; IVIG, intravenous immunoglobulin; LBW, low birth weight; PLT, platelet; PRBC, peripheral red blood cell; RCT, randomized controlled trial; RDS, respiratory distress syndrome.
  [a] The meta-analysis of these 3 studies showed no significant difference in mortality rate.[15]
  [b] The meta-analysis of these 2 studies found a nonsignificant trend to reduce any grade of IVH.[15]

Table 3
Controlled studies comparing the efficacy of different solutions used for partial exchange transfusion

Study	Design	Inclusion Criteria	Intervention	Outcome
Deorari et al,[24] 1995	Single-center RCT	Venous Ht >65% with symptoms	Plasma vs normal saline	Similar changes in postexchange Ht and viscosity values
Roithmaier et al,[25] 1995	Single-center RCT	Venous Ht >65% with symptoms	Virus-inactivated human plasma serum vs Ringer solution	Similar reduction in postexchange Ht, PV increase in serum group, BV reduction in Ringer group
Krishnan et al,[26] 1997	Single-center RCT	Venous Ht >65% with symptoms or Ht >70% alone	Plasma vs normal saline	Similar reduction in postexchange Ht

Abbreviations: BV, blood volume; Ht, hematocrit; PV, plasma volume; RCT, randomized controlled trial.

was 16 mL/kg. Preinfusion and postinfusion assessment of coagulation tests showed a significant reduction of both PT and APTT, suggesting that the infused volume of FFP was sufficient to affect clotting times.[6]

Puetz and colleagues[2] dosed FFP at 10 mL/kg, 20 mL/kg, and greater than 20 mL/kg in 71%, 23%, and 2% of cases, respectively. In 40% of cases, the FFP administration reduced prolonged coagulation tests, which were assessed considering specific age-related reference ranges, into the normal range for gestational age. Altuntas and colleagues[3] reported that 44% of neonates received an FFP infusion of 10 mL/kg and 56% received 20 mL/kg. After FFP infusion, the PT normalized in 42% of cases and the APTT normalized in 60%. In the UK National Comparative Audit of the use of FFP, the median dose of FFP administered to infants was 14 mL/kg, with 20% receiving a dose less than 10 mL/kg.[4] In a subsequent report,[30] the investigators outlined that considering only infants in whom FFP was administered to correct abnormal coagulation values, and using the Andrew and colleagues[31] reference ranges for coagulation tests (Table 4),[30] normalization of the PT and APTT occurred in 15% and 10% of cases, respectively. Using the reference ranges suggested by Christensen and colleagues[33] (see Table 4), a correction of coagulation tests after FFP administration was obtained in 68% of infants of less than 28 weeks' gestation, and in 59% of infants of 28 to 34 weeks' gestation.

Assuming that FFP has an average clotting factor and inhibitor potency of 1 IU/mL, a dose of 10 mL/kg should increase clotting factors and inhibitor levels by approximately 10 IU/dL (10%).[34] Hence, the infusion of 10 mL/kg of FFP should increase the plasma coagulations levels significantly. Taking into account available clinical and pharmacokinetic data, an effective dose of FFP should be 10 to 15 mL/kg. Higher doses (>20 mL/kg) might be warranted in some situations involving the underlying disease process, the half-life of the factor being replaced. Intravascular volume overload also should be a consideration when deciding on the proper dose of FFP.

IMPLICATIONS OF HEMOSTASIS ASSESSMENT IN THERAPEUTIC DECISION-MAKING FOR FRESH FROZEN PLASMA ADMINISTRATION

Understanding physiologic hemostasis and interpreting coagulation tests are both needed to optimize neonatal FFP management. The dynamic and evolving process of the hemostatic system that occurs during infancy and childhood was first described by

Table 4
Defining coagulopathy in the premature and term neonate, at birth (A) and during the first 3 months of life (B), according to PT, APTT, and fibrinogen values

(A) Gestational Age at Birth (wk)	PT, Upper Limit[a] (s)	APTT, Upper Limit[a] (s)	Fibrinogen, Lower Limit[a] (mg/dL)
<28[33]	>21	>64	<71
28–34[33]	>21	>57	<87
30–36[32]	>16	>79	<150
≥37[31]	>16	>55	<167

(B) Gestational Age at Birth (wk)	PT, Upper Limit[a] (s)	APTT, Upper Limit[a] (s)	Fibrinogen, Lower Limit[a] (mg/dL)
30–36[32] and postnatal age of			
5 d	>15	>74	<160
30 d	>14	>62	<150
90 d	>15	>51	<150
≥37[31] and postnatal age of			
5 d	>15	>60	<162
30 d	>14	>55	<162
90 d	>14	>50	<150

Abbreviations: APTT, activated partial thromboplastin time; PT, prothrombin time.
[a] The upper limit of PT and APTT, and the lower limit of fibrinogen are defined for values outside the 95% confidence limits of the age-related reference ranges.

Andrew[35] and was termed "developmental hemostasis." The fundamental principle underlying developmental hemostasis is that the levels of most coagulation proteins vary significantly with age. These age-related changes lead to corresponding changes in the standard coagulation screening tests, such as the PT and the APTT. Given the age-dependent specificities, the evaluation and interpretation of coagulation tests in neonates should be based on reference ranges that are appropriate for gestational and postnatal age.[31–33] Moreover, because the PT and APTT are measured on citrated platelet-poor plasma with the addition of exogenous reagents, the times of clot formation will vary depending on the reagents and methodology used. A consensus statement of the International Society on Thrombosis and Hemostasis recommends the use of age-appropriate, analyzer-appropriate, and reagent-appropriate reference ranges.[36]

Abnormal coagulation tests, defined as results outside the 95% confidence limits of the age-related hemostatic parameter, are shown in **Table 4**. In neonates, the presence of abnormal coagulation tests have significant limitations as predictors of bleeding, and do not necessarily correlate with a clinically relevant disease.[2,6,33,37] In addition, there is a lack of data demonstrating that FFP administration to nonbleeding neonates with abnormal coagulation tests reduces their risk of a subsequent hemorrhage.[38,39] Therefore, the most appropriate use of FFP should be the treatment of active bleeding in neonates who have laboratory confirmation of coagulopathy. Prophylactic use of FFP in nonbleeding neonates, on the basis that their coagulation test is abnormal, cannot be considered an evidence-based practice (see **Table 1**).

Catford and colleagues[30] reported that the practice of drawing routine clotting tests on admission to the NICU increases the prophylactic use of FFP administered to correct isolated abnormal coagulation values without associated bleeding. We are of the opinion that routine coagulation testing on NICU admission is not indicated because this it leads to FFP administration without evidence of benefit (See Best Practices).

Concerns have been raised about the risk of bleeding in neonates with perinatal asphyxia undergoing therapeutic hypothermia.[40] Coagulopathy is one of the consequences of perinatal asphyxia, and the use of hypothermia might worsen hemostatic dysfunction.[41–45] Reduction in procoagulation and anticoagulation proteins has been reported in asphyxiated and cooled neonates, resulting in abnormal clotting tests.[46] However a meta-analysis evaluating the effect of therapeutic hypothermia in asphyxiated encephalopathic newborns showed no significant difference in coagulopathy, thrombosis, or hemorrhage in cooled versus noncooled neonates.[47] In a recent retrospective study, Forman and colleagues[48] reported on 76 neonates treated with hypothermia for hypoxic ischemic encephalopathy, 54% of whom had bleeding episodes. Thirty-three (43.4%) neonates received FFP transfusion (28.9% and 14.5% for bleeding associated with coagulopathy and for isolated abnormal clotting tests without bleeding, respectively). In this study, neonates with bleeding, compared with nonbleeding neonates, had statistically longer coagulation times, including international normalized ratio and APTT, and lower platelet counts and lower fibrinogen levels. However, receiver operating characteristic curve analyses found low specificity and sensitivity of these tests for predicting bleeding episodes. Although there are no officially accepted guidelines, current evidence does not support FFP administration to asphyxiated cooled neonates with isolated abnormal clotting tests in the absence of bleeding (see **Table 1**). Therapeutic hypothermia is the current standard of care for hypoxic ischemic encephalopathy after perinatal asphyxia, thus further studies are needed to evaluate the issues of coagulopathy and its treatment in this specific group of neonates.

Because of the complexity of the in vivo coagulation process, standard laboratory tests cannot accurately measure all the individual elements involved in hemostatic function. Consequently, the standard coagulation tests of neonates must be interpreted with caution. A key limitation of the standard coagulation tests is that they are poor predictors of bleeding. Viscoelastic tests of coagulation, such as thromboelastography (TEG; Haemanetics Corp, Braintree, MA, USA) and rotational thromboelastometry (ROTEM; TEM international, Munich, Germany) may be able to overcome some of these limitations.[49] Those tests differ significantly from conventional coagulation tests, as they evaluate the kinetics of the entire process of coagulation from initial clot formation through to fibrin polymerization and final clot strength. These dynamic tests provide a composite picture reflecting the interaction of plasma, blood cells, and platelets, and more closely reflect the in vivo condition than conventional tests.

The study of coagulation viscoelastic tests in neonates is limited. Radicioni and colleagues[50] measured the thromboelastographic profiles of 49 premature neonates with and without intracranial hemorrhage. No significant differences of TEG and standard coagulation test values between the 2 groups were observed at birth. In addition, newborns with intracranial hemorrhage showed increased thromboelastogram-defined thrombin generation from birth to 21 days of life, suggesting a state of hypercoagulation. In a study by Forman and colleagues[51] of 24 neonates undergoing therapeutic hypothermia for perinatal asphyxia, TEG results were affected by temperature, indicating more impaired coagulation at lower temperature. In addition, TEG parameters were more predictive of clinical bleeding with temperature-dependent cutpoints.

STRATEGIES TO IMPROVE COMPLIANCE WITH FRESH FROZEN PLASMA ADMINISTRATION GUIDELINES IN THE NEONATAL INTENSIVE CARE UNIT

Although the use of transfusion guidelines improves transfusion practice, poor adherence to FFP transfusion guidelines continues to be documented.[1,2,4–6,52] Transfusion medicine is an excellent example of where benefits of the electronic health record can improve blood product utilization by applying real-time clinical decision support systems. For instance, Baer and colleagues,[53] implemented a program of electronic transfusion ordering in 4 NICUs of a multihospital health care institution and reported a significant reduction in transfusion rates, including FFP administration, as well as improved compliance with transfusion guidelines. These changes were safe, with no increase in NICU length of stay or mortality rate. In a systematic review evaluating the effects of electronic decision support systems on blood product ordering practices, evidence of improved red blood cell usage was observed.[54] The effect of decision support systems on plasma, platelets, and cryoprecipitate usage is less clear, probably because fewer studies have focused on these blood products.

Considering that the best evidence for use of FFP in neonatology is in a neonate with hemorrhage and coagulopathy, the assessment of bleeding is a critical point in the decision-making process. A neonatal bleeding assessment tool (NeoBAT) has been developed, with the aim of standardizing the clinical recording of bleeding in high-risk neonates.[55] During the study period, bleeding occurred in 25% of neonates overall and was most common in preterm neonates. Double-blinded assessment of bleeding severity showed a 98% concordance. The study investigators suggested that because bleeding is a common complication of high-risk neonates, the NeoBAT could be useful to determine bleeding risk and transfusion outcomes. Transfusion decisions could be strengthened by the use of an objective bleeding assessment tool in association with laboratory tests of hemostasis.

SUMMARY

Current evidence support the administration of FFP to neonates in limited conditions, including the treatment of bleeding associated with coagulopathy, disseminated intravascular coagulation, and inherited deficiencies of coagulation factors when replacement products are not available. However, clinical audits continue to report a common use of FFP in neonates outside evidence-based recommendations, raising questions about cost and risk. The 2 main reasons for poor adherence to guidelines are the lack of clinical trials evaluating FFP efficacy in many specific circumstances, and the limitation of standard coagulation tests as predictors of bleeding. The use of health information technology may improve transfusion practice by minimizing unnecessary FFP administrations. In addition, preliminary experience in neonates in whom hemostasis is assessed by using viscoelastic tests of clot formation suggest that these methods have potential advantages over standard coagulation tests. Prospective epidemiologic studies focused on clinical outcomes in high-risk neonates are needed to inform studies aimed at evaluating the efficacy of FFP in specific conditions.

Best Practices

What is the current practice in the use of FFP in the NICU?

- A significant number of neonates continue to receive FFP outside recommendations.
- In neonates, standard coagulation tests are poor predictors of bleeding risk, thus they do not form a firm basis for FFP administration decisions.

What changes in practice are likely to improve outcomes?

- NICUs should implement evidence-based guidelines for the use of FFP to minimize the adverse effects of transfusion and wastage of products (C1).
- The dose of FFP should be at least 10 to 15 mL/kg of body weight (C1).

- The use of FFP should be guided by the results of coagulation tests (grading of recommendations related to specific conditions is reported in **Table 1**), which should be interpreted with appropriate reference ranges for gestational and postnatal age (B1).
- Routine coagulation testing on NICU admission is not indicated because it leads to increased FFP transfusion without evidence of benefit (C2).
- Safe and appropriate uses of FFP are facilitated by transfusion information technology (C1).

Level of evidence and strength of recommendations, according to the GRADE system,[7] for changes suggested in FFP transfusion practice are reported in parentheses.

REFERENCES

1. Baer VL, Lambert DK, Schmutz N, et al. Adherence to NICU transfusion guidelines: data from a multihospital healthcare system. J Perinatol 2008;28:492–7.
2. Puetz J, Darling G, McCormick KA, et al. Fresh frozen plasma and recombinant factor VIIa use in neonates. J Pediatr Hematol Oncol 2009;31:901–6.
3. Altuntas N, Yenicesu I, Beken S, et al. Clinical use of fresh-frozen plasma in neonatal intensive care unit. Transfus Apher Sci 2012;47:91–4.
4. Stanworth SJ, Grant-Casey J, Lowe D, et al. The use of fresh-frozen plasma in England: high levels of inappropriate use in adults and children. Transfusion 2011; 51:62–70.
5. Puetz J, Witmer C, Huang YS, et al. Widespread use of fresh frozen plasma in US children's hospitals despite limited evidence demonstrating a beneficial effect. J Pediatr 2012;160:210–5.e1.
6. Motta M, Del Vecchio A, Perrone B, et al. Fresh frozen plasma use in the NICU: a prospective, observational, multicentred study. Arch Dis Child Fetal Neonatal Ed 2014;99:F303–8.
7. Atkins D, Best D, Briss PA, et al. Grading quality of evidence and strength of recommendations. BMJ 2004;328:1490–4.
8. Gross SJ, Filston HC, Anderson JC. Controlled study of treatment for disseminated intravascular coagulation in the neonate. J Pediatr 1982;100:445–8.
9. Yuen P, Cheung A, Lin HJ, et al. Purpura fulminans in a Chinese boy with congenital protein C deficiency. Pediatrics 1986;77:670–6.
10. Branson HE, Katz J, Marble R, et al. Inherited protein C deficiency and coumarin-responsive chronic relapsing purpura fulminans in a newborn infant. Lancet 1983;2:1165–8.
11. Hambleton G, Appleyard WJ. Controlled trial of fresh frozen plasma in asphyxiated low birthweight infants. Arch Dis Child 1973;48:31–5.
12. Beverley DW, Pitts-Tucker TJ, Congdon PJ, et al. Prevention of intraventricular haemorrhage by fresh frozen plasma. Arch Dis Child 1985;60:710–3.
13. Ekblad H, Kero P, Shaffer SG, et al. Extracellular volume in preterm infants: influence of gestational age and colloids. Early Hum Dev 1991;27:1–7.
14. A randomized trial comparing the effect of prophylactic intravenous fresh frozen plasma, gelatin or glucose on early mortality and morbidity in preterm babies. The Northern Neonatal Nursing Initiative (NNNI) Trial Group. Eur J Pediatr 1996;155:580–8.
15. Osborn DA, Evans N. Early volume expansion for prevention of morbidity and mortality in very preterm infants. Cochrane Database Syst Rev 2004;(2):CD002055.
16. Randomised trial of prophylactic early fresh-frozen plasma or gelatin or glucose in preterm babies: outcome at 2 years. The Northern Neonatal Nursing Initiative (NNNI) Trial Group. Lancet 1996;348:229–32.

17. Acunas BA, Peakman M, Liossis G, et al. Effect of fresh frozen plasma and gammaglobulin on humoral immunity in neonatal sepsis. Arch Dis Child Fetal Neonatal Ed 1994;70:F182–7.
18. Krediet TG, Beurskens FJ, van Dijk H, et al. Antibody responses and opsonic activity in sera of preterm neonates with coagulase-negative staphylococcal septicemia and the effect of the administration of fresh frozen plasma. Pediatr Res 1998;43:645–51.
19. Gottuso MA, Williams ML, Oski FA. The role of exchange transfusion in the management of low-birth-weight infants with and without severe respiratory distress syndrome. J Pediatr 1976;89:279–85.
20. Emery EF, Greenough A, Gamsu HR. Randomised controlled trial of colloid infusions in hypotensive preterm infants. Arch Dis Child 1992;67:1185–8.
21. Mou SS, Giroir BP, Molitor-Kirsch EA, et al. Fresh whole blood versus reconstituted blood for pump priming in heart surgery in infants. N Engl J Med 2004;351:1635–44.
22. Ozment C. Prospective, randomized pilot study of prophylactic fresh frozen plasma administration during neonatal-pediatric extracorporeal membrane oxygenation. Available at: https://clinicaltrials.gov/ct2/show/NCT01903863?term=fresh+frozen+plasma&rank=2. Accessed January 20, 2015.
23. Ozek E, Soll R, Schimmel MS. Partial exchange transfusion to prevent neurodevelopmental disability in infants with polycythemia. Cochrane Database Syst Rev 2010;(1):CD005089.
24. Deorari AK, Paul VK, Shreshta L, et al. Symptomatic neonatal polycythernia: comparison of partial exchange transfusion with saline versus plasma. Indian Pediatr 1995;32:1167–71.
25. Roithmaier A, Arlettaz R, Bauer K, et al. Randomized controlled trial of Ringer solution versus serum for partial exchange transfusion in neonatal polycythaemia. Eur J Pediatr 1995;154:53–6.
26. Krishnan L, Rahim A. Neonatal polycythemia. Indian J Pediatr 1997;64:541–6.
27. Dempsey EM, Barrington K. Crystalloid or colloid for partial exchange transfusion in neonatal polycythemia: a systematic review and meta-analysis. Acta Paediatr 2005;94:1650–5.
28. de Waal KA, Baerts W, Offringa M. Systematic review of the optimal fluid for dilutional exchange transfusion in neonatal polycythaemia. Arch Dis Child Fetal Neonatal Ed 2006;91:F7–10.
29. Johnson CA, Snyder MS, Weaver RL. The effects of fresh frozen plasma infusions on coagulation screening tests in neonates. Arch Dis Child 1982;57:950–2.
30. Catford K, Muthukumar P, Reddy C, et al. Routine neonatal coagulation testing increases use of fresh-frozen plasma. Transfusion 2014;54:1444–5.
31. Andrew M, Paes B, Milner R, et al. Development of the human coagulation system in the full-term infant. Blood 1987;70:165–72.
32. Andrew M, Paes B, Milner R, et al. Development of the human coagulation system in the healthy premature infant. Blood 1988;72:1651–7.
33. Christensen RD, Baer VL, Lambert DK, et al. Reference intervals for common coagulation tests of preterm infants (CME). Transfusion 2014;54:627–32.
34. Hellstern P, Muntean W, Schramm W, et al. Practical guidelines for the clinical use of plasma. Thromb Res 2002;107(Suppl 1):S53–7.
35. Andrew M. The relevance of developmental hemostasis to hemorrhagic disorders of newborns. Semin Perinatol 1997;21:70–85.
36. Ignjatovic V, Kenet G, Monagle P. Developmental hemostasis: recommendations for laboratories reporting pediatric samples. J Thromb Haemost 2012;10:298–300.

37. Venkatesh V, Khan R, Curley A, et al. How we decide when a neonate needs a transfusion. Br J Haematol 2013;160:421–33.
38. Van de Bor M, Briet E, Van Bel F, et al. Hemostasis and periventricular-intraventricular hemorrhage of the newborn. Am J Dis Child 1986;140:1131–4.
39. Tran TT, Veldman A, Malhotra A. Does risk-based coagulation screening predict intraventricular haemorrhage in extreme premature infants? Blood Coagul Fibrinolysis 2012;23:532–6.
40. Bauman ME, Cheung PY, Massicotte MP. Hemostasis and platelet dysfunction in asphyxiated neonates. J Pediatr 2011;158:e35–9.
41. Shah P, Riphagen S, Beyene J, et al. Multiorgan dysfunction in infants with post-asphyxial hypoxic-ischaemic encephalopathy. Arch Dis Child Fetal Neonatal Ed 2004;89:F152–5.
42. Sarkar S, Barks JD, Bhagat I, et al. Effects of therapeutic hypothermia on multi-organ dysfunction in asphyxiated newborns: whole-body cooling versus selective head cooling. J Perinatol 2009;29:558–63.
43. Rohrer MJ, Natale AM. Effect of hypothermia on the coagulation cascade. Crit Care Med 1992;20:1402–5.
44. Wolberg AS, Meng ZH, Monroe DM 3rd, et al. A systematic evaluation of the effect of temperature on coagulation enzyme activity and platelet function. J Trauma 2004;56:1221–8.
45. Mitrophanov AY, Rosendaal FR, Reifman J. Computational analysis of the effects of reduced temperature on thrombin generation: the contributions of hypothermia to coagulopathy. Anesth Analg 2013;117:565–74.
46. Oncel MY, Erdeve O, Calisici E, et al. The effect of whole-body cooling on hematological and coagulation parameters in asphyxic newborns. Pediatr Hematol Oncol 2013;30:246–52.
47. Jacobs SE, Berg M, Hunt R, et al. Cooling for newborns with hypoxic ischaemic encephalopathy. Cochrane Database Syst Rev 2013;(1):CD003311.
48. Forman KR, Diab Y, Wong EC, et al. Coagulopathy in newborns with hypoxic ischemic encephalopathy (HIE) treated with therapeutic hypothermia: a retrospective case-control study. BMC Pediatr 2014;14:277.
49. Radicioni M, Mezzetti D, Del Vecchio A, et al. Thromboelastography: might work in neonatology too? J Matern Fetal Neonatal Med 2012;25(Suppl 4):18–21.
50. Radicioni M, Bruni A, Bini V, et al. Thromboelastographic profiles of the premature infants with and without intracranial hemorrhage at birth: a pilot study. J Matern Fetal Neonatal Med 2014;17:1–5.
51. Forman KR, Wong E, Gallagher M, et al. Effect of temperature on thromboelastography and implications for clinical use in newborns undergoing therapeutic hypothermia. Pediatr Res 2014;75:663–9.
52. Motta M, Testa M, Tripodi G, et al. Changes in neonatal transfusion practice after dissemination of neonatal recommendations. Pediatrics 2010;125:e810–7.
53. Baer VL, Henry E, Lambert DK, et al. Implementing a program to improve compliance with neonatal intensive care unit transfusion guidelines was accompanied by a reduction in transfusion rate: a pre-post analysis within a multihospital health care system. Transfusion 2011;51:264–9.
54. Hibbs SP, Nielsen ND, Brunskill S, et al. The impact of electronic decision support on transfusion practice: a systematic review. Transfus Med Rev 2015;29(1):14–23.
55. Venkatesh V, Curley A, Khan R, et al. A novel approach to standardised recording of bleeding in a high risk neonatal population. Arch Dis Child Fetal Neonatal Ed 2013;98:F260–3.

Thrombosis in the Neonatal Intensive Care Unit

Matthew A. Saxonhouse, MD

KEYWORDS

- Neonatal thrombosis • Anticoagulation • Prothrombotic disorder • Thrombolysis
- Perinatal arterial ischemic stroke • Cerebral sinovenous thrombosis

KEY POINTS

- Thrombosis is a significant problem affecting both term and preterm neonates.
- Most neonates that develop thrombosis have acquired risk factors or prothrombotic disorders.
- Proper imaging is essential for accurately identifying thromboses.
- The use of central venous/arterial catheters significantly increases a neonate's risk for thrombosis.
- Recommendations for neonatal treatment are based on expert opinion and data from case studies/series.

INTRODUCTION

Neonates have the highest risk for thrombosis among Pediatric patients (**Box 1**).[1,2] The placement of central venous and arterial catheters significantly increases this risk. Many prothrombotic disorders have been implicated in the pathogenesis of neonatal thrombosis, yet their exact role remains unclear. Despite treatment recommendations, there is a significant lack of randomized controlled trials demonstrating the efficacy of these treatments. Management of neonatal thromboses should occur at an experienced tertiary center that has proper support in place. This review focuses on a brief discussion of the neonatal hemostatic system highlighting why neonates are at risk for thrombosis, discusses the most common locations of neonatal thromboses and how to accurately image for them, reviews prothrombotic disorders' role in neonatal thrombosis, and discusses possible treatment modalities.

Division of Neonatology, Levine Children's Hospital at Carolinas Medical Center, 1000 Blythe Boulevard, 7th Floor, Charlotte, NC 28203, USA
E-mail address: Matthew.saxonhouse@carolinashealthcare.org

Clin Perinatol 42 (2015) 651–673
http://dx.doi.org/10.1016/j.clp.2015.04.010
0095-5108/15/$ – see front matter © 2015 Elsevier Inc. All rights reserved.

> **Box 1**
> **Incidence of neonatal thrombosis**
>
> - Incidence of symptomatic neonatal thrombosis is 5.1 per 100,000 live births[1] and 2.4–6.8 per 1000 neonatal intensive care admissions[2,7]
> - Term and preterm and male and female neonates are affected equally.[1,2,25]

NEONATAL HEMOSTASIS

The neonatal coagulation system (anticoagulation and fibrinolytic systems) differs from those of children and adults (**Table 1**).[7,8] These differences shift the neonate into a somewhat prothrombotic state, which is balanced by other factors preventing spontaneous thromboses in well neonates.[9] However, numerous acquired and prothrombotic disorders may disrupt this balance, placing a neonate at risk for developing a clinically significant thrombosis (**Table 2**).[3–6,9] Age-appropriate reference ranges of coagulation and anticoagulation proteins are published.[3,5,6]

TYPES AND LOCATIONS OF NEONATAL THROMBOSES

Common locations, presenting signs and symptoms, and imaging modalities recommended for different types of thromboses are presented in **Table 3**.

Arterial Thromboses

Perinatal arterial ischemic stroke

Perinatal arterial ischemic stroke (PAIS), which affects both preterm and term infants, mainly occurs in the left hemisphere within the distribution of the middle cerebral artery, with multifocal cerebral infarctions usually being of embolic origin.[12]

The exact pathophysiologic mechanisms responsible for PAIS are unknown. A patent foramen ovale allowing thrombi from the placental circulation to pass into the cerebral arterial vasculature resulting in vessel occlusion has been one suggested theory.[32] Pathologic examination of the placenta from any high-risk delivery may

Table 1
Anticoagulant and procoagulant protein levels in neonates compared with adults

	Protein	Neonatal Level Compared with Adult Level
Neonatal Procoagulant proteins	Factor VIII von Willebrand factor activity	Increased
Neonatal anticoagulant proteins	Factor II Factor VII Factor IX Factor X Factor XI Factor XII Protein C Protein S Antithrombin Heparin cofactor II	Decreased

Adapted from Manco-Johnson M. Controversies in neonatal thrombotic disorders. In: Ohls RY, editor. Hematology, immunology and infections disease: neonatology questions and controversies. Philadelphia: Saunders Elsevier; 2008. p. 59; with permission.

Table 2
Risk factors implicated in the development of neonatal thromboses

Maternal Risk Factors	Delivery Risk Factors	Neonatal Risk Factors
Infertility	Emergent cesarean	CVCs[a]
Oligohydramnios	section	Arterial catheters
Prothrombotic disorder	Fetal heart rate	CHD
Preeclampsia	abnormalities	Sepsis
Diabetes	Instrumentation	Meningitis
Intrauterine growth	Meconium-stained	Birth asphyxia
restriction	fluid	Respiratory distress syndrome
Chorioamnionitis		Dehydration
Prolonged rupture of		Congenital nephritic/nephrotic syndrome
membranes		Necrotizing enterocolitis
Autoimmune disorders		Polycythemia
		Pulmonary hypertension
		Prothrombotic disorders (see **Box 3**)
		Surgery
		Extracorporeal membrane oxygenation
		Medications (steroids)

[a] Greatest risk factor for thrombosis.
From Saxonhouse MA, Manco-Johnson MJ. The evaluation and management of neonatal coagulation disorders. Semin Perinatol 2009;33:56; with permission; and *Data from* Refs.[2,10–24]

assist with supporting this theory. Other risk factors implicated in the cause of PAIS are listed in **Table 2**, with prothrombotic disorders being reported in more than half of the population studied with PAIS.[32]

- Current guidelines recommend anticoagulation treatment *only* for neonates with proven cardioembolic stroke or recurrent PAIS.[27]

Iatrogenic arterial thrombosis
The use of indwelling arterial catheters is frequent in the neonatal intensive care unit (NICU) and has significant clinical benefits for managing critically ill neonates. Unfortunately, the presence of these catheters coupled with other risk factors in the ill neonate (see **Table 2**) may increase the risk for a symptomatic arterial thrombosis. Iatrogenic arterial thromboses have been associated with umbilical arterial catheters (UACs), peripheral arterial catheters (PALs), and femoral arterial catheters (**Box 2**).[33]

High UAC positioning may have fewer complications,[27,34] whereas continuous heparin infusion at 1 unit/mL may prolong catheter patency without reducing the risk for thrombosis.[34,35] The longer a UAC remains in place, the higher the probability for thrombus formation (80% incidence if used for 21 days).[36]

Spontaneous arterial thrombosis
Spontaneous arterial thromboses are rare (see **Table 3**) and warrant an evaluation for a prothrombotic disorder (**Box 3**).[38] Treatment depends on the clinical symptoms and location of the thrombus.

Venous Thromboses

Central venous catheter–related thrombosis (excluding intracardiac)
Umbilical venous catheters (UVCs) and percutaneous intravenous central catheters (PICCs) are routinely used in the NICU; however, occlusion and infection remain the 2 most commonly reported long-term problems (**Box 4**).[48] An analysis of 3332 neonates with central venous catheters (CVCs; including UVCs, PICCs, and surgically

Table 3
Types of neonatal thromboses, presenting signs/symptoms, and best imaging modalities to diagnose them

	Type of Thromboses (Vessels Potentially Involved)	Presenting Signs/Symptoms	Imaging Modality
Arterial	PAIS (left middle cerebral artery,[a] anterior cerebral artery, posterior cerebral artery)	Seizures,[b] lethargy, hypotonia, apnea, feeding difficulties	Diffusion-weighted MRI/magnetic resonance angiography
	Iatrogenic[c] (abdominal aorta, radial artery, renal artery, mesenteric artery, popliteal artery)	Line dysfunction,[b] extremity blanching or cyanosis,[b] persistent thrombocytopenia, sepsis, other symptoms depending on location	
	Spontaneous (iliac artery, left pulmonary artery, aortic arch, descending aorta)	Symptoms depend on location	
Venous	Iatrogenic[c]/spontaneous vessel occlusion (superior vena cava, inferior vena cava, hepatic vein, subclavian vein, abdominal veins, peripheral veins)	Line dysfunction, persistent thrombocytopenia, persistent infection, pericardial tamponade, symptoms of right heart failure, superior vena cava syndrome	Doppler ultrasound (limited in low-birth-weight infants; 27-g catheters are not consistently visualized during ultrasound examinations[c,26])
	Renal vein	Triad of (1) macroscopic hematuria, (2) palpable abdominal mass, and (3) thrombocytopenia; acute hypertension	
	Portal venous	Thrombocytopenia, elevations of liver enzymes	
	Cerebral sinovenous (superior sagittal sinus, transverse sinuses of the superficial venous system, straight sinus of the deep system)	Seizures,[b] respiratory distress, poor feeding, irritability, fever, apnea, lethargy, jitteriness	Diffusion-weighted MRI with venography
	CHD-related (right/left atria, right/left ventricle, superior vena cava, inferior vena cava)	Pericardial tamponade, symptoms of right heart failure, superior vena cava syndrome	Echocardiography

a Most common vessel involved.
b Most common symptom.
c Catheter related.
Data from Refs.[12,20,23,27-31]; and Adapted from Saxonhouse MA. Management of neonatal thrombosis. Clin Perinatol 2012;39:192-3; with permission.

Box 2
Key points: iatrogenic arterial thrombosis

- Complications from UAC-associated thromboses include mesenteric ischemia, renal failure, tissue necrosis, hypertension, septicemia, and even death.[36,37]

- Suspicion or confirmation of an arterial thrombosis due to catheter placement should warrant prompt removal of the catheter.

- Imaging should be performed before catheter removal, and careful consideration should be given to whether local thrombolysis via the catheter may be indicated.[27]

---

placed CVCs) demonstrated an incidence rate of thrombosis of 9.2% (1.1%–66.7%).[48] Other studies have reported the thrombosis rate for PICC lines to range from 2.2% to 33.6%.[49] Autopsies have estimated that 20% to 65% of infants who die with a UVC in situ have microscopic evidence of thromboses.[50–52]

Small-for-gestational-age, polycythemic neonates requiring central venous access may represent a significantly high-risk population for thrombosis.[48] The site of insertion does not seem to affect the incidence and morbidity of CVC-related thrombosis.[48]

Removal of a CVC should follow the diagnosis of a thrombosis; however, because of the risk for emboli, current recommendations are to delay CVC removal until 3 to 5 days after anticoagulant therapy has been started, although no clinical studies exist to support this practice.[27] The treatment of CVC-related thrombosis depends on the

---

Box 3
Prothrombotic disorders implicated in the development of neonatal thrombosis

Factor V Leiden mutation[a,b,c]

Factor II G20210A gene mutation[a,c]

Increased apolipoprotein (a)

Methylenetetrahydrofolate reductase gene mutation (MTHFR C677T) genotype[b,c]

Hyperhomocysteinemia

Protein C deficiency[a,c]

Protein S deficiency[a,c]

Antithrombin deficiency[a,b]

Heparin cofactor II deficiency

Dysfibrinogenemia

PAI-1 4G/5G gene mutation[c]

Increased levels of factor VIIIC, IX, XI, or fibrinogen

Antiphospholipid antibodies (including anticardiolipin antibodies, lupus anticoagulant)

Chromosome 2q

Chromosome 2q13 deletion

Either a single disorder, or more commonly, the combination of multiple disorders may result in a prothrombotic phenotype.
[a]May follow autosomal-dominant inheritance model.
[b]Increased risk for spontaneous arterial thrombosis.
[c]Implicated with development of RVT.[39,40]
Data from Refs.[13,15–17,25,41–47]

> **Box 4**
> **Key points: central venous catheter–related thrombosis**
>
> - Long-term complications of CVC-related thromboses include venous chronic venous obstruction with cutaneous collateral circulation, chylothorax, portal hypertension (see discussion in text), and postthrombotic syndrome.[53–56]
> - The Centers for Disease Control and Prevention currently recommend that UVCs be limited to 14 days.[57]

presence of clinical symptoms, the location of the thrombus, and whether the thrombus is stagnant or propagating following detection.[48] Further specific management guidelines are presented later.

Intracardiac thromboses not associated with congenital heart disease

The placement of CVCs in the right atrium remains controversial because of the risks for pericardial tamponade or intracardiac thrombi.[41,58] Intracardiac (mainly right atrial thrombi) thrombi is a life-threatening condition due to the risk for dissemination of emboli into the lungs or obstruction of the right pulmonary artery.[59,60] Please refer to the treatment section for specific details.

Renal vein thrombosis

Symptoms of renal vein thrombosis (RVT), not always present in triad, are presented in **Table 3**. Most neonatal RVTs are unilateral (70%) and tend to involve the left kidney, with a male predominance (**Box 5**).[10] Current treatment recommendations for RVT are presented in **Table 4**.

Portal vein thrombosis

Spontaneous regression of neonatal PVT may occur,[64,65] and recanalization occurs more frequently in cases with partial thrombi (70%–77%) than in cases with occlusive thrombi (31%–48%)[26,66] with a mean time of resolution of 63 days (2–626 days; median 25 days).[66]

The major concern with neonatal PVT is the development of portal hypertension, although this long-term complication is uncommon, especially if the thrombus remains in the left portal vein and does not propagate into the main or right portal vein (**Box 6**).[26,67–71] One study demonstrated portal hypertension occurring at a mean of 5.7 years after the acute event; therefore, routine follow-up is recommended for any neonate diagnosed with PVT.[72] Another complication of neonatal PVT is liver lobe atrophy. Although no evidence for anticoagulation or thrombolysis exists for cases of neonatal PVT, there are circumstances wherein treatment may be warranted (**Table 5**).[67]

> **Box 5**
> **Key points: renal vein thrombosis**
>
> - Complications of RVT include adrenal hemorrhage, extension into the inferior vena cava, hypertension, renal failure, and death.[10]
> - Most infants with RVT will suffer either complete, cortical, or segmental infarction of the affected kidneys.[63]
> - Prothrombotic disorders have been found in 43% to 67% of patients with RVT (see Box 3).[10,11,61,62]

Table 4 Management options for neonates with renal vein thrombosis		
	Unilateral RVT	Bilateral RVT
Absence of renal impairment or extension into the inferior vena cava	Supportive care with monitoring of the RVT for extension If extension occurs, anticoagulation for 6 wk to 3 mo[a]	Supportive care with monitoring of the RVT for extension If extension occurs, anticoagulation for 6 wk to 3 mo[a]
Extension into the inferior vena cava	Anticoagulation[a]	Anticoagulation[a]
Renal failure	N/A	Initial thrombolytic[b] therapy with rTPA, followed by anticoagulation[a]

[a] See Tables 9 and 10 for dosing options.
[b] See Tables 10 and 11 for dosing options and appropriate monitoring.
   Data from Refs.[10,11,27,61,62] and Adapted from Saxonhouse MA. Management of neonatal thrombosis. Clin Perinatol 2012;39:195; with permission.

Cerebral sinovenous thrombosis

Most neonates with cerebral sinovenous thrombosis (CSVT) will present on the day of birth or within the first week of life (Box 7).[76–78] Impaired or absent venous drainage in one of the cerebral sinuses leads to increased venous pressure, vasogenic edema, and secondary infarction.[32] Hemorrhagic infarction may be present in 50% to 60% of newborns on first imaging.[79] A spontaneous intraventricular or thalamic hemorrhage in a late-preterm or full-term neonate warrants evaluation for CSVT.

The primary goal in the management of CSVT is to treat the underlying cause that may have predisposed the infant to develop CSVT (see Table 2).[79] Studies in infants with CSVT demonstrate that in the supine position, compression of the occipital bone occurs, which may reduce cerebral blood flow. Adjusting the infant's positioning to decompress the occipital bone has been shown to increase flow in the sigmoid and superior sagittal sinuses, offering a noninvasive therapy.[80]

Thrombosis in Infants with Congenital Heart Disease

Neonates with congenital heart disease (CHD), especially those undergoing cardiac surgery, represent a high-risk group for thrombosis (Box 8). Blood flow disturbances

Box 6 Key points: portal vein thrombosis
• Sepsis, omphalitis, and UVCs have been specifically implicated in the development of neonatal PVT.[67]
• Other than placement in the portal vein, UVC position does not seem to be significantly associated with PVT.[67]
• Most neonates with PVT remain asymptomatic during the neonatal period (see Table 3).[67]
• Acute complications include liver necrosis, cerebral infarction from paradoxic emboli, hepatic hematoma, hemorrhagic ascites, intrapulmonary bleeding, and death.[73–75]
• Neonatologists must continue to understand the risks associated with UVC placement and the potential complications of PVT.
• Proper placement must be confirmed and should only occur if the placement of a UVC outweighs its risks.

Table 5
Management options for neonates with portal venous thrombosis

Treatment Plan	Description of PVT	Recommended Ultrasound (US) Follow-Up
Observation	No extension observed and infant clinically stable	7–10 d
Anticoagulation	Extension into the IVC, RA, or RV but no end-organ compromise	10 d If thrombus resolved, may stop therapy. If still present, treat for 6 wk to 3 mo depending on US follow-up
Thrombolytic therapy	End-organ compromise with extension of the thrombosis into the IVC, RA, or RV	Daily May stop thrombolysis when symptoms improve but would transition to anticoagulation

Abbreviations: IVC, inferior vena cava; RA, right atrium; RV, right ventricle.
Adapted from Williams S, Chan AK. Neonatal portal vein thrombosis: diagnosis and management. Semin Fetal Neonatal Med 2011;16:337; with permission.

due to hypoplastic ventricles with limited inflow/outflow, dilated atria, arterial or femoral venous catheters, and surgically placed shunts all create an environment conducive to thrombus formation.[81] Cardiac surgery is associated with platelet dysfunction/activation, inflammation, and blood hypercoagulability.[81,82]

RISK FACTORS FOR NEONATAL THROMBOSES INCLUDING APPROPRIATE LABORATORY EVALUATION

The combination of acquired risk factors (see **Table 2**) and prothrombotic disorders (see **Box 3**) may represent the perfect storm for the development of clinically significant neonatal thromboses. Registry data and case series have demonstrated that most symptomatic neonatal thromboses either are associated with multiple prothrombotic disorders or are a combination of prothrombotic disorders and acquired risk factors.[1,2,10,11,13–17,42–45,61,88–90] Therefore, it is recommended that neonates with clinically significant thromboses (regardless of acquired risk factors) be tested for prothrombotic disorders.[18]

- Homozygous or compound heterozygous disorders, such as severe protein C, protein S, or antithrombin III deficiency, usually present in newborns with severe clinical manifestations (purpura fulminans).[27]

Laboratory Evaluation

Important points to remember when performing the laboratory evaluation for a prothrombotic disorder in a neonate are presented in **Box 9**. The timing of the evaluation

Box 7
Key points: cerebral sinovenous thrombosis

- Management algorithm for neonatal CSVT is presented in **Fig. 1**.
- Mortality from CSVT ranges from 2% to 24% with disabilities such as epilepsy, cerebral palsy, and cognitive impairments ranging from 10% to 80% of patients.[79]

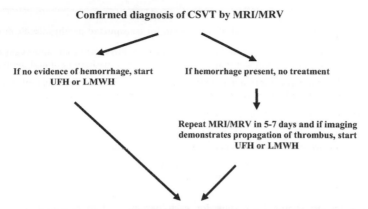

Confirmed diagnosis of CSVT by MRI/MRV

If no evidence of hemorrhage, start UFH or LMWH

If hemorrhage present, no treatment

Repeat MRI/MRV in 5-7 days and if imaging demonstrates propagation of thrombus, start UFH or LMWH

Repeat MRI/MRV in 6 weeks for vessel recanalization. If complete, stop therapy. If not, consider additional 6 weeks of treatment

Fig. 1. Management of neonatal CSVT. The figure displayed represents the current recommendations for appropriate evaluation, management, and follow-up of neonates diagnosed with CSVT. If either UFH or LMWH is provided, dosing guidelines are provided in **Tables 9** and **10**, respectively. MRV, magnetic resonance venography. (*Data from* Yang JY, Chan AK, Callen DJ, et al. Neonatal cerebral sinovenous thrombosis: sifting the evidence for a diagnostic plan and treatment strategy. Pediatrics 2010;126:e693–700.)

should be based on the severity of the thrombosis, presence of other acquired risk factors, and treatment plan.[13] Further details are outlined in **Tables 6** and **7**.

MANAGEMENT OF THROMBOSIS

Management of neonates with clinically significant thromboses should take place at a tertiary referral center that has an experienced Neonatologist or Pediatric Hematologist. The center should also have adequate laboratory, radiology, pharmacy, transfusion medicine, and pediatric surgical support.[9,27] Treatment options include observation, nitroglycerin ointment (vasospasm), anticoagulant or thrombolytic therapy, or surgery.

Withholding therapy and monitoring sequentially for alterations in the size of the thrombus in infants with asymptomatic thrombi associated with CVCs is a reasonable plan.[27]

Recommendations and dosing regimens for anticoagulant/thrombolytic therapy in neonates are based on uncontrolled studies, extrapolation from adult and pediatric data, small case series, cohort studies, and expert opinion.[27] There are situations

---

Box 8
Key points: thrombosis in infants with congenital heart disease

- Lower levels of antithrombin in neonates with CHD may predispose aortopulmonary shunt thrombosis.[83]

- Complications of thrombosis in neonates with CHD include pulmonary embolism, stroke, hemorrhage, and cardiac failure.[84,85]

- Occurrence of thrombosis after pediatric cardiac surgery has been linked to a 3.4-fold increase in mortality.[86,87]

Box 9
Key points to remember in the laboratory evaluation for a suspected prothrombotic disorder

- Due to many of the pro-/anticoagulation protein levels being lower than adult values, the diagnosis of a coagulation disorder may be difficult in the immediate neonatal period.

- Certain protein-based assays may aid in treatment during the neonatal period (antithrombin and plasminogen assays) and may be performed during the neonatal period.

- DNA-based assays are accurate and may be obtained at any time.

- The different evaluations listed in the text are based on the presence of acquired risk factors, type of thrombosis, severity of thrombosis, and treatment regimen (if indicated).

- The initiation of long-term anticoagulation will usually not occur during the neonatal period and, therefore, the complete evaluation for a prothrombotic disorder may take place at 3 to 6 months of age.

- Laboratory testing should be unique for each patient and in concordance between Neonatology and Pediatric Hematology at an experienced tertiary referral center that has either a reference laboratory or a reliable referral center limiting blood loss in neonates.

- Baseline complete blood count, prothrombin time (PT), activated partial thromboplastin time (aPTT), and fibrinogen levels should be performed before any evaluation.

---

when neonatal thromboses are life-, organ-, or limb-threatening. Efficacy has been demonstrated from case studies/series on the use of recombinant tissue plasminogen activator (rTPA) or anticoagulation with limited side effects.[27] Therefore, it is reasonable to assume that a randomized trial demonstrating the effectiveness of rTPA or anticoagulation for limb-/life-threatening neonatal thromboses may never be done because the risk to withhold such treatment may far outweigh the benefit of a controlled trial.[63] Still, serious complications (intracranial hemorrhage, ICH) must be considered in any

Table 6
Evaluation for prothrombotic disorder: presence of acquired risk factors

Laboratory Testing	Collection Tube
Antiphospholipid antibody panel, anticardiolipin, and lupus anticoagulant[a] (immunoglobulin G, immunoglobulin M)	Citrated plasma
Protein C activity[b] Protein S activity[b] Plasminogen level[b] (if considering thrombolytic therapy) Antithrombin (activity assay)[b]	Citrated plasma
Factor V Leiden Prothrombin G[c]	EDTA (Ethylenediaminetetraacetic acid)

The evaluation presented may be performed in its entirety during the neonatal period or may be performed at 3–6 months of age. The entire evaluation listed may be done in 1–2 mL of blood.
[a] May be performed from maternal serum during first few months of life.
[b] Protein-based assays are affected by the acute thrombosis and must be repeated at 3–6 months of life, before a definitive diagnosis may be made.[13,91] If anticoagulation is being administered, then these assays should be obtained 14–30 days after discontinuing the anticoagulant.
[c] DNA-based assays.
Adapted from Saxonhouse MA, Manco-Johnson MJ. The evaluation and management of neonatal coagulation disorders. Seminars in Perinatology 2009;33:59; with permission.

Table 7
Evaluation for prothrombotic disorder: no acquired risk factors present

Laboratory Testing	Collection Tube
Antiphospholipid antibody panel, anticardiolipin, and lupus anticoagulant (immunoglobulin G, immunoglobulin M)[a]	Citrated plasma
Protein C activity[b] Protein S activity[b] Antithrombin (activity assay)[b]	Citrated plasma
Factor V Leiden[c] Prothrombin G[c] Methylenetetrahydrofolate reductase[c] PAI-1 4G/5G mutation[c]	EDTA
Homocysteine[b] Lipoprotein a[b]	Citrated plasma
FVIII activity[b] FXII activity[b] Plasminogen activity[b] Heparin cofactor II[b]	Citrated plasma

The evaluation presented may be performed in its entirety during the neonatal period or may be performed at 3–6 months of age. The entire evaluation listed may be done in 5–6 mL of blood.

A possible limitation to this approach is the amount of blood required for adequate testing, especially when evaluating a premature or anemic infant.

[a] May be performed from maternal serum during the first few months of life.

[b] Protein based-assays are affected by the acute thrombosis event and must be repeated at 3–6 months of life, before a definitive diagnosis may be made.[13,91] If anticoagulation is being administered, then these assays should be obtained 14–30 days after discontinuing the anticoagulant.

[c] DNA-based assays.

Adapted from Saxonhouse MA, Manco-Johnson MJ. The evaluation and management of neonatal coagulation disorders. Seminars in Perinatology 2009;33:59; with permission.

neonate before initiating antithrombotic therapy. Absolute and relative contraindications for thrombolytic and anticoagulant therapy in neonates are displayed in **Table 8**.

- Clinicians may use 1-800-NO CLOTS to receive up-to-date management guidance from expert consultants over the phone.[27]

Table 8
Absolute and relative contraindications for initiating thrombolytic/anticoagulant therapy in neonates

	Absolute	Relative
Medical conditions	1. Central nervous system surgery or ischemia (including birth asphyxia) within 10 d 2. Active bleeding 3. Invasive procedures within 3 d 4. Seizures within 48–h	1. Platelet count <50 × 10^4/μL (100 × 10^4/μL for ill neonates) 2. Fibrinogen concentration <100 mg/dL 3. INR (international normalized ratio) >2 4. Severe coagulation deficiency 5. Hypertension

Adapted from Manco-Johnson M. Controversies in neonatal thrombotic disorders. In: Ohls RY, editor. Hematology, immunology and infections disease: neonatology questions and controversies. Philadelphia: Saunders Elsevier; 2008. p. 68; with permission; and *Data from* Refs.[21,27,33,53,91]

Nitroglycerin

Management of peripheral vasospasm following UAC or PAL placement is presented in **Fig. 2**. Nitroglycerine is a nitric oxide donor that may have a direct effect on vascular smooth muscle producing local vasodilatation of veins and arteries.[93–95] Resultant increased blood flow, due to this acute dilatation, may overcome the vasospasm, allowing flow around microthrombi or improving collateral circulation to the affected areas.[96,97]

Anticoagulation

Low-molecular-weight heparins (LMWHs) are the most commonly used anticoagulants in infants and children, with enoxaparin being the most frequently used.[100–103] Enoxaparin has the best factor Xa/factor IIa inhibition ratio and has demonstrated fewer bleeding complications in clinical trials, the longest half-life, and the most consistent pharmacokinetic and pharmacodynamic pediatric data.[104–106]

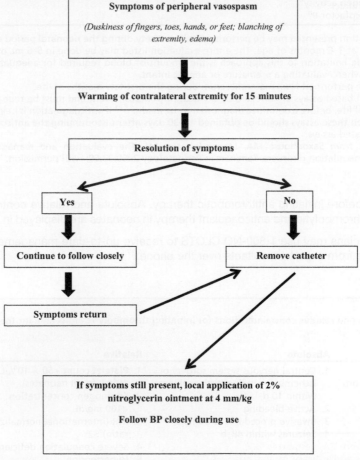

Fig. 2. Management of peripheral vasospasm. The figure displayed represents the current recommendations for the evaluation and management for neonates with peripheral vasospasm most likely due from complications from PALs or UACs. Nitroglycerin dosing is provided. BP, blood pressure. (*Data from* Refs.[27,96–99])

Antithrombin levels are lower in neonates compared with adults.[3,5,6] Because of these lower levels and an increased rate of heparin clearance, neonates tend to require higher doses of anticoagulation to achieve therapeutic levels.[77] Antithrombin concentrate has been used to optimize heparin therapy and provide a more consistent state of anticoagulation during extracorporeal membrane oxygenation, cardiopulmonary bypass, and aortopulmonary shunt placement, without increasing the risk for excessive bleeding.[83,107–111] Anticoagulation dosing in neonates is based on lower levels of antithrombin; therefore, if antithrombin concentrate is administered to achieve anticoagulation and the anticoagulant dose is not adjusted, significant bleeding complications may occur.

Unfractionated Heparin

Dosing and monitoring guidelines are displayed in **Table 9**. Unfractionated heparin (UFH) therapy is usually continued for 2 to 30 days,[27] but data to support this

Table 9
Clinical indications and recommended dosing guidelines for unfractionated heparin therapy in neonates

Clinical Indication	Traditional Dosing	Other Recommended Dosing[a,112]	Appropriate Monitoring (Applied to All Dosing Regimens)
Asymptomatic or symptomatic thrombus but non-limb-threatening	Any GA Bolus dose: 75 units/kg IV over 10 min Maintenance dose: 28 units/kg/h	<28-wk GA Bolus dose: 25 units/kg IV over 10 min Maintenance dose: 15 units/kg/h 28–37-wk GA Bolus dose: 50 units/kg over 10 min Maintenance dose: 15 units/kg/h >37-wk GA Bolus dose: 100 units/kg over 10 min Maintenance dose: 28 units/kg/h	Maintain anti-factor Xa level of 0.03–0.7 units/mL (aPTT of 60–85 s) Check anti-factor Xa level 4 h after loading dose and 4 h after each change in infusion rate Dosing adjustments based on anti-factor Xa levels are published elsewhere[27,113] Complete blood count, platelet count, and coagulation screening (including aPTT, PT, and fibrinogen) should be performed before starting UFH therapy Recommendations are that platelet count and fibrinogen levels should be repeated daily for 2–3 d once therapeutic levels are achieved and at least twice weekly thereafter[27]

Abbreviation: GA, gestational age.
[a] Safety and efficacy of this dosing have not been confirmed by clinical studies; use with caution.[112]
Data from Refs.[27,91,112] and *Adapted from* Armstrong-Wells JL, Manco-Johnson MJ. Neonatal thrombosis. In: de Alarcon P, Werner EJ, Christensen RD, editors. Neonatal Hematology. New York: Cambridge University Press; 2013. p. 282; with permission.

recommendation are lacking. The major complication of UFH in neonates is bleeding, with one registry reporting a 2% major hemorrhage rate.[2] UFH has a short half-life and cessation of the infusion usually resolves any excessive bleeding. If cessation of the infusion does not control bleeding, then a full coagulation assessment should be performed and hemostatic deficiencies replaced. Protamine may be considered in the setting of an anti-Xa activity level greater than 0.8 U/mL with active bleeding. One unit of protamine will neutralize 100 units of UFH. The plasma heparin burden can be estimated by multiplying estimated plasma volume by anti-Xa concentration.[9] Protamine dosing should be conservative, and one-half the calculated dose is generally given initially (excess protamine is an anticoagulant).

Heparin-induced thrombocytopenia (HIT) is rare in neonates[114,115]; however, a drop in the platelet count by 50% or persistent platelet counts less than 70 to 100,000/mm[3] occurring 5 to 10 days after the first exposure to heparin should alert the clinician to the possibility of HIT.

Low-Molecular-Weight Heparin

Dosing and management guidelines are displayed in **Table 10**. Although adverse effects from LMWH are rare, several major complications have been described.[93–95,116]

Table 10
Clinical indications and recommended dosing guidelines for low-molecular weight heparin (enoxaparin) therapy in neonates

Clinical Situation	Traditional Dosing	Other Recommended Dosing[a,112]	Prophylactic Dose	Appropriate Monitoring
Asymptomatic or symptomatic thrombus but non-limb-threatening	Any GA 1.5 mg/kg SQ every 12 h	<28 wk gestation 1.25 mg/kg SQ every 12 h 28–37 wk gestation 1.5 mg/kg SQ every 12 h >37 wk gestation 1.625 mg/kg SQ every 12 h	0.75 mg/kg SQ every 12 h	Goal of anti-FXa levels of 0.5 to 1.0 U/mL Check level 4 h after second dose and then every few days or weekly[104] Dosing adjustments based on anti-FXA levels are published elsewhere[27,113] If infant with high hemorrhagic profile, use dosing regimen of 1 mg/kg SQ every 12-h[27]

Enoxaparin must be withheld for 24-h before any invasive procedure.

LMWH may be administered either by subcutaneous injection or through an indwelling subcutaneous catheter (Insuflon;Unomedical, Birkerod, Denmark). Studies have demonstrated up to 56% in incidence of local adverse effects with Insuflon usage and caution should be used in very low birth weight infants.[27,91,93,94,116–118]

Abbreviations: GA, gestational age; SQ, subcutaneous.

[a] Safety and efficacy of this dosing has not been confirmed by clinical studies; use with caution.[112]

Adapted from Armstrong-Wells JL, Manco-Johnson MJ. Neonatal thrombosis. In: de Alarcon P, Werner EJ, Christensen RD, editors. Neonatal Hematology. New York: Cambridge University Press; 2013. p. 282; with permission.

Overall, LMWH therapy has been effective in the NICU and centers have reported partial or complete resolution of thromboses in 59% to 100% of cases.[93,117]

Thrombolysis

Thrombolytic therapy, mainly rTPA, for use in neonates, should be reserved for limb-, organ-, or life-threatening thromboses, including catheter-related right atrial thromboses.[27,33,63,119–121] The safety and efficacy of rTPA treatment in neonates have been demonstrated in limited reports, but these have demonstrated either complete or partial clot lysis.[91,119–121]

rTPA has also been used in the management of premature infants with infective endocarditis[122]; however, one must use caution when administering thrombolytics to premature infants because of the high incidence of intracranial hemorrhage (ICH).

- Extensive discussion with an infant's family should occur before the use of rTPA in neonates because of its serious risks.

Dosing recommendations are displayed in **Table 11**, and appropriate careful monitoring for thrombolytic therapy is presented in **Table 12**.

Surgery

The use of microsurgical techniques with thrombolysis has been reported in patients with peripheral arterial occlusion.[124] One center has reported their experience with 11 patients with arterial vascular access-associated thrombosis secondary to peripheral arterial line complications. Five patients required arteriotomy, embolectomy, and subsequent microvascular reconstruction.[124] When faced with limb-/life-threatening arterial or venous thrombosis and antithrombotic therapy is absolutely contraindicated, surgery may be a viable option.

Table 11
Clinical indications and recommended dosing guidelines for recombinant tissue plasminogen activator therapy in neonates

Clinical Situation	Gestational Age	Recommended Dosing	Appropriate Monitoring
Limb-/life-threatening thrombus	<28 wk	0.03 mg/kg/h or 0.06 mg/kg/h Infuse UFH[a] at 10 units/kg/h	Dose escalation up to 0.24 mg/kg/h can be considered, but has to be
	>28 wk	May use same as for <28-wk or 0.1–0.5 mg/kg/h for 6–12 h and repeat daily for up to 3 d[112] Infuse UFH[a] at 10 units/kg/h	done slowly with continuing monitoring of the patient[b] (see **Table 12**) Supplementation with plasminogen (FFP) before commencing therapy is recommended to ensure adequate thrombolysis[27]

[a] rTPA does not inhibit clot propagation or directly affect hypercoagulability; therefore, simultaneous infusion of UFH is recommended.[27,119]
[b] See **Table 12**.
    Abbreviation: FFP, fresh frozen plasma.
    Data from Refs.[91,119]. *Adapted from* Armstrong-Wells JL, Manco-Johnson MJ. Neonatal thrombosis. In: de Alarcon P, Werner EJ, Christensen RD, editors. Neonatal Hematology. New York: Cambridge University Press; 2013. p. 282; with permission.

Table 12
Monitoring recommendations for thrombolytic therapy in neonates

Testing	When Performed	Levels Desired (If Applicable)[a]
Imaging of thrombosis	Before initiation of treatment Every 12–24 h during treatment	—
Fibrinogen level	Before initiation of treatment 4–6 h after starting treatment Every 12–24 h	Minimum of 100 mg/dL[123] Supplement with cryoprecipitate
Platelet count	Before initiation of treatment 4–6 h after starting treatment Every 12–24 h	Minimum of 50–100 × 10^4/μL,[92] dependent on bleeding risk
Cranial imaging	Before initiation of treatment Daily	—
Coagulation testing	Before initiation of treatment 4–6 h after starting treatment Every 12–24 h	—
Plasminogen	Before initiation of treatment 4–6 h after starting treatment Every 12–24 h	Adequate to achieve thrombolysis Supplementation with plasminogen (FFP) before commencing therapy is recommended to ensure adequate thrombolysis[27,119]
Line associated or mucosal oozing	All clinical assessments	Topical thrombin as needed

[a] Levels should be obtained before the initiation of treatment, 4–6 hours after starting treatment, and every 12–24 hours during treatment.
Adapted from Saxonhouse MA. Management of neonatal thrombosis. Clin Perinatol 2012;39:191–208; with permission; and *Data from* Refs.[33,119,120]

SUMMARY

Neonatal thrombosis represents an increasing problem affecting some of our most fragile patients. The lack of randomized clinical trials addressing the management of neonatal thrombosis forces neonatologists to base their medical decisions on limited evidence. As more data are obtained from centers specializing in neonatal thrombosis, more knowledge will be gained on how to optimize therapy. Current guidelines have been presented to assist Neonatologists and Pediatric Hematologists to make the most educated medical decisions. Despite numerous acquired risk factors implicated in the development for neonatal thrombosis, prothrombotic disorders continue to be reported in neonates. Neonatologists and others caring for high-risk infants with thromboses should continuously refer to the literature because new guidelines are recommended and others are updated. For now, the ultimate goal is to treat effectively without causing additional harm.

Best Practices

What is the current practice for thrombosis in the NICU?

Evaluation and treatment of any neonate with a clinically symptomatic thrombosis should occur at a tertiary referral center that has proper neonatology, pediatric hematology, pharmacy, radiology, and laboratory support. The use of central catheters is a major risk factor for the development of a clinically significant thrombosis. Most recommendations for treatment are based on expert opinion, case series, and data registries.

What changes in current practice are likely to improve outcomes?

Further clinical studies and data collection will enhance what the best treatment strategies should be for neonates with clinically significant thromboses. Proper imaging modalities should be performed based on the type of thrombosis that one is concerned about. Laboratory evaluations for prothrombotic disorders should be performed at specific time periods, allowing for proper diagnosis, and should be sent to specific referral laboratories, limiting blood volumes needed for these evaluations.

Is there a clinical algorithm?

Treatment algorithms are presented for peripheral vasospasm, renal vein thromboses, portal vein thromboses, and cerebral sinovenous thromboses. However, most recommendations for treatment and management are grade 2C. The use of rTPA and anticoagulation in neonates is based on limited evidence.

1. Monagle P, Chan AK, Goldenberg NA, et al. Antithrombotic therapy in neonates and children: antithrombotic therapy and prevention of thrombosis, 9th ed: American College of Chest Physicians Evidence-based Clinical Practice Guidelines. Chest 2012;141:e737S–801S.

2. Manco-Johnson MJ. How I treat venous thrombosis in children. Blood 2006;107:21–9.

Summary

Neonatal thrombosis represents an increasing problem affecting some of our most fragile patients. As more data are obtained from centers specializing in neonatal thrombosis, more knowledge will be gained on how to optimize therapy and minimize complications. Neonatologists and others caring for high-risk infants with thromboses should continuously refer to the literature because new guidelines are recommended and others are updated. For now, the ultimate goal is to treat effectively without causing additional harm.

REFERENCES

1. Schmidt B, Andrew M. Neonatal thrombosis: report of a prospective Canadian and international registry. Pediatrics 1995;96:939–43.
2. Nowak-Gottl U, von Kries R, Gobel U. Neonatal symptomatic thromboembolism in Germany: two year survey. Arch Dis Child Fetal Neonatal Ed 1997;76: F163–7.
3. Andrew M, Paes B, Milner R, et al. Development of the human coagulation system in the healthy premature infant. Blood 1988;72:1651–7.
4. Manco-Johnson MJ. Development of hemostasis in the fetus. Thromb Res 2005; 115(Suppl 1):55–63.
5. Andrew M, Paes B, Milner R, et al. Development of the human coagulation system in the full-term infant. Blood 1987;70:165–72.
6. Andrew M, Paes B, Johnston M. Development of the hemostatic system in the neonate and young infant. Am J Pediatr Hematol Oncol 1990;12:95–104.
7. van Elteren HA, Veldt HS, Te Pas AB, et al. Management and outcome in 32 neonates with thrombotic events. Int J Pediatr 2011;2011:217564.
8. Ries M. Molecular and functional properties of fetal plasminogen and its possible influence on clot lysis in the neonatal period. Semin Thromb Hemost 1997;23:247–52.
9. Saxonhouse MA, Manco-Johnson MJ. The evaluation and management of neonatal coagulation disorders. Semin Perinatol 2009;33:52–65.
10. Lau KK, Stoffman JM, Williams S, et al. Neonatal renal vein thrombosis: review of the English-language literature between 1992 and 2006. Pediatrics 2007;120: e1278–84.

11. Kosch A, Kuwertz-Broking E, Heller C, et al. Renal venous thrombosis in neonates: prothrombotic risk factors and long-term follow-up. Blood 2004;104:1356–60.

12. Chalmers EA. Perinatal stroke–risk factors and management. Br J Haematol 2005;130:333–43.

13. Nowak-Gottl U, Duering C, Kempf-Bielack B, et al. Thromboembolic diseases in neonates and children. Pathophysiol Haemost Thromb 2003;33:269–74.

14. van Ommen CH, Heijboer H, Buller HR, et al. Venous thromboembolism in childhood: a prospective two-year registry in the Netherlands. J Pediatr 2001;139:676–81.

15. Boffa MC, Lachassinne E. Infant perinatal thrombosis and antiphospholipid antibodies: a review. Lupus 2007;16:634–41.

16. Kenet G, Nowak-Gottl U. Fetal and neonatal thrombophilia. Obstet Gynecol Clin North Am 2006;33:457–66.

17. Alioglu B, Ozyurek E, Tarcan A, et al. Heterozygous methylenetetrahydrofolate reductase 677C-T gene mutation with mild hyperhomocysteinemia associated with intrauterine iliofemoral artery thrombosis. Blood Coagul Fibrinolysis 2006;17:495–8.

18. Manco-Johnson MJ, Grabowski EF, Hellgreen M, et al. Laboratory testing for thrombophilia in pediatric patients. On behalf of the Subcommittee for Perinatal and Pediatric Thrombosis of the Scientific and Standardization Committee of the International Society of Thrombosis and Haemostasis (ISTH). Thromb Haemost 2002;88:155–6.

19. Lee J, Croen LA, Backstrand KH, et al. Maternal and infant characteristics associated with perinatal arterial stroke in the infant. JAMA 2005;293:723–9.

20. Wasay M, Dai AI, Ansari M, et al. Cerebral venous sinus thrombosis in children: a multicenter cohort from the United States. J Child Neurol 2008;23:26–31.

21. Beardsley DS. Venous thromboembolism in the neonatal period. Semin Perinatol 2007;31:250–3.

22. Raju TN, Nelson KB, Ferriero D, et al, NICHD-NINDS Perinatal Stroke Workshop Participants. Ischemic perinatal stroke: summary of a workshop sponsored by the National Institute of Child Health and Human Development and the National Institute of Neurological Disorders and Stroke. Pediatrics 2007;120:609–16.

23. Golomb MR, Dick PT, MacGregor DL, et al. Neonatal arterial ischemic stroke and cerebral sinovenous thrombosis are more commonly diagnosed in boys. J Child Neurol 2004;19:493–7.

24. Wu YW, Lynch JK, Nelson KB. Perinatal arterial stroke: understanding mechanisms and outcomes. Semin Neurol 2005;25:424–34.

25. Kenet G, Lutkhoff LK, Albisetti M, et al. Impact of thrombophilia on risk of arterial ischemic stroke or cerebral sinovenous thrombosis in neonates and children: a systematic review and meta-analysis of observational studies. Circulation 2010;121:1838–47.

26. Kim JH, Lee YS, Kim SH, et al. Does umbilical vein catheterization lead to portal venous thrombosis? Prospective us evaluation in 100 neonates. Radiology 2001;219:645–50.

27. Monagle P, Chan AK, Goldenberg NA, et al. Antithrombotic therapy in neonates and children: antithrombotic therapy and prevention of thrombosis, 9th ed: American College of Chest Physicians Evidence-based Clinical Practice Guidelines. Chest 2012;141:e737S–801S.

28. Sharathkumar AA, Lamear N, Pipe S, et al. Management of neonatal aortic arch thrombosis with low-molecular weight heparin: a case series. J Pediatr Hematol Oncol 2009;31:516–21.

29. Nagel K, Tuckuviene R, Paes B, et al. Neonatal aortic thrombosis: a comprehensive review. Klin Padiatr 2010;222:134–9.
30. Tridapalli E, Stella M, Capretti MG, et al. Neonatal arterial iliac thrombosis in type-I protein C deficiency: a case report. Ital J Pediatr 2010;36:23.
31. Elhassan NO, Sproles C, Sachdeva R, et al. A neonate with left pulmonary artery thrombosis and left lung hypoplasia: a case report. J Med Case Rep 2010;4:284.
32. van der Aa NE, Benders MJ, Groenendaal F, et al. Neonatal stroke: a review of the current evidence on epidemiology, pathogenesis, diagnostics and therapeutic options. Acta Paediatr 2014;103:356–64.
33. Thornburg C, Pipe S. Neonatal thromboembolic emergencies. Semin Fetal Neonatal Med 2006;11:198–206.
34. Barrington K. Umbilical artery catheters in the newborn: effects of position of the catheter tip. Cochrane Database Syst Rev 2000;(2):CD000505.
35. Barrington K. Umbilical artery catheters in the newborn: effects of heparin. Cochrane Database Syst Rev 2000;(2):CD000507.
36. McAdams RM, Winter VT, McCurnin DC, et al. Complications of umbilical artery catheterization in a model of extreme prematurity. J Perinatol 2009;29: 685–92.
37. Sandal G, Duman L, Ayata A. A newborn case of intestinal infarction with homozygous MTHFR C677T and heterozygous of factor V Leiden G1691A, PAL-1 4G/5G mutations. Genet Couns 2014;25:81–4.
38. Piersigilli F, Auriti C, Landolfo F, et al. Spontaneous thrombosis of the abdominal aorta in two neonates. J Perinatol 2014;34:241–3.
39. Sandal G, Kuybulu AE, Ayata A. Unilateral renal vein thrombosis in a newborn heterozygous of the factor II G20210A and PAI-1 4G/5G gene mutation. Genet Couns 2013;24:455–8.
40. Brandao LR, Simpson EA, Lau KK. Neonatal renal vein thrombosis. Semin Fetal Neonatal Med 2011;16:323–8.
41. Cartwright DW. Placement of neonatal central venous catheter tips: is the right atrium so dangerous? Arch Dis Child Fetal Neonatal Ed 2002;87:F155 [discussion: F155–6].
42. Bucciarelli P, Rosendaal FR, Tripodi A, et al. Risk of venous thromboembolism and clinical manifestations in carriers of antithrombin, protein C, protein S deficiency, or activated protein C resistance: a multicenter collaborative family study. Arterioscler Thromb Vasc Biol 1999;19:1026–33.
43. Saxonhouse MA, Burchfield DJ. The evaluation and management of postnatal thromboses. J Perinatol 2009;29:467–78.
44. Nowak-Gottl U, Junker R, Hartmeier M, et al. Increased lipoprotein(a) is an important risk factor for venous thromboembolism in childhood. Circulation 1999;100:743–8.
45. Nowak-Gottl U, Dubbers A, Kececioglu D, et al. Factor V Leiden, protein C, and lipoprotein (a) in catheter-related thrombosis in childhood: a prospective study. J Pediatr 1997;131:608–12.
46. Rosendaal FR. Venous thrombosis: the role of genes, environment, and behavior. Hematology Am Soc Hematol Educ Program 2005;1–12.
47. Dahlback B, Hillarp A, Rosen S, et al. Resistance to activated protein C, the FV:Q506 allele, and venous thrombosis. Ann Hematol 1996;72:166–76.
48. Park CK, Paes BA, Nagel K, et al. Neonatal central venous catheter thrombosis: diagnosis, management and outcome. Blood Coagul Fibrinolysis 2014;25: 97–106.

49. Pettit J. Assessment of infants with peripherally inserted central catheters: Part 1. Detecting the most frequently occurring complications. Adv Neonatal Care 2002;2:304–15.

50. Tanke RB, van Megen R, Daniels O. Thrombus detection on central venous catheters in the neonatal intensive care unit. Angiology 1994;45:477–80.

51. Schmidt B, Zipursky A. Thrombotic disease in newborn infants. Clin Perinatol 1984;11:461–88.

52. Khilnani P, Goldstein B, Todres ID. Double lumen umbilical venous catheters in critically ill neonates: a randomized prospective study. Crit Care Med 1991;19: 1348–51.

53. Greenway A, Massicotte MP, Monagle P. Neonatal thrombosis and its treatment. Blood Rev 2004;18:75–84.

54. Le Coultre C, Oberhansli I, Mossaz A, et al. Postoperative chylothorax in children: differences between vascular and traumatic origin. J Pediatr Surg 1991; 26:519–23.

55. Barnes C, Newall F, Monagle P. Post-thrombotic syndrome. Arch Dis Child 2002; 86:212–4.

56. Siu SL, Yang JY, Hui JP, et al. Chylothorax secondary to catheter related thrombosis successfully treated with heparin. J Paediatr Child Health 2012;48: E105–7.

57. O'Grady NP, Alexander M, Dellinger EP, et al. Guidelines for the prevention of intravascular catheter-related infections. The Hospital Infection Control Practices Advisory Committee, Center for Disease Control and Prevention, U.S. Pediatrics 2002;110:e51.

58. Cartwright DW. Central venous lines in neonates: a study of 2186 catheters. Arch Dis Child Fetal Neonatal Ed 2004;89:F504–8.

59. Torres-Valdivieso MJ, Cobas J, Barrio C, et al. Successful use of tissue plasminogen activator in catheter-related intracardiac thrombus of a premature infant. Am J Perinatol 2003;20:91–6.

60. Bose J, Clarke P. Use of tissue plasminogen activator to treat intracardiac thrombosis in extremely low-birth-weight infants. Pediatr Crit Care Med 2011;12: e407–9.

61. Marks SD, Massicotte MP, Steele BT, et al. Neonatal renal venous thrombosis: clinical outcomes and prevalence of prothrombotic disorders. J Pediatr 2005; 146:811–6.

62. Messinger Y, Sheaffer JW, Mrozek J, et al. Renal outcome of neonatal renal venous thrombosis: review of 28 patients and effectiveness of fibrinolytics and heparin in 10 patients. Pediatrics 2006;118:e1478–84.

63. Saxonhouse MA. Management of neonatal thrombosis. Clin Perinatol 2012;39: 191–208.

64. Schwartz DS, Gettner PA, Konstantino MM, et al. Umbilical venous catheterization and the risk of portal vein thrombosis. J Pediatr 1997;131:760–2.

65. Stringer DA, Krysl J, Manson D, et al. The value of Doppler sonography in the detection of major vessel thrombosis in the neonatal abdomen. Pediatr Radiol 1990;21:30–3.

66. Morag I, Shah PS, Epelman M, et al. Childhood outcomes of neonates diagnosed with portal vein thrombosis. J Paediatr Child Health 2011;47:356–60.

67. Williams S, Chan AK. Neonatal portal vein thrombosis: diagnosis and management. Semin Fetal Neonatal Med 2011;16:329–39.

68. Sarin SK, Agarwal SR. Extrahepatic portal vein obstruction. Semin Liver Dis 2002;22:43–58.

69. Yadav S, Dutta AK, Sarin SK. Do umbilical vein catheterization and sepsis lead to portal vein thrombosis? A prospective, clinical, and sonographic evaluation. J Pediatr Gastroenterol Nutr 1993;17:392–6.
70. Guimaraes H, Castelo L, Guimaraes J, et al. Does umbilical vein catheterization to exchange transfusion lead to portal vein thrombosis? Eur J Pediatr 1998;157: 461–3.
71. Mitra SK, Kumar V, Datta DV, et al. Extrahepatic portal hypertension: a review of 70 cases. J Pediatr Surg 1978;13:51–7.
72. Alvarez F, Bernard O, Brunelle F, et al. Portal obstruction in children. II. Results of surgical portosystemic shunts. J Pediatr 1983;103:703–7.
73. Devlieger H, Snoeys R, Wyndaele L, et al. Liver necrosis in the new-born infant: analysis of some precipitating factors in neonatal care. Eur J Pediatr 1982;138: 113–9.
74. Parker MJ, Joubert GI, Levin SD. Portal vein thrombosis causing neonatal cerebral infarction. Arch Dis Child Fetal Neonatal Ed 2002;87:F125–7.
75. Ries M, Zenker M, Kandler C, et al. Severe bleeding diathesis in a premature baby with extensive hepatic necrosis due to portal vein thrombosis of prenatal onset. Ann Hematol 1999;78:339–40.
76. deVeber G, Andrew M, Adams C, et al. Cerebral sinovenous thrombosis in children. N Engl J Med 2001;345:417–23.
77. Berfelo FJ, Kersbergen KJ, van Ommen CH, et al. Neonatal cerebral sinovenous thrombosis from symptom to outcome. Stroke 2010;41:1382–8.
78. Fitzgerald KC, Williams LS, Garg BP, et al. Cerebral sinovenous thrombosis in the neonate. Arch Neurol 2006;63:405–9.
79. Yang JY, Chan AK, Callen DJ, et al. Neonatal cerebral sinovenous thrombosis: sifting the evidence for a diagnostic plan and treatment strategy. Pediatrics 2010;126:e693–700.
80. Tan MA, Miller E, Shroff MM, et al. Alleviation of neonatal sinovenous compression to enhance cerebral venous blood flow. J Child Neurol 2013;28:583–8.
81. Manlhiot C, Menjak IB, Brandao LR, et al. Risk, clinical features, and outcomes of thrombosis associated with pediatric cardiac surgery. Circulation 2011;124: 1511–9.
82. Gruenwald CE, Manlhiot C, Crawford-Lean L, et al. Management and monitoring of anticoagulation for children undergoing cardiopulmonary bypass in cardiac surgery. J Extra Corpor Technol 2010;42:9–19.
83. Niebler RA, Mitchell ME, Scott JP. Repeated aortopulmonary shunt thrombosis in a neonatal patient with a low antithrombin level. World J Pediatr Congenit Heart Surg 2014;5:94–6.
84. Chan AK, Deveber G, Monagle P, et al. Venous thrombosis in children. J Thromb Haemost 2003;1:1443–55.
85. Monagle P. Thrombosis in pediatric cardiac patients. Semin Thromb Hemost 2003;29:547–55.
86. Brown KL, Ridout DA, Goldman AP, et al. Risk factors for long intensive care unit stay after cardiopulmonary bypass in children. Crit Care Med 2003;31:28–33.
87. Gillespie M, Kuijpers M, Van Rossem M, et al. Determinants of intensive care unit length of stay for infants undergoing cardiac surgery. Congenit Heart Dis 2006; 1:152–60.
88. Nowak-Gottl U, Strater R, Heinecke A, et al. Lipoprotein (a) and genetic polymorphisms of clotting factor V, prothrombin, and methylenetetrahydrofolate reductase are risk factors of spontaneous ischemic stroke in childhood. Blood 1999;94:3678–82.

89. Nowak-Gottl U, Junker R, Kreuz W, et al. Risk of recurrent venous thrombosis in children with combined prothrombotic risk factors. Blood 2001;97:858–62.

90. Brenner B. Thrombophilia and adverse pregnancy outcome. Obstet Gynecol Clin North Am 2006;33:443–56, ix.

91. Manco-Johnson MJ. How I treat venous thrombosis in children. Blood 2006;107: 21–9.

92. Manco-Johnson M. Controversies in neonatal thrombotic disorders. In: Ohls RY, editor. Hematology, immunology and infections disease: neonatology questions and controversies. Philadelphia: Saunders Elsevier; 2008. p. 58–74.

93. Malowany JI, Knoppert DC, Chan AK, et al. Enoxaparin use in the neonatal intensive care unit: experience over 8 years. Pharmacotherapy 2007;27:1263–71.

94. Obaid L, Byrne PJ, Cheung PY. Compartment syndrome in an ELBW infant receiving low-molecular-weight heparins. J Pediatr 2004;144:549.

95. van Elteren HA, Te Pas AB, Kollen WJ, et al. Severe hemorrhage after low-molecular-weight heparin treatment in a preterm neonate. Neonatology 2011; 99:247–9.

96. Abrams J. Glyceryl trinitrate (nitroglycerin) and the organic nitrates. Choosing the method of administration. Drugs 1987;34:391–403.

97. Bogaert MG. Clinical pharmacokinetics of glyceryl trinitrate following the use of systemic and topical preparations. Clin Pharmacokinet 1987;12:1–11.

98. Baserga MC, Puri A, Sola A. The use of topical nitroglycerin ointment to treat peripheral tissue ischemia secondary to arterial line complications in neonates. J Perinatol 2002;22:416–9.

99. Varughese M, Koh TH. Successful use of topical nitroglycerine in ischaemia associated with umbilical arterial line in a neonate. J Perinatol 2001;21:556–8.

100. Raffini L, Huang YS, Witmer C, et al. Dramatic increase in venous thromboembolism in children's hospitals in the United States from 2001 to 2007. Pediatrics 2009;124:1001–8.

101. Kerlin BA, Blatt NB, Fuh B, et al. Epidemiology and risk factors for thromboembolic complications of childhood nephrotic syndrome: a Midwest Pediatric Nephrology Consortium (MWPNC) study. J Pediatr 2009;155:105–10, 110.e1.

102. Young G. Old and new antithrombotic drugs in neonates and infants. Semin Fetal Neonatal Med 2011;16:349–54.

103. Chan AK, Monagle P. Updates in thrombosis in pediatrics: where are we after 20 years? Hematology Am Soc Hematol Educ Program 2012;2012:439–43.

104. Molinari AC, Banov L, Bertamino M, et al. A practical approach to the use of low molecular weight heparins in VTE treatment and prophylaxis in children and newborns. Pediatr Hematol Oncol 2015;32(1):1–10.

105. Bounameaux H. Unfractionated versus low-molecular-weight heparin in the treatment of venous thromboembolism. Vasc Med 1998;3:41–6.

106. Samama MM, Gerotziafas GT. Comparative pharmacokinetics of LMWHS. Semin Thromb Hemost 2000;26(Suppl 1):31–8.

107. Avidan MS, Levy JH, Scholz J, et al. A phase III, double-blind, placebo-controlled, multicenter study on the efficacy of recombinant human antithrombin in heparin-resistant patients scheduled to undergo cardiac surgery necessitating cardiopulmonary bypass. Anesthesiology 2005;102:276–84.

108. Niebler RA, Christensen M, Berens R, et al. Antithrombin replacement during extracorporeal membrane oxygenation. Artif Organs 2011;35:1024–8.

109. Wong TE, Delaney M, Gernsheimer T, et al. Antithrombin concentrates use in children on extracorporeal membrane oxygenation: a retrospective cohort study. Pediatr Crit Care Med 2015;16(3):264–9.

110. Wong TE, Huang YS, Weiser J, et al. Antithrombin concentrate use in children: a multicenter cohort study. J Pediatr 2013;163:1329–34.e1.
111. Perry R, Stein J, Young G, et al. Antithrombin III administration in neonates with congenital diaphragmatic hernia during the first three days of extracorporeal membrane oxygenation. J Pediatr Surg 2013;48:1837–42.
112. Armstrong-Wells JL, Manco-Johnson MJ. Neonatal thrombosis. In: de Alarcon P, Werner EJ, Christensen RD, editors. Neonatal hematology. New York: Cambridge University Press; 2013. p. 277–85.
113. Michelson AD, Bovill E, Monagle P, et al. Antithrombotic therapy in children. Chest 1998;114:748S–69S.
114. Spadone D, Clark F, James E, et al. Heparin-induced thrombocytopenia in the newborn. J Vasc Surg 1992;15:306–11 [discussion: 311–2].
115. Martchenke J, Boshkov L. Heparin-induced thrombocytopenia in neonates. Neonatal Netw 2005;24:33–7.
116. Streif W, Goebel G, Chan AK, et al. Use of low molecular mass heparin (enoxaparin) in newborn infants: a prospective cohort study of 62 patients. Arch Dis Child Fetal Neonatal Ed 2003;88:F365–70.
117. Malowany JI, Monagle P, Knoppert DC, et al. Enoxaparin for neonatal thrombosis: a call for a higher dose for neonates. Thromb Res 2008;122(6):826–30.
118. Michaels LA, Gurian M, Hegyi T, et al. Low molecular weight heparin in the treatment of venous and arterial thromboses in the premature infant. Pediatrics 2004; 114:703–7.
119. Wang M, Hays T, Balasa V, et al. Low-dose tissue plasminogen activator thrombolysis in children. J Pediatr Hematol Oncol 2003;25:379–86.
120. Nowak-Gottl U, Auberger K, Halimeh S, et al. Thrombolysis in newborns and infants. Thromb Haemost 1999;82(Suppl 1):112–6.
121. Caner I, Olgun H, Buyukavci M, et al. A giant thrombus in the right ventricle of a newborn with Down syndrome: successful treatment with RT-PA. J Pediatr Hematol Oncol 2006;28:120–2.
122. Marks KA, Zucker N, Kapelushnik J, et al. Infective endocarditis successfully treated in extremely low birth weight infants with recombinant tissue plasminogen activator. Pediatrics 2002;109:153–8.
123. Elbers J, Viero S, MacGregor D, et al. Placental pathology in neonatal stroke. Pediatrics 2011;127:e722–9.
124. Coombs CJ, Richardson PW, Dowling GJ, et al. Brachial artery thrombosis in infants: an algorithm for limb salvage. Plast Reconstr Surg 2006;117:1481–8.

Index

Note: Page numbers of article titles are in **boldface** type.

A

Absolute monocyte counts, in necrotizing enterocolitis, 576
Adhesions, platelet, 627
Afibrinogenemia, 629
Age of Red Blood Cells in Premature Infants (ARIPI), 502
Aggregometry, platelet, 631–632
Anemia
    in necrotizing enterocolitis, 574–575
    prevention of, darbepoietin for, 560–561
Antibody screen, umbilical cord blood for, 549–550
Anticoagulant proteins, 652
Anticoagulant therapy, for thrombosis, 661–665
Antiphospholipid antibody panel, 660–661
Antithrombin, measurement of, 660–661
Apoptosis
    biomarkers for, 532–534
    neuroprotection from, 471–473
ARIPI (Age of Red Blood Cells in Premature Infants), 502
Arterial thromboses, 652–654
Arteriotomy, for thrombosis, 665
Aspirin, platelet dysfunction due to, 628, 630
Autophagy, neuroprotection from, 471–473

B

B cells, in necrotizing enterocolitis, 570–571
Bacterial overgrowth, in necrotizing enterocolitis, 568
Basophils, in necrotizing enterocolitis, 576
Beclin 1 protein, in necrosis, 472
Bernard-Soulier syndrome, 628–629
Biomarkers, of oxidative stress, **529–539**
Bite cells, in hemolysis, 519–520
Bleeding time, for platelet evaluation, 632–634
Blister cells, in hemolysis, 519–520
Blood culture, of umbilical cord blood, 548, 550
Blood pressure, maintenance of, after delayed cord clamping/milking, 545
Brain Imaging and Developmental Follow-up of Infants Treated with Erythropoietin or Placebo (BRITE), 475
Brain injury
    neuroprotection for, 469–481
    oxidative stress in, **529–539**
    stem cell transplantation for, 602–604

Moving?

Make sure your subscription moves with you!

To notify us of your new address, find your **Clinics Account Number** (located on your mailing label above your name), and contact customer service at:

Email: journalscustomerservice-usa@elsevier.com

800-654-2452 (subscribers in the U.S. & Canada)
314-447-8871 (subscribers outside of the U.S. & Canada)

Fax number: 314-447-8029

Elsevier Health Sciences Division
Subscription Customer Service
3251 Riverport Lane
Maryland Heights, MO 63043

ELSEVIER

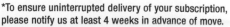

Printed and bound by CPI Group (UK) Ltd, Croydon, CR0 4YY

03/10/2024

01040490-0003